Successfully Choosing Your EMR

MSP Self-Disclosure

Arthur Gasch and Betty Gasch are principals of Medical Strategic Planning, Inc. (MSP), an privately-held, NJ business-intelligence company. All MSP stock is held by its employees. MSP is an impartial and unbiased source of information about the U.S. EMR/EHR market, which it has been tracking for decades.

This book is based on original research conducted by MSP and data collected from 104 EMR developers that is available to all EMR stakeholders (patients, care providers in various in-patient and out-patient settings, public policy officials, hospital CIOs, quality advocates and others) to help them understand the Crucial Decisions involved in successfully choosing an EMR that fits practice needs, workflow and budgets.

Neither the authors nor other MSP employees participate on the boards of any companies selling Electronic Medical Records (EMRs) or Computer Practice Management (CPM) systems. MSP does not sell, market, lease or otherwise distribute any EMR products or receive any commissions or finder's fees from any EMR developers or their marketing organizations.

Successfully Choosing Your EMR:

15 Crucial Decisions

Arthur Gasch
Medical Strategic Planning Inc., Lincroft, NJ, USA

Betty Gasch
President/CEO, Medical Strategic Planning Inc., Lincroft, NJ, USA

WILEY-BLACKWELL

A John Wiley & Sons, Ltd., Publication

Endorsements

The selection of an electronic medical record systems (EMRS – the computer system which clinicians routinely use to capture and document clinical encounters with patients which completely replaces paper-based medical records) is truly one of the most crucial decisions that a practice will ever make. The EMRS is the system that clinicians and staff will come to rely on as it completely replaces archaic, paper-based medical records. You're really "betting the farm" when making this decision! EMRS' are truly a disruptive technology because the EMRS will impact virtually every facet within a practice and it will definitely change the way you practice. This book represents the most pragmatic work yet on preparations essential to selecting an EMRS. The book focuses on real world issues surrounding the selection of an EMRS. It provides an impressive array of useful, even insightful information concerning the selection of an EMRS for clinician practices. I recommend that clinicians everywhere utilize this book to help mitigate risks associated with this most crucial decision.

RICHARD DICK, PH.D.,
FORMER CHAIRMAN, IOM COMMITTEE ON CPR REQUIREMENTS

The move toward electronic medical records is important to improve patient health outcomes, to enhance patient safety, to study the effectiveness of different treatments, and to lower health care costs. Not all protocols, procedures, and organization of these electronic records are equal. This book provides new insight into the advantages and drawbacks of these different electronic medical record systems.

CONGRESSMAN RUSH HOLT, (D. NJ),
MEMBER CHILDREN'S ENVIRONMENTAL HEALTH CAUCUS

This book opened my eyes to several crucial issues I had overlooked. It has offered us an education and unbiased approach to EMR/EHR system selection. This book, in conjunction with the MSP EHR Selector, allows us to compare the available CCHIT-certified EMRs to those that best fit our practice needs. I am glad we found it and recommend it to my colleagues looking to adopt EMR systems.

RADU KRAMER, M.D.,
INTERNAL MEDICINE AND NEPHROLOGY

Table of Contents

Acknowledgements

It is with deep appreciation that we acknowledge the many individuals who have encouraged us and then devoted their time and assistance in helping us compile the material for this book, proof and refine it.

This work would not have been accomplished without the years of labor of William F. Andrew, originator of the Andrew & Associates EMR Survey, which ultimately became the MSP/Andrew EMR Benchmark. Bill created the survey in 1994 after an Institute of Medicine (IOM) Committee issued the Computer-Based Patient Record (CPR) criteria report. He conducted the survey for a decade, almost single-handedly, and it became a landmark measurement of how well EMR technology was advancing and implementing IOM and subsequent standards. In later years, we had the privilege of helping Bill put the survey online. Bill helped to proof this text, which was a tedious chore, and offered many insights and suggestions for the book.

This work was also aided by Reed Gelzer, MD, and his organization, DocIntegrity. Reed is the author of Chapter 13 on the legal aspects of the EMR. Indeed, Patricia A. Trites and Reed collaborated on a fine book, *How to Evaluate Electronic Health Record (EHR) Systems,* which is available from AHIMA. We suggest that any readers who wish to explore the legal aspects of medical records obtain a copy of Patricia and Reed's book ($129). Reed has been a tireless champion for the adoption of criteria that would make EMR-generated documents admissible legal evidence and overcome issues in some EMRs that allow them to be intentionally or unintentionally adulterated.

We also thank Caroline Samuels, MD, the originator of what became the EHR Selector, which MSP hosts for physicians and collaborating medical groups seeking a way to match EMR products to practice needs and budgets. Caroline's insights on Chapter 9 was particularly helpful in conceptualizing workflow as information flow for decision support, and not simply mechanical screen automation and optimization.

We were also aided in Chapter 9 by Charles Webster, MD, a frequent HIMSS speaker, who graciously permitted us to repurpose some material MSP had previously published with his help in the Industry Alert™ newsletter. Dr. Webster is Vice President of the Encounter Pro EMR, which is based upon a user-accessible workflow engine of his design.

Thanks also to Annie Carter, CNS, RN at Riverview Medical Center's (Red Bank) Emergency Department for her feedback on workflow and for her real-life experiences working with their EMR.

Thanks to Allen Wenner, MD for his enthusiasm and helpful suggestions, as well as his specific input on using structured patient interview tools to capture patient-contributed aspects of the history of present illness and chief complaints. He also provided some of the graphics showing EMR deployment in his offices, which helped in our coverage of that topic.

We also appreciate the advice, encouragement and assistance of Linda Rastelli, the editor of Wiley's *Understanding Autism for Dummies*, who guided us in the search for a publisher, and provided the idea for the practice vignettes that we wrote for the book. Thanks to all of the personnel at Wiley for their abundant support and encouragement in this endeavor.

We thank Robert Bruegel, PhD who provided advice and suggested the Crucial Decisions overall organization of the book.

Our thanks to our friends, Jim and Leila Armstrong for their ongoing encouragement of this project and a place to rest in the midst of the writing.

The authors' special thanks and deep gratitude goes to Karen Gasch, who handled graphic design and manuscript formatting services through various rewrites of many chapters and numerous revisions to the text that created text reflows, necessitating additional formatting changes.

Finally, thanks to other MSP team members for their picking up some of our daily workload that made time for writing this book possible.

Introduction

If you are a physician or other healthcare provider, who is overwhelmed by the thought of converting your practice from paper-based to Electronic Medical Record (EMR) based[1], or deploying an EMR in your hospital clinical area, or a hospital CIO trying to piece together a Stark "Safe Harbor" program for your attending physicians, you've probably discovered few practical books published on the subject. This is particularly true if you are looking for timely coverage of EMRs/EHRs/PHRs in relation to recent 2009 American Recovery & Reinvestment Act (ARRA) legislation, how EMR fits into the Nationwide Health Information Network (NHIN) or the proposed remaking of the entire U.S. healthcare system. This book shows you how to successfully choose and adopt an EMR.

Why This Book is Needed

This book is informed by the HITECH section of the ARRA, which provides significant government funds for the adoption of EMRs for U.S. physician practices and hospitals, and is changing the direction of EMR system adoption. It's especially needed because of the serious flaws in the U.S. healthcare system that need to be addressed and the stakes are only getting higher. According to the Institute of Medicine (IOM), in its famous *"To Err is Human"* report, 98,000 preventable deaths occur annually in the U.S. alone due to human mistakes, many of which are prescription errors; a startling statistic indeed. In fact, more recent studies reveal that the original IOM data underestimated the extent of deaths due to medical mistakes.

Medical errors have claimed many more lives around the world than have all of the terrorist attacks from 1999 (the year the first IOM statistics were published) to the present day. This includes the victims from the World Trade Center, the Pentagon and Pennsylvania on 9/11/2001; the Bali nightclub bombings of 2/12/2002; the Chechen rebel seizure of a Moscow theater on 10/23/2002, the Madrid train bombings of 3/11/2004; the London bombings of 7/7/2005 and too many countless other terrorist attacks combined. America and other countries went to war after those attacks and spent hundreds of billions of dollars to prevent reoccurrences, yet the U.S. has, until recently, not significantly addressed the mounting death toll from medical errors. Since

---

[1] Nearly 62% of surveyed physician group practice administrators consider selecting and implementing a new electronic health records system as a considerable or an extreme challenge according to an MGMA survey of practice managers reported in August 12, 2009 HDM Breaking News

1999, more than 900,000 lives have been lost due to preventable medical errors (based on the IOM study cited above).

Since EMRs can help reduce mistakes, shouldn't physicians around the world be clamoring for the adoption of Electronic Medical Records (EMRs), instead of dragging their feet? Shouldn't physicians want to manage that change, rather than be victims of it?

Electronic medical record systems can reduce errors of all sorts, yet of the more than 873,233 physicians practicing in the United States today, (of which 654,000 work in group practices), the American Medical Association (AMA) estimates that only about 73,000 are using fully deployed electronic health record systems in their practices, while a smaller group has partially deployed EMR-Lite systems. A more current estimate, released at HIMSS 2009 conference, indicates that 33 percent of medical offices with four or fewer physicians currently use some sort of EMR or EMR-Lite software.[2] While the totals vary depending upon practice specialty, the vast majority of American physicians have not yet adopted EMR systems.

EMR penetration of U.S. hospitals is not much better. According to the March 25, 2009 issue of the New England Journal of Medicine, an article entitled, *Use of Electronic Health Records in U.S. Hospitals*, by Ashish K. Jha, MD, MPH et al., revealed that, *"Only 1.5 percent of U.S. hospitals have a comprehensive electronic records system (i.e., present in all clinical units), and an additional 7.6 percent have a basic system (i.e., present in at least one clinical unit). Computerized provider-order entry (CPOE) for medications has been implemented in only 17 percent of hospitals. Larger hospitals, those located in urban areas, and teaching hospitals were more likely to have electronic records systems."* [3]

EMR Adoption Has Become a National Priority

The migration from paper-based charts to electronic patient information stored in EMR databases is a foundational priority for healthcare reform in the U.S. – primarily because it has the potential to save money, reduce mistakes and improve quality of care. Electronic transformation is an issue in all care settings, from hospital inpatient areas to clinics, physician offices, rehab and long-term care settings and even into patients' homes. This is due in part to the fact that the government continues to push patients as quickly as possible out of higher cost-of-care settings into lower ones that are often more sparsely staffed. Indeed, the U.S. is far behind other countries like New Zealand, the Netherlands, the U.K., Australia, Germany and even Canada in adoption of EMRs.

Like the stethoscope when it was first invented, the EMR currently remains a departure from the medical status-quo. Similar to the stethoscope today, the

---

[2] *67% of Physician Offices Do Not Use Electronic Medical Record (EMR) Software.* By Jack Schember, Director of Marketing for SK&A. Press Release of April 6, 2009

[3] *Use of Electronic Health Records in U.S. Hospitals,* By Ashish K. Jha, et al. Published March 25, 2009 at www.nejm.org, (10.1056/NEJMsa0900592)

EMR will also become an essential tool and the symbol of medicine practiced in the 21st century. Our children and grandchildren will look back on the pre-EMR era and wonder how medicine was practiced without this powerful decision support tool!

If you would like to learn about EMRs, whether you are ready to select and deploy one or are just starting up the EMR learning curve, this book is written for you. It is not only written as a dialog to physicians, but also to nurses, practice managers, receptionists, hospital CIOs, and even patients who seek insight into how healthcare can be transformed by widespread EMR deployment, done properly – and how it may be ruined if it is not done properly. Every American who has the potential to become a patient in the current healthcare system is a stakeholder in the adoption of EMR.

Finally, the government has become serious about funding the Nationwide Healthcare Information Network (NHIN) and the conversion to EMR via the American Recovery and Reinvestment Act of 2009 (ARRA), and the HITECH section it contains, which covers EMR deployment. This legislation makes over $35 billion available, anticipates savings of $14B, having a net budget impact of approximately $21B, or a net of $19B after $2B in funding for the Office of the National Coordinator (ONC) is deducted. This reimbursement depends on EMR implementations that are "certified" as achieving certain Meaningful Use functionality (Meaningful Use will be defined shortly).

When the government decides to pay for something, it is a serious indication that whatever that "something" is, it will come to fruition. The government is serious about seeing EMR implementation happen in the next five years. Therefore, it's no longer a question of whether EMR implementation will happen, but simply what the time frame will be and what form it will take. Practices that procrastinate in adopting EMRs cheat themselves out of government reimbursement today and will experience future reductions in reimbursement for care of CMS patients beginning in 2015. More significantly, they will also experience a reduction in total reimbursement for EMR deployment expenses starting in 2011 because the total payments from ARRA will be made over a five-year period.

The Early Bird Gets the Most Reimbursement

Physicians may not realize that practices that begin the EMR process late will receive significantly less reimbursement overall than those who start in 2009 or 2010. Incentives per physician of up to $44K will be available starting in 2011 for practices that have adopted EMRs. Timing is everything because the later physicians get into the program, the less their reimbursement will be. If a physician has adopted an EMR and can show Meaningful Use by 2011 or 2012, they can receive up to $18K per physician per year in additional CMS reimbursement. In the second year, the reimbursement drops to $12K, in the third year to $8K, in the fourth year to $4K, and in the fifth year to $2K.

In signing the ARRA legislation on Feb. 17, 2009, President Barack Obama described it by saying, "*It's an investment that will take the long overdue step of computerizing America's medical records, to reduce the duplication and waste that costs billions of health care dollars and (reduce) the medical errors that every year cost thousands of lives."*

If you are a physician or other healthcare provider, selecting and deploying Electronic Medical Records (EMRs) will impact the success of your practice over the next decade more than anything else you do (for better or worse). EMRs facilitate 2 percent incremental reimbursement for practices meeting Electronic Prescribing (eRx) requirements, 2 percent incremental reimbursement for practices complying with Physician Quality Reporting Initiative (PQRI) requirements, and reductions in malpractice insurance premiums (in some states). ARRA has now made funds available to reimburse the costs of adopting EMR solutions by physician group practices!

Physicians, what will your practice be worth (to sell) in 5 years if you haven't successfully adopted EMRs? Who will be enthusiastic about buying a paper-based practice? If you want to ensure the highest return on investment when selling your practice, read this book carefully.

Impact of Meaningful Use (MU)
The 2009 ARRA legislation links EMR reimbursement to something called "Meaningful Use." Meaningful Use (MU) is not directly a measure of EMR functionality, rather it's a measure of outcomes that depend on EMR functionality. It is essential to have an EMR that can capture, track and report the data necessary to document the achievement of Meaningful Use results. The MU term will not be fully defined until later in 2009; that creates a tight schedule for EMR selection and planning, which should not be hurried.

This book will help physicians expedite their EMR process without rushing it. Additional tools that can expedite your EMR vendor functionality search are available, such as the MSP EHR Selector (www.ehrselector.com). See Appendix III for information.

This book provides insights from the April 28 & 29 (2009) testimony before the subcommittee established to define Meaningful Use, and from the June 16, 2009 clarifications subsequently released. Final clarification will occur December 31, 2009, after this book has gone to press. Check the Office of the National Coordinator (ONC) for the final MU standards. MU will be a moving target. There are the initial requirements for 2011, another set effective 2013 and a final set effective 2015. The MU requirements are updated every two years, to allow the industry time to integrate them into EMR product engineering schedules.

Impact of ARRA (HITECH) is Mixed
The ARRA legislation is already working in the healthcare arena. The 2008 HIMSS conference drew over 26,000 attendees and over 900 exhibitors when conducted in its normal (February 2008) time slot. In 2009, the date was moved to April because the conference was held in Chicago; interestingly, that date change saved the 2009 HIMSS conference. In February 2009,

registration for the HIMSS conference was way off and the conference looked like a financial disaster for the first time in decades. Then the ARRA was passed and immediately both attendee and exhibitor registrations skyrocketed. When the conference kicked off, total attendance was down less than 5 percent and exhibitor levels were only off by 30 companies compared to year-ago levels. This was all the benefit of the ARRA legislation, which restored provider confidence that the government was serious about both EMR and economic stimulus. HIMSS 2009 Conference was a huge success and a money maker because of the impact of ARRA legislation! That success translated into action as attendees returned to their hospitals/offices and also as the media in attendance wrote up the findings from the speakers at HIMSS.

The ARRA legislation also had a negative effect. Since it was passed in February 2009 throughout the remainder of 2009, the EMR market has languished and sales of EMR systems have dropped, due to uncertainty in the market over MU requirements. It is not likely to recover until at least one quarter of 2010 after the final MU requirements are actually issued.

The General Approach to EMR Adoption

Adopting an EMR and successfully deploying it is not rocket science, but it's not to be approached casually either. Successful selection and deployment of an EMR requires a systematic process that may require a minimum of 6-9 months, but take up to a year or more to accomplish in some cases. Therefore, starting the planning process is highly recommended for practices desiring to show Meaningful Use by 2011. How long it takes and how much work it requires will depend on three things:

1 Your level of knowledge about computers;
2 Your time spent trying to discover an effective EMR search process; and
3 Time spent finding reliable data on a cross-section of EMR developers.

Even with all their benefits, EMRs are no panacea; they introduce some novel and unique issues of their own. EMRs connect doctors to patients in new ways, providing them access to their patients' Personal Health Records (PHRs) and to the Nationwide Healthcare Information Network (NHIN) that is being developed by the U.S. government. The wrong EMR can easily kill office workflow efficiency, increase exposure to record theft and create other new risks of practicing medicine. Indeed, about 20 percent of EMRs deployed today do not meet the full expectations of those who deployed them. In preparing for your initial EMR, you need to plan for your second-generation EMR also, in particular how you will get data out of your first-generation product and into its replacement. Interoperability is about more than simply getting lab and other test results into your first EMR. That's something that no government standard yet covers.

Short-circuiting the EMR decision process is risky. One major complaint voiced by unhappy EMR adopters was that their EMR made their overall work process slower or it was hard-to-use. There were various complaints;

sometimes it was the number of screens displayed by the EMR, other times it was information organization and display, for some, the menus seemed too deep and hard to navigate quickly, and some felt there were too many pick list choices. This can be summed up as poor usability. When you boil usability down, the three key ingredients are:

1 Workflow optimization;
2 EMR customization;
3 Menu depth and organization.

One important measure of success in deploying an EMR is whether or not an encounter summary documenting the patient's visit is available for the patient when he/she leaves your office. Obviously the results of some tests done by remote labs or other third parties will not be available, but the summary should document all tests ordered and the rest of the patient encounter. Today, an EMR encounter summary can document the transmission of all patient prescriptions to the patient's pharmacy of choice, the acknowledgment by that pharmacy that the order has been received, the problem list, chief complaints, the physician's instructions or plan of care and so on. When results become available electronically from the labs, they should be electronically integrated into the lab section of the patient's EMR, but some EMRs don't support this.

The EMR should automate the process of seeing patients, enhancing workflow rather than crippling it. Many EMRs do not yet achieve such objectives, but some do. Many EMRs impose static, pre-configured workflow on their users, a workflow that differs from their paper-based workflow. This is such an important topic, it is covered extensively in two separate chapters.

Empowering Patients and Their Families

One could argue that the Congressional mandate in creating the ARRA funding is not to empower medical institutions to adopt EMR products, as much as it is to empower *"every American to have an electronic health record by 2014 (actual Congressional wording)."*[4] If one follows this line of reasoning, it could be argued that Meaningful Use denotes "regular use by the American patient of their electronic medical records to aid in their maintenance of wellness."

Nowhere in this logic is the notion that Meaningful Use indicates "adoption by every healthcare provider of an EMR that makes some of the patient's data available to the individual MD at the point of care, to better enhance decision making." In fact, these are two entirely different approaches, a contrast between what might be termed a patient-controlled, individual health record, and a centralized approach involving a Health Information Exchange (HIE) of medical information to create Electronic Health Records (EHRs). The EHR approach is a cobbled-together consolidation of medical information concerning one patient that a participating EMR system can exhibit on demand.

---

[4] *Meaningful Use: A Definition, Recommendations from the Meaningful Use Workgroup to the Health IT Policy Committee.* Posted June 16, 2009

We don't pursue the individual health record line of reasoning in this book because it appears that this novel view (controlled by the patient of all people) has much less political influence (and money behind it) than the more complex notion of a solution based on rigid standards, with data transfer rules that are rigorously enforced upon all healthcare providers who participate in the government-financed, patient care program, even though logic would argue for the first, not the second approach to the problem.

Success of Government-Mandated Healthcare Change in the U.K.

In that regard, the U.S. could be plodding down the path taken by the National Health Service (NHS) in the U.K. a decade ago, which wasted almost $16B, only to end up failing to get physicians to genuinely embrace the approach. Several of the current U.S. healthcare EMR and I.T. companies were the players in the U.K. fiasco (at least the ones that are still in business and have not merged with their competitors).

However, there is no evidence that the individual health record approach would be any more successful since WebMD has had such a personal health record for sometime, and only a small percent of its users have adopted it. Most likely, the data in the WebMD PHR is too general and not very actionable, which may be why the adoption is so low.

Recently, the Kaiser Foundation reported information in Health Affairs that showed that use of an individual health record in their system reduced doctor's office visits by 25 percent per year for patients with chronic diseases.[5] That is a remarkable accomplishment, and an indicator of what might be achieved with automation. However, it seems to depend on two assumptions. First, that each patient/member maintains their membership in a single program for multiple years. Second, that physicians and other caregivers are compensated in a manner that is independent of the number of patients being seen.

The first objective might actually be met, if the Obama Administration is able to get the 31 or 46 million currently uninsured Americans into some sort of government-financed healthcare group. But the second criterion of physicians caring for that group being incentivized independently of the number of such patients they see and care for, is unlikely to be achieved. Indeed, with reimbursement per patient under the CMS programs constantly dropping, many physicians are closing their practices to new CMS patients, and probably would not take on new ones, whether or not they come with a government-financed individual health record that was accessible to the average physician.

---

[5] *The Kaiser Permanente Electronic Health Record: Transforming and Streamlining Modalities of Care.* By Catherine Chen et al. Published March 2009 by Health Affairs, Vol. 28, No. 2 (2009): pp. 323-333 doi: 10.1377/hlthaff.28.2.323

Product Diversity is Essential

Assuming America pursues the approach of financing the adoption of EMRs by all caregivers as the intermediate step to creating a health record for all Americans, then the diversity of the EMR is crucial to the plan, as no one EMR (or functionality set) will meet the needs of the 46 different medical practice specialties that will be required to adopt it. Beyond diversity is the matter of control. Healthcare providers will continue to control the health records they create for their patients, and no one of them will have the patient's entire history, nor any real incentive to sustain the patient's records (and make them available to EHRs or HIOs that might want to consolidate them), once the patient is no longer active in their practices. Thus, there are likely to be gaps in the health records created for individual Americans, as their caregivers change. In contrast, if the patient is seen as the keeper of his/her own health records, then he or she always has an incentive for it to be as complete as possible, and to include entries by all who have provided episodes of care.

Purchasing an EMR is Like Buying a Car

The current EMR decision process from the physician's perspective is not unlike the approach to purchasing an automobile. No one would suggest that every consumer in America should buy a one-size-fits-all automobile. No one brand or model would suit everyone's diverse needs very well. A family with seven children could not practically use a two-seater sports car, neither could a rancher use a limousine as a work vehicle on his 1,000-acre spread.

This analogy is equally true for EMR purchases. A pediatric practice needs an EMR that includes growth charts and immunization records, but such features are irrelevant for podiatry, dental, mental health, oncology, obstetrical, and most other practice specialties. The EMR you adopt must match your unique practice and workflow.

Most physicians/clinicians are much more familiar with the automobile decision process than with the EMR one. For that very reason, this book discusses the 15 Crucial Decisions tree and the "branches" to be considered before you start talking to EMR developers. It provides you with pointers on assessing EMR developer stability and a table of EMR developers and their products is provided in Appendix I. Conferences you can attend to view EMR products are listed in Appendix II. This book also helps you understand how to determine if an EMR right out-of-the-box will enhance or cripple your current office workflow. There are Scorecards located at the end of most chapters to assist you in documenting the answers to your Crucial Decisions. These Scorecards can also be downloaded from the Web site, www.ehrselector.com. We encourage everyone involved in your practice to use these Scorecards to document how you are progressing.

This book will guide you through "the EMR jungle of more than 200 EMR developers located in the U.S., Canada and Australia." By the time you're ready to call in EMR developers, you'll have made the Crucial Decisions that will reduce your EMR search to a short list of those that match your preferences.

Who This Book is For

While we have written for those deploying their first EMR, the material is just as valuable to those ready to replace their existing EMR with a new one, or an integrated EMR/CPM (Computer Practice Management) solution, or an EMR that also offers a patient-portal. The earliest EMR adopters who purchased their systems 6-13 years ago are facing a host of migration issues, transferring data from those old systems, into their next-generation, integrated EMR/CPM solutions. Many older EMRs run on now obsolete hardware and software platforms, and some are not CCHIT certified or have not kept up with current quality, safety and patient privacy standards.

While the book uses the example of EMR deployment to U.S. medical practices or other outpatient care settings, it also applies to the U.S. inpatient hospital setting and medical practices in other countries. Unlike CPM deployment across such settings that vary dramatically based on billing issues, EMR systems address the same key questions in any country still using paper-based medical records. The book uses the motif of a dialog personalized to physicians and their staffs, but is also a good read for practice managers, physician organizations, EMR consultants, EMR developers, insurers, government policy makers, or anyone else interested in understanding this cutting-edge medical technology from the care provider's point of view.

The book directs readers to other information needed in the EMR selection process, and to reliable sources of that information on the Web that won't compromise physician identity or practice anonymity.

15 Crucial Decisions

What is an EMR Crucial Decision? It is one that has so many consequences, that you can't simply (or inexpensively) change your mind about it.

Many EMR decisions are not crucial and can be easily changed. For example, the decision of whether to scan all of your patients' charts when you deploy your new EMR, or scan active patient records the day before each has their next appointment, can be changed. You can start with a just-in-time approach, and if it doesn't work, scan in every chart in the place.

An example of an EMR Crucial Decision is whether to deploy an EMR in your office or via a remote, Web server Software-as-a-Service approach. Once you have bought your EMR and hardware for the in-office deployment, switching to the Web server route leaves you stuck with extra hardware and in need of additional legal services. Or, if you have decided on an approach that does not structure data, switching to one that does is quite difficult. Obtaining legal help or not, is an EMR Crucial Decision. If your contract (or licensing) agreement is unbalanced, trying to fix it after you have purchased and deployed may be impossible. This book guides you through the factors that affect these decisions; it is both practical and fairly thorough. These 15 Crucial Decisions are the branches of a "Crucial Decision Tree" that must be navigated in order for the end result to be the correct EMR for you and those who will use it in your office.

The 15 EMR Crucial Decisions™ Covered in This Book:

1 **Crucial Decision:** The most fundamental question concerning EMRs – Is now the right time to adopt? (Chapter 1).

2 **Crucial Decision:** What method will you use to build staff consensus to adopt an EMR in your practice? (Chapter 2).

3 **Crucial Decision:** What level of EMR functionality will you deploy? (Chapter 3).

4 **Crucial Decision:** Will a freeform or a structured clinical patient data approach serve you better today? What about in 5 years? (Chapter 4).

5 **Crucial Decision:** How does everyone in your office prefer to interact with an EMR? Should it be accessible to patients to enter data? Do you want to implement multiple user interfaces? (Chapter 5).

6 **Crucial Decision:** Do you want an in-office (client-server) or a Web-based (Software-as-a-Service) EMR deployment? What are the fundamental implications of each choice? (Chapter 6).

7 **Crucial Decision:** What level of data structuring will meet your needs today and 5 years from now? (Chapter 7).

8 **Crucial Decision:** What is your preferred level of interoperability with other EMRs, EHRs, HIOs, PHRs, Registries and Public Health Agencies? (Chapter 8).

9 **Crucial Decision:** Do you want a WfME EMR or a conventional EMR? How can you document your current paper-based workflow so you'll better know what you need in an EMR? (Chapters 9 & 10).

10 **Crucial Decision:** What core medical record content do you need and what specialty-specific features do you require? (Chapter 11).

11 **Crucial Decision:** What makes an EMR developer a stable business partner? (Chapter 12).

12 **Crucial Decision:** Do you need legal advice to mitigate the risks of EMR purchasing or licensing agreements? (Chapters 13 & 18).

13 **Crucial Decision:** Can someone in-house support your EMR, or do you need an outside contractor for local support services? (Chapter 14).

14 **Crucial Decision:** What must you do to keep from having an EMR Emergency? What must you do to protect your patient records from loss or theft and make them HIPAA-compliant? (Chapters 15 & 16).

15 **Crucial Decision:** What will you spend transforming your practice from paper to an EMR system? Do you need legal assistance to get the EMR contract right? If so, where do you find it? (Chapters 17 & 18).

Finally, we underscore that these 15 Crucial Decisions form the roots of a "Crucial Decision Tree," which has many branches. Some of these branches/

decisions are mutually exclusive, and at the end of your decision process you will find yourself in one of the following situations:

1 A small group of EMR developers meet all your Crucial Decision requirements, and you have the funding, so you are ready to move ahead.

2 Only one EMR developer meets all your Crucial Decision requirements, so you are ready to proceed with that EMR developer.

3 No EMR developers meet all your Crucial Decision requirements, but you have the funding and wish to proceed. In this case you will need to reevaluate your requirements until at least one EMR developer qualifies.

4 You have decided this isn't the time for you to select and deploy an EMR, in which case this book will have been a great investment.

What is Important to Healthcare Providers

Most readers considering EMR deployment are looking for a small group of EMR developers that are worthy of further and more in-depth consideration. Problem is, if you aren't sure what's important, it's hard to achieve that objective. This book will enable you to figure out what's important to you.

This book is based upon current data taken from the MSP/Andrew EMR Benchmark™, an independent survey of EMR developers. It discusses EMR products supporting 46 practice specialties (URL www.ehrselector.com). You do not need to use the MSP EHR Selector to benefit from this book, but if you choose to subscribe, indicate "Wiley" as the group and "15Crucial" (case sensitive) as the password to obtain a significant discount.

Americans as Healthcare Consumers

Americans are increasingly interested in the U.S. healthcare system and its dysfunctions, and are trying to understand its conflicted incentives. Sites like www.floridahealthfindings.gov and others yield data on hospital readmission rates and other parameters. Examining the data highlights the fragmented nature of the healthcare system, which does not provide good communication among caregivers, nor good coordination of care when a patient moves from one care setting to another. The current system provides little money or incentive to prevent avoidable acute admissions. If there is to be any productive and effective change in healthcare delivery, that must change. Preventable readmission rates reflect poor care and misaligned government payment priorities. A 2007 study of CMS patients found the readmission rate at 15 days to be 8.8 percent and at 30 days to be 13.3 percent, reflecting over $20B in excess cost.[6] Such problems are within the government's power to fix without new legislation, yet are ignored. EMRs provide one tool that could improve continuity of care, particularly across transitions of care, assuming that EMR data can be exchanged among all caregivers. This is particularly

---

[6] *Readmission Rates Come Under Increased Scrutiny.* By Charlotte Huff. Published September 2008 by H&HN Magazine, p. 10

important for patients with chronic conditions that account for 75 percent of America's $2.3B dollar healthcare bill.

About the Authors, MSP & EMRs

Arthur Gasch and Betty Gasch, BSN, RN, principals of Medical Strategic Planning, Inc. (MSP), a New Jersey based, employee-owned corporation established in 1992, each bring a unique focus to this book.

Arthur Gasch has tracked U.S. and Canadian healthcare markets since the 1970s. Arthur, and a colleague, Ed Winters, created the first Hewlett-Packard customer computer application seminars in 1975. In 1992, Arthur was Manager of Market Research for the Electromedical Group of Siemens Corporation. Arthur was a presenter at the 1999 Symposium on the ICU 2010. He has been a presenter at various TEPR, AHIMA, AGA (Digestive Week) and World Congress conferences conducted from 2002 to 2008. Arthur was the EMR session moderator (and a presenter) at the 6th Annual NJ U.N. Consular Program for Biotechnology and Life Sciences, held October 16, 2009 at Raritan Community College in NJ.

Betty Gasch writes from a nursing and clinical perspective. Betty worked as patient care coordinator for a NJ home care agency and learned first hand the frustrations of EMRs that impose inefficient workflow. Betty has worked in hospital ICUs and as a critical care nursing educator. She developed programs for nurses on invasive hemodynamic monitoring, arrhythmias and other topics. Betty believes that appropriately-chosen and deployed EMR technologies can empower physicians, nurses, and other healthcare providers to better meet patient and family needs.

MSP develops highly-granular and actionable, medical business intelligence data on U.S. and Canadian medical device and information systems. MSP publishes the Industry Alert and md2eMD™ newsletters that include much EMR content. MSP is the ongoing developer of the MSP ESP Web portal.

Regarding Trademarks

The ™ symbol is generally used on the first occurrence of a term in the book, or the first occurrence in a chapter, and is not thereafter appended. The same is true for ® the Registered trade mark symbol.

CHAPTER 1

Why Adopt Electronic Medical Records Now?

> **Crucial Decision**
> **The most fundamental question concerning EMRs: Is now the right time to adopt?**
> This chapter also addresses the following questions:
> - If yes, do you want an EMR-Lite, open system or proprietary EMR approach?
> - What do EMR, EHR, RHIO, HIE and other relevant terms mean?
> - How do you start the adoption process?

EMR Adventures

Dr. David Rodriguez, a 55-year-old physician who works in a four-member practice in Denver, Colorado, is having a hectic morning. One of the other doctors, Brian Goldstein, is on vacation, and that means the rest of the staff has to pick up the slack. After having to juggle an office jammed with patients plus several emergency phone calls from Brian's patients (and his own), he is overdue for a break. When his last patient of the morning tells him that he thinks he's having side effects from his medication, Dr. Rodriguez immediately knows just what to substitute. This will be an easy visit, he thinks.

David used to write out his prescriptions by hand, and having to type the information into the clinic's new electronic prescribing system takes him a little longer. He wonders if "Brian's new toy," as the others have been calling it, is worth what it cost. Brian had argued that an Electronic Medical Record (EMR) was a great idea, but it was definitely going to cut into the year's profits. David types in the name of the medication quickly, looking forward to lunch.

"So Mr. Short, give this new medication a try and we'll see you next month," David starts to say, but on his screen something is flashing. He hopes it isn't a software glitch. He looks closer. "Allergy Alert," it says.

David scrolls down to the "Allergies/Adverse Reactions" box in Mr. Short's electronic record. Many documents had been scanned in to create this record. And long weekends of work had been required of their already overworked staff to bring the office's paper records online. Sure enough, the drug he had quickly (too quickly!) prescribed, is listed as one of his patient's allergens. Mr. Short hadn't said anything about being allergic to ibuprofen, but the man is

Successfully Choosing Your EMR: 15 Crucial Decisions. By © Arthur Gasch and Betty Gasch.
Published 2010 by Blackwell Publishing

nearing 80 and probably forgot. Or maybe he misheard the doctor when he said the medication's name. But there it was on the screen.

David realized that the new system had just stopped him from prescribing the wrong drug, one that would have created in his trusting patient a serious and possibly fatal allergic reaction. If he hadn't been notified by the EMR's set of medication and allergy alerts, Mr. Short would soon have been at his pharmacy picking up a drug that could have brought on a stroke or cardiac event, especially in a man of his age. David blamed himself for being tired and for allowing himself to miss this key information. But fortunately, the EMR wasn't tired and had automatically caught the mistake.

When Brian returned from vacation, David thought as he typed in another medication choice, there would be no more snarky comments from him about the new EMR. He was going to thank Brian for pushing the practice to select and deploy one. The other doctors had wanted to delay, not feeling comfortable with the technology, but the technology had just proved its usefulness. While the new EMR would still take some getting used to, David knew now that it was the right decision. In fact, he asked himself, why had they waited so long?

Why Hasn't EMR Been More Widely Embraced?

Dr. David Rodriguez is fictitious, but his predicament is quite real. Medication errors are common in the vast majority of group practices across the country (and in other countries as well). And EMRs with electronic prescription (e-Rx) capabilities can help to resolve this situation.

When the discussion turns to EMR adoption, physicians sometimes ask, "If the EMR is so good, why isn't it more widely adopted?" That's a very good question. MSP has been involved in EMR benchmarking for the past 13 years. This research identifies the top four reasons physicians have not adopted EMRs as: "Too much change is involved," "Lack of funding," "Difficulty evaluating the myriad of EMR products," and "Lack of office staff support." Figure 1.1 catalogs additional reasons that physicians haven't adopted EMRs according to EMR developers, who were asked to list the top seven barriers to EMR adoption.

Most EMR system users are glad to have them. A 2008 New England Journal of Medicine survey of 2,758 practicing physicians found that, of the small minority who had already adopted EMR systems, most were happy with their impact on patient care.[1] Those with fully functional systems reported higher satisfaction than those with more basic systems, although the majority with only basic system deployments were also pleased with the results.

---

[1] *Electronic Health Records in Ambulatory Care – A National Survey of Physicians.* By Catherine M. DesRoches, Dr.P.H, et al. Published July 3, 2008, Vol. 359, pp. 50-60 by the New England Journal of Medicine

Figure 1.1 Major Barriers to Adoption of EMR as Stated by EMR Developers

Stated Barrier to Adoption	% Believing to Be True
Too Much Change Involved	63%
Lack of Funding	58%
Difficulty Evaluating EMRs	43%
Lack of Office Staff Support	40%
No One Solution for All MDs	39%
EMRs Don't Meet Needs	39%
Lack of I.T. People	37%
No Reasonable ROI	32%
Concern About Amount of Training Needed	28%
Unwillingness to Change to Structured Terminology	24%
Migration Headache from Paper to Electronic Charting	24%
Difficulties of EMR/CPM Integration	21%
Consolidating EMR Market	18%
HIPAA Compliance	18%
Want a Mature EMR	17%
Too Much Investigation Time Involved	14%

People, including physicians, have trouble accommodating significant change, and adopting an EMR imposes a significant change. The adjustments involved seem overwhelming to many physicians, particularly those who are not already familiar with computers (whose total daily experience with them may be limited to checking their e-mail, if they even use e-mail).

Fear of failure is also a very significant issue, and has been well-founded, as 1-in-5 EMRs failed to live up to the expectations of those who deployed them. However, failure is mostly the result of inadequate planning, lack of thorough product evaluation or overlooking crucial issues that should have been addressed in the purchase or license agreement. These concerns are addressed in this book. Doctors are reluctant to deploy a tool that they feel uncomfortable using and fear might cause them to "fail" in front of their patients. Doctors are also reluctant to deploy a tool they themselves cannot fix when it's acting up, and most smaller practices don't have qualified Information Technology (I.T.) staff to handle EMR repair and management.

The cost objection is being addressed by the U.S. government putting more money on the table for EMR adoption. The Stark "Safe Harbor" exemptions make it legal for hospital I.T. personnel to assist in the deployment and maintenance of EMR technology for attending physicians. Whether doctors are comfortable with that arrangement is another matter. Indeed, organizations in each state are emerging to support I.T. deployment in physician offices. Sites like www.ehrselector.com are increasingly listing these organizations in the various states around the country. The government has also put financial reimbursement for the adoption of EMR on the table.

The final need is concise, task-specific technology information. You and your staff don't have time to take general computer courses that don't specifically relate to questions about deploying and maintaining an EMR. You want educational/technical materials that are highly focused and very specific to the diverse aspects of successful EMR planning and deployment. Hopefully, the contents of this book and information in the appendices will prove useful in that respect. The technically-focused chapters can give you a basis for understanding EMR support issues and set expectations about them. These chapters are a practical, on-going resource to you; or to whomever you choose to support the EMR you deploy in your practice (or clinical area).

The Benefits of Adopting EMR Systems

In the research cited earlier, MSP asked EMR developers to state what their EMRs' major benefits were. Figure 1.2 shows the consolidated responses mentioned by more than 100 EMR developers. Many listed more than one benefit expected. Not all of these benefits might be achieved by the adoption of any one particular EMR solution or in any one practice specialty.

Figure 1.2 Major Benefits of Adopting EMRs as Seen by EMR Developers

Benefits of EMR Adoption	% Believing to Be True
Reducing Medication Errors/Managing Medication Allergies	74%
Charting Compliance/Increased Reimbursement	68%
Computer Provider Order Entry (CPOE)	65%
Access to Charts from Multiple Offices	63%
Templates that are Specialty Specific	63%
Managing Patient Charts	63%
Charting Legibility	61%
E&M Coding	59%
Reducing Documentation Time	57%
Obtain Clinical Alerts Based on Test Results	57%
Simultaneous Chart Access in One Office	55%
Improved Workflow Management	52%
Move to Highly Structured Charting	47%
Real-Time Diagnosis and Decision Support	47%
Reducing FTEs and Payroll	44%
Disease Management	40%
Inform Drug Therapies Based on Lab Values	36%

Continued

Figure 1.2 Major Benefits of Adopting EMRs as Seen by EMR Developers

Benefits of EMR Adoption	% Believing to Be True
Load Patient-Specific Drug Formularies	34%
Transforming Paper Chart via Scanning/Indexing	33%
Interface to HIS	29%
Deploying an EMR that Accommodates Each Specialist's Needs	28%
Obtaining Pay-for-Performance Incentives	27%
Interfacing with Practice CPM System	21%
Tracking/Managing Patient Advanced Directives	17%
Providing a Patient Prescription Refill Portal	17%
Appointment Scheduling Through EMR	15%

There are also land mines associated with EMR adoption, which are discussed in later chapters of this book, so you can hopefully avoid them.

Everyone's Top Priority – Reducing Medication Errors

The number one benefit cited by the developers (and discovered by Dr. Rodriguez in our opening vignette) is the patient-focused benefit of reducing medication errors and preventing allergic reactions. The right EMR can also improve chart completion, improve work documentation thus allowing appropriate E&M coding, reduce the number of employees (and therefore payroll), improve workflow, facilitate CPOE, eliminate labor and space associated with the manual management of paper charts and provide access to charts in every office by multiple staff involved in the patient encounter - all things that cannot be achieved with a paper-based charting approach.

It is our belief that reducing the number of employees may not be an appropriate objective in smaller physician offices. If your EMR can enhance workflow, plan to increase staff to accommodate some of the 31 million newly insured Americans that the health reform legislation will ultimately create. Local physician offices are precisely where these newly insured patients should look for care. You can often create an extra exam room by re-purposing an old paper chart storage area, so don't be too quick to plan to reduce staff and payroll.

A less frequently emphasized benefit of EMR adoption is better support of disease management. In order to meet Meaningful Use, hospitals where you have admitting privileges, may also push you to interface with their HIS (Health Information System). An EMR gives you the tool to document care that qualifies for both the quality measure and e-Rx incremental CMS reimbursements. With an EMR you can better track and manage advanced directives, engage in e-mail dialog with patients (if you care to) and have the data required to analyze physician practice patterns, and receive/send disease outbreak or bioterrorism data once the Nationwide Health Information Network (NHIN) becomes fully operational.

At the end of the day, it doesn't matter what any EMR developer's goals are, it matters what your goals are. The trick is to find the EMR that best matches your goals and is easy to use so it enhances your office workflow.

Many Other Priorities – What Are Yours?

If you can't decide what your goals are, you will have difficulty sorting through the various EMR developers' products. Some benefits can be achieved without a full-featured EMR. Many physicians are concerned about having specific enough documentation to justify submitting higher paying E&M codes. Separate E&M coding tools are already available without full EMR functionality. If your goal is only to increase reimbursement, then look for an EMR that includes a good E&M coding module that can integrate with your CPM system. If your practice involves mostly capitated care for patients with chronic diseases, then look for an EMR developer with a strong disease management focus or that interfaces to specific disease registries you'll need to access.

In the case of medication errors, most of the developers' EMRs address this issue somewhat. The New England Journal of Medicine survey cited at the beginning of this chapter found that 86 percent of doctors with fully-functional electronic record systems (those with clinical decision support and order entry features, including electronic prescribing) reported having a reduced incidence of medical errors as a result. Patient diagnostic accuracy and quality of patient care were also improved.

Medical misdiagnosis rates are high, ranging widely in various studies from 8 to 42 percent, depending upon specialty and point of encounter with the medical system. EMRs with decision support functionality can help physicians and medical staffs improve that statistic in almost all practices, but EMRs vary in their decision support capabilities.

Deciding on an initial goal for your EMR, most of these benefits are not only applicable to U.S. physicians, but to medical practitioners around the world. In fact, the largest U.S. EMR developers (GE, McKesson, Cerner, Allscripts, Siemens and others) are also major international EMR suppliers involved in advancing paperless practices in the U.K., Canada, Australia, India, the Middle East and China.

Why is Timely Action Imperative?

Five major reasons to automate your clinical charting now:

1   The American Recovery and Reinvestment Act of 2009 (ARRA) legislation provides reimbursement of funds spent to adopt EMRs that achieve Meaningful Use (also see Introduction for details), but the longer you wait, the less money you will get back. Malpractice insurers and third-

party payers are strongly encouraging practices to adopt as well. Indeed, you will need to start soon to avoid being caught in the avalanche of physicians waiting for the clarification of Meaningful Use. After that there will be a scarcity of all types of services. Within 5 years EMRs will essentially be mandated, so why wait?.

2 An EMR will help your practice reduce medication and other preventable errors, and facilitate your adoption of evidence-based medicine. There are already incremental reimbursement incentives (up to 4 percent) for practices that report PQRI (Physician Quality Reporting Initiative) data and utilize electronic prescription checking. So EMRs enhance practice revenue today.

3 Your practice is worth less if it isn't successfully automated. EMRs not only improve your practice's bottom line today, but make your practice more valuable when it comes time for you to sell it and retire. Without an EMR, you will find reimbursement continuing to decline in relation to your ever-escalating costs.

4 The challenge of continued patient satisfaction as more people seek healthcare makes improving workflow and reducing errors essential steps.

5 Practices that do not adopt EMR by 2014 will see a one-percent-per-year reduction in the payments they receive for CMS patients (to a total of 5%). That penalty is likely to increase in subsequent years.

Government and Others Value Quality & Evidence-Based Medicine

Electronic Medical Record (EMR) solutions are on the Obama healthcare reform agenda to improve quality, reduce administrative costs and help move the U.S. to an evidence-based practice methodology. President Obama's are not the only initiatives, but they help and the early adopter gets the bulk of the incentives being offered.

"The 2006 Tax Relief and Health Care Act (TRHCA) (P.L.109-432) required the establishment of a physician quality reporting system, including an incentive payment for eligible professionals (EPs) who satisfactorily report data on quality measures for covered services furnished to Medicare beneficiaries during the second half of 2007 (the 2007 reporting period). CMS named this program the Physician Quality Reporting Initiative (PQRI).

2009 PQRI Payment Incentives: The Medicare Improvements for Patients and Providers Act of 2008 (MIPPA) (Pub. L. 110-275) made the PQRI program permanent, but only authorized incentive payments through 2010. EPs who meet the criteria for satisfactory submission of quality measures data for services furnished during the reporting period, January 1, 2009 – December 31, 2009, will earn an incentive payment of 2.0 percent of their total allowed charges for Physician Fee Schedule (PFS) covered professional services furnished during that same period (the 2009 calendar year)."[2]

---

[2]The standard list of 153 quality measures and 7 measures groups can be found online at http://www.cms.hhs.gov/PQRI/Downloads/2009_PQRI_MeasuresList_030409.pdf.

According to a report by the Congressional Budget Office (CBO), in an analysis requested by Rep. Henry Waxman, (D-CA), left to itself, the market would take until 2019 for half of the U.S. hospitals and two-thirds of physicians to deploy EMRs. That same report suggested that if policy was amended to provide financial and other policy incentives, hospital adoption would be boosted to 70 percent and physician adoption to 90 percent levels in that same period.

The Obama Administration has now provided those incentives in the ARRA (and HITECH) legislation. EMR prices are relatively low right now, and most of the cost will ultimately be offset by government incentives. The EMR adoption process takes about a year, so practices need to seriously consider starting it now, particularly if they want to get in on reimbursement starting in 2011. When the EMR market heats up and adoption rates increase, so will prices, and deployment and training times will also lengthen.

Lately, hospitals and other organizations with their own agendas for promoting EMRs have become engaged. If you wait to adopt an EMR, more payors, malpractice insurers, employer groups, hospital CIOs, and others will want a say in controlling the EMR you select. These groups, while well-meaning, are not in a position to understand how their suggestions will impact your practice's workflow efficiency or fit other practice needs. Beware of third-parties (Trojan horses) bearing EMR financial reimbursement gifts – if they come with any strings attached. Be certain you don't sacrifice the best solution for your office to placate another organization's needs. After you adopt any EMR, you will have to live with the results it provides. If an EMR doesn't meet your needs and improve your workflow, it is not a bargain, even if it is apparently "free". Remember that you will pay the software maintenance costs every year after you adopt an EMR, which are based on its list price, no matter what you initially paid for it. That cost will be anywhere from 16 to 26 percent of the list price.

What About Open Source EMR Solutions?

Open source EMRs[3], such as PatientOS, which a one of the various incantations of the Veterans Health Information Systems and Technology Architecture (VistA), are an alternative to be considered – just like any other proprietary EMR alternative. VistA is an enterprise-wide information system built around an electronic health record that was once used throughout the United States Department of Veterans Affairs (VA) medical system. In fact, there are several flavors of VistA.

These open source systems have one major advantage over many proprietary EMRs; the source code for the entire application is available to all users. This openness is usually not available with proprietary EMR alternatives,

---

[3] See the Open Source EMR Organization (OEMR), www.oemr.org, for more information. The group has developers in the United States, Puerto Rico, Australia, Sweden, Holland, Israel, India, Malaysia, Nepal, Indonesia, Bermuda, Armenia and Kenya.

particularly from larger, more established EMR developers. Making the EMR source code available to physicians in case of potentially disruptive events in the EMR developer's life (such as bankruptcy or the acquisition of the developer by another vendor that decides not to make the acquired product their "go ahead" version) is something that should be negotiated in all purchasing and licensing agreements; as it is the only leverage that a small group practice has in assuring that their system is supported in such events. In the open system approach, every user has access to the application source code (which is the meaning of open source), and can develop (or hire someone to develop) any variations they want to for "their version" of the application.

Open source raises two questions. Are you interested in maintaining (or developing) your application in the event of the failure of the EMR developer? And, are open source EMR developers more likely to fail than their proprietary EMR counterparts?

While access to source code is one important issue, it's not the overriding issue. Any EMR you seriously consider deploying must be a good overall fit, e.g. it must work well. It's like a suit; if the jacket fits your shoulders perfectly, but the arms are 4 inches too short, and the rise of the trousers is 4 inches longer than needed, then you'll look like a monkey wearing a nice suit – even if it's free! In the same way, any open source EMR must be evaluated against every criteria that's important to you, and not simply touted because it's open source.

On the MSP EHR Selector Web site, only one open source EMR has been willing to be listed and compared to the dozens of commercially available EMR alternatives and you can see how it compares. There are two main reasons that any EMR developer would not want to list their EMR on the this Web site. First, the EMR developer can't afford the modest product vetting fee to have critical product features independently vetted. Second, they feel their EMR product(s) don't compare well across the 700+ criteria covered by the MSP EHR Selector. That would not be a problem at other EMR information sites, because these sites do not catalog as many product features; rather their comparisons can be based as few as 15-25 very basic and non-specific EMR criteria that don't accentuate important product differences.

Proprietary EMRs

Physicians want to know what they are buying in an EMR and how it will work in their practice specialty. One can conclude from the current 20 percent failure/dissatisfaction rate that just because Brand-X EMR (even if CCHIT – Commission for the Certification of Health Information Technology – certified) works well in mental health, it may be a terrible fit in pediatrics, or cardiology, or oncology – all with vastly different EMR functionality needs. Working well is much more than simply complying with CCHIT certification criteria. It's about practice-specific templates, EMR user interfaces that are easy-to-use and intuitive, and about inherent design that enhances workflow rather than layering so much nonessential functionality on the EMR, that it becomes a complex, difficult-to-learn behemoth. EMRs can be certified and yet not fit the needs of any specific practice specialty very well. CCHIT criteria do not address many of these other important issues.

There are over 220 EMR products that we track in the market at any one time, 100+ of which can be dismissed rather quickly due to their size and functionality characteristics. Of the 120 or so remaining, over 40 of them can easily be compared in-depth. If EMRs are to be adopted and succeed on a wide scale, across all practice specialty types, then EMR developers are going to have to allow physicians to compare critical functionality for specific practice specialties, and that makes tools that enable such comparisons fairly and impartially, more critical than ever to the EMR evaluation and selection process.

No static information resource can provide such a comparison – not this book and not an EMR features CD because EMR products are not static entities; and static information quickly becomes outdated information. Major changes occur every 6-9 months, and the rate of change in 2010 and 2011 will be enormous in response to Meaningful Use requirements being published and new guidelines being issued by liability insurance and medical specialty organizations. Physicians need to find current and comprehensive sources of information concerning EMR products. Even though there are 220+ EMR developers in the market, no single EMR currently supports all 46 major practice specialties included in the MSP EHR Selector; indeed, two-thirds of all EMRs support fewer than 10 practice specialties. This is desirable, because it means they support them effectively – something that the larger EMR developers supporting 20 or 30 specialties, don't necessarily do adequately, as their KLAS Research[4] rating clearly demonstrate.

ONCHIT and CCHIT: Government Certification of EMRs

The Bush Administration tried to accelerate EMR adoption by creating the Office of the National Coordinator of Healthcare Information Technology (ONCHIT or now ONC). That office then established CCHIT (Commission for Certification of Health Information Technology) to promote standardizing minimal functions for the EMR and to certify EMR products (unfortunately they referred to it as EHR certification, which created confusion).

If an EMR vendor sells three EMRs, they each need to be separately certified. Not all EMRs conform to CCHIT standards, but currently over 90 EMRs have received certification in the last 2.5 years. Also, not all of them have maintained their certification. If reducing malpractice insurance premiums or obtaining financing for your EMR under the Stark Safe Harbors legislation matters to you, be sure to select from only those EMR products that are CCHIT-certified in the current year.

---

[4] KLAS Research rates EMR vendors for physician and hospital satisfaction after they are installed. KLAS ratings are integrated into the MSP EHR Selector (www.ehrselector.com) and can also be found at the KLAS Research Web site, www.klasresearch.com.

EMR Terminology and Conceptual Evolution

The conceptual underpinnings of electronic medical and health records is being defined and redefined as these systems continue to be deployed. Even the terminology is evolving, making it difficult to follow the topic in the literature. There are three essential terms and concepts that are important to understanding electronic medical records as you begin your EMR search.

- The first is the Personal Health Record (PHR), which is a repository of information collected by patients about themselves, which includes anything from self-entered data to Electronic Medical Record (EMR) data they have collected from various providers. There are about 130 PHR products available at this time. Many are islands unto themselves.
- The second term is Electronic Medical Record (EMR), which is the topic of this book. It refers to electronic data implemented to support one medical care provider/practice, such as a physician office, or home healthcare agency, or skilled nursing facility or clinical department in a hospital. The EMR is not specific to how the data is stored, and covers both the storage of information at the care site (e.g. physician office) by an EMR that is deployed there, and also an EMR that is deployed on the Internet by an EMR Application Service Provider (ASP) located somewhere on the World Wide Web, where records are stored and maintained at their site and not in the physician office.
- The third term is Electronic Health Record (EHR), which is a longitudinal repository of information assembled for a point-of-care from any EMR or PHR sources known to exist for the patient. The point-of-care could be an emergency department (ED) that requests patient data from a hospital EMR, several physician office EMRs and the patient's own PHR. The EHR record created at the point-of-care may not have previously existed before the ED request processed by a Regional Health Information Organizations (RHIOs) that supports health information exchanges (HIEs). Patient records available through RHIOs are generally not persistent. There is much variation in EHR usage. Some also define EHRs as systems that support semantic interoperability. Figure 1.3 provides a simplified picture.

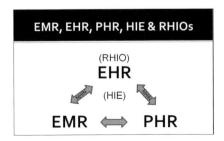

Figure 1.3 PHR, EMR, EHR Relationship

For the purposes of this book, we'll use the term Electronic Medical Record (EMR) exclusively to mean an electronic equivalent of the paper chart located in one healthcare provider's office/location, which they created and control the access to.

The ability of the EMR to be interoperable and bidirectionally exchange data with the EHR (upon request) and the PHR in a way that these other computer systems "understand" the information being received, can be properly integrated into the receiving record, and be independently acted upon by the receiving system, is important. This is our layman's definition of "bidirectional semantic interoperability". It is likely to become a requirement for Meaningful Use, if not initially, in subsequent years. To achieve it requires structured data that supports standards. This is not achieved by many EMRs or PHRs. In reality, it is state-of-the-art if an EMR can even get structured data from a patient's PHR – forget bidirectional exchange.

Older Terms Used Create Confusion

In some literature and Web articles, you may find the EMR referred to (incorrectly) as an EHR. If fact the government has been careless about differentiating the two terms. As shown in the previous diagram, Electronic Health Records (EHRs) are composed of data from two or more EMRs or from an EMR and a patient's Personal Health Record (PHR).

The Institute of Medicine (IOM), in 1991, referred to current-day EMR systems as CPRS (Computer-based Patient Record Systems). The Medical Records Institute (MRI) coined the term EPR (Electronic Patient Record), initiating a national conference called TEPR (Toward the Electronic Patient Record), which is now defunct. The term EMR (Electronic Medical Record) system was then substituted for these terms in various outpatient settings. EPR is not a widely used term anymore, but where it is used, it can be thought of as synonymous with EMR.

Later, the term EHR (Electronic Health Record) was introduced. Initially it did not have the notion of being a longitudinal repository of ALL patient information, so many individual EMR developers adopted the term, and so unfortunately did the Commission for the Certification of Health Information Technology (CCHIT, see box). This further blurred the distinction between EMR and EHR terms.

Elsewhere, federal legislation refers to an EHR as a repository of consumer health status information in computer-readable form used for clinical diagnosis and treatment for a broad array of clinical conditions. This is ambiguous enough to be a correct definition of EHR, but CCHIT uses it in the context of ONE care provider, so they really mean EMR. This appeared in the Federal Register for purposes of clarifying federal reimbursement under the recent Stark "Safe Harbor" law passed in 2008. We'll use the term EMR in this book and advise you when we are really talking about EHR.

The term Health Information Organization (HIO) has now emerged as well. HIOs provide the capability to electronically move clinical information among disparate health care information systems over the NHIN while maintaining the meaning of the information being exchanged. Regional Health Information Organizations (or RHIOs) are the organizations that will be responsible for encouraging and causing integration and information exchange in the U.S. healthcare system, again over the NHIN. Confusing isn't it? See Chapter 8, *Interoperability Beyond EMRs* for clarification and elaboration.

What's EMR-Lite?

You may also come across the term, EMR-Lite. An EMR-Lite is a new approach to deploying some of the most basic functions of EMRs – functions such as drug-drug interactions, e-prescription or CPOE (Computerized Provider Order Entry), without deploying all of the other functionality of a general purpose EMR. Due to their limited functionality, EMR-Lite products cannot yet be CCHIT certified, which may create issues getting deployment expenses reimbursed under ARRA/ HITECH (as it is now written). The term can be applied to electronic records that are less structured and depend heavily on document scanning, dictation and speech recognition that create free-form text entry, or other approaches that are only partially structured. Many EMR-Lite products can chart some clinical data. Such systems can be very user-friendly and inexpensive but consider data structuring, the upgrade path to full-featured EMRs and evolving government requirements before committing to this approach.

The EMR-Lite idea is to pick the low hanging fruit from the EMR deployment tree. It's not a bad approach under certain circumstances; the deployment cost is less, the learning curve is not as steep and thus deployment is easier, it addresses some of the key EMR functionality and is a technology that most physicians feel comfortable managing. In days of yore, this was the venue of companies like Epocrates and PatientKeeper, but now mainstream, integrated EMR and CPM developers like Henry Schein and others are offering EMR-Lite alternatives to their fully integrated, top-end solutions. The idea is to draw in physicians to their branded EMR-Lite product, and then keep the account when the physician is ready to use full EMR product functions. To differentiate their EMR-Lite products from Epocrates and others, many EMR developers have added E&M codes and other extras that some of the more mature CPOE and handheld devices don't offer. It's not a bad approach, but if it appeals to you, here's what to look for:

- The EMR-Lite product must have an inexpensive, simple upgrade path to full EMR functionality, which maintains all patient records created by the EMR-Lite version. If you decide on the EMR-Lite approach, make sure all records created with the EMR-Lite product will be 100 percent compatible with the records created by the full featured EMR product.
- The EMR-Lite product must be upgradable to an EMR that meets minimum Meaningful Use requirements, so that you can be reimbursed for deploying it. Be cautious here. It doesn't seem like Uncle Sam is going to reimburse you twice, so if Meaningful Use does cover your EMR-Lite product, it probably won't cover your upgrade costs to the fully functional EMR (or

integrated EMR+CPM) product. By opting for the less sophisticated EMR-Lite product, you may be letting your rich Uncle off the hook for the cost of any upgrades.

- Finally, make sure that the full EMR product that you can ultimately upgrade to is an excellent fit for your specific needs, since that's the ultimate goal. If the full EMR product is not a good fit for any reason, deploying the EMR-Lite version makes no sense. If the EMR-Lite locks you into a migration path to the wrong type of EMR, it won't be a good starter alternative.

This means you must evaluate the complete EMR product, and only when you have found one that meets your full EMR needs, look at any EMR-Lite the EMR developer offers before deciding which to implement.

As long as you take the above considerations into account, deployment of an EMR-Lite solution may be a way of putting your toes into the EMR waters. But it is definitely a short-term solution.

Thoughts for Smaller, Rural Hospitals

Special challenges apply to hospitals looking to adopt EMR at the point of care, particularly smaller and rural ones. Given the financial challenges of being small and the difficulty of attracting physicians to rural areas, the prospect and cost of adopting hospital-wide EMRs is daunting. Over one out of three American hospitals operate in non-urban or metropolitan areas and 66 percent of these (about 1,306) have downsized to 25 beds[5] or less in order to qualify for the Critical Access Hospital (CAH) program offered by the government. Under the CAH program the government reimburses the actual costs of operations rather than paying on a DRG basis.

Being 25 beds in size makes small hospitals no larger than a large group practice and means that they will struggle with the same implementation issues. While the cost of adoption may be off the table thanks to ARRA, the ability to find and keep the information technology staff necessary to deploy and operate an EMR is certainly not. Hospitals in this category may need to seek alliances with larger systems in order to ease issues such as: physician attraction, collaboration, and EMR planning and deployment.

Physicians admitting to small hospitals or CAHs, aren't likely to find financial assistance through the Stark Safe Harbor legislation and need to look to ARRA (HITECH) funding to cover EMR deployment costs. Moreover, don't expect much information technology support from small hospitals or CAHs either. Approaching the hospital administration to host a meeting of all area physicians to discuss a collaborative EMR support approach may prove fruitful. As a group, community physicians and their small hospital represent a value proposition that could be interesting to computer support organizations.

---

[5] Critical Access Hospitals (CAHs) can also have up to 10 additional psych beds and 10 additional rehab beds, so could have a total of 45 beds related to some type of care that an EMR might have to support.

We would be pleased to conduct an EMR informational Webinar for such hospitals and their attending physicians as well.

Thoughts for Solo Practitioners

The ARRA (HITECH) legislation changes the playing field of solo practitioners and potentially puts your practice (without an EMR) at risk. ARRA ups the ante of expectations for all physician practices but particularly for solo practices. It does this by creating a critical mass of technology requirements that may be beyond what you personally have time to do. It isn't about the money, it's about the time. You can't see patients and wait on hold for 10 to 30-minutes for remote technical support from inside or outside of the U.S. Adoption of an EMR will mean adding (or contracting with) I.T. support staff. Collaboration with other solo practitioners is a good alternative for you and may be essential to make EMR adoption realistic for your practice.

Can EMRs Improve Patient Satisfaction?

Satisfaction surveys show that patients are increasingly frustrated with their medical office experience in paper-based practices, but often remain silent. One way to uncover hidden patient frustrations is to ask patients how you can improve their experience in your office. An anonymous survey works best. You could provide a card with a Web address where your patients can take a satisfaction survey online or give them a survey form and a pre-posted, business-reply envelope to mail it back for tabulation. You may be surprised at the responses you get to a satisfaction survey that asks questions such as:

- "How friendly is the office staff?"
- "Would you prefer to have your information on file or continue to fill out paper forms at each office visit?"
- "Would you prefer your doctor know which pharmacy you use and send your prescriptions over for you?"

Surveys have already shown that increasing numbers of patients expect conveniences such as medication refills that are automated, or the ability to schedule appointments via the Internet. Technologically-savvy, younger patients have concerns about the way care is delivered today, so don't mistake silence for satisfaction. Patients respect their caregivers but frequently have some level of dissatisfaction with how they are treated and how much of their time is wasted waiting for care. If your patients affirm any of these common frustrations via your survey, your practice is definitely a candidate for conversion to an EMR system, and maybe a replacement of your current CPM system as well. A patient portal or office kiosk may also be part of the solution.

We suggest running two patient satisfaction surveys, one before you adopt your EMR and another one-year afterwards. Compare the results and you have a direct measure of how the deployment of an EMR has changed your practice and your patient satisfaction levels. Don't start the second survey until your EMR has been in place for nine months, so that things are running smoothly.

Not all patients like practices that have deployed EMRs. If the implementation is poorly conceived or executed, it can lead to patients feeling that, "the doctor spends more time looking at the computer than he/she does looking at me." That's not a good outcome and it's not a necessary one either. Redesign your exam room to accommodate your EMR carefully. Don't chart with your back to the patient, use the right tool, probably a medical tablet PC. Engage the patient in looking at the screen with you at some points, so the patient is drawn into the EMR charting process you are conducting.

It Has to Be the Ideal EMR for You!

Is all this information on EMRs perhaps beginning to make your head spin? How will you ever discover your ideal EMR? Listed below are some EMR adoption basics, but keep in mind that your ideal EMR is like that suit referenced earlier – it needs to fit both you and your other office personnel well, not the practice across the hall, not what the CCHIT Commission mandates or what the government would like to see, or you local hospitals wants you to adopt so they can share test results. The ideal EMR is a very personal matter. This book, and the resources it identifies, will help you to discover what "ideal" is to you. However, here are some common denominators that everyone needs in an EMR.

It must be secure, work in real-time, and be a patient-centric information resource designed for clinicians to use at the point-of-care. Secure because patient data is protected; real-time means it's used during the patient encounter, not entered later; and patient-centric means it's organized around your patients' needs, not secondary stakeholders' needs. It should enhance your diagnostic skills, improve your decision-making and care plan processes by providing access to diagnostic information while the patient is present in your exam room.

Some EMRs excel at streamlining workflow, others allow customization of patient encounter tasks. The ideal EMR would support the collection of data for uses other than direct clinical care, such as billing, quality management, outcomes reporting, resource planning, public health disease surveillance and reporting and supporting claims made during meetings with CMS Recovery Audit Contractors (RACs).

The ideal EMR is also a tool that delivers encounter documentation to the patient before they leave the physician's office and whenever possible engages the patient in providing some of their own information, even if that requires some staff assistance.[6] That's not original to us, nor is it something that every provider agrees with, but we encourage you to wrestle with the concept.

---

[6] *The Patient-Computer Interview: A Neglected Tool That Can Aid the Clinician.* By John W. Bachman. Published January 2003, Vol. 78, No. 1, pp. 67-78, Mayo Clinic Proceedings

Broaching the EMR Adoption Subject

Given the benefits, isn't it time to incorporate an EMR into your practice? How can you broach the EMR adoption conversation with your office staff? Dismiss any inclinations to make this decision alone – lest you become the "lone-EMR-ranger". That's a guaranteed failure approach. Broaching uncomfortable topics is always challenging. A good plan helps, waiting for the right timing does also. Who in your office is frustrated with the status-quo and likely to become an ally in making a change? Who is likely to oppose any change from the status-quo, whether change is needed or not?

If you handle difficult conversations well, and succeed in winning over the skeptics, skip the rest of this chapter, do what works for you and don't let us mess you up. On the other hand, if you frequently wonder why the outcome you hoped for isn't the outcome you typically end up with – read on.

Both authors believe that because an EMR will affect everyone in your office, you need to begin by speaking to all staff about the general idea of adopting an EMR. All staff means your receptionist, billing people, nursing, advanced practice nursing or physician assistants, and physicians – we believe you need to include them all! Use this book as an excuse and suggest that everyone read it as a prelude to a discussion of the pros and cons of adopting an EMR. Pass a few copies around, so that this preliminary step doesn't take forever.

If you are the one most interested in an EMR but are not the one who usually brings up new topics, get a copy of *Crucial Conversations*[7] and *Crucial Confrontations*[8] and read these excellent books yourself. These are two of the best books available, and they will help you to manage this change as a crucial conversation. Today, with the ARRA (HITECH) incentives on the table and healthcare on the verge of a massive overhaul, this is a crucial moment and EMR adoption truly requires a crucial conversation. Both books are available at any large bookstore or on Amazon.

EMRs not only benefit the physician adopters, but often their staff even more. It is essential that all stakeholders understand how an EMR will affect them in their roles and why adopting this technology makes sense from an overall practice perspective. Consider talking to your colleagues and staff at your next office meeting about the current situation your practice faces in the new healthcare climate, and how EMRs could help. If you decide to go ahead, have all involved staff members read a chapter at a time and then discuss each chapter. By working through it together, everyone stays on the same page – and it will build a sense that you are all in this together.

---

[7] *Crucial Conversations: Tools for Talking When Stakes are High*. By Kerry Patterson et al. Published 2002 by McGraw-Hill Publishing, ISBN: 13: 9780071401944

[8] *Crucial Confrontations: Tools for Talking about Broken Promises, Violated Expectations, and Bad Behavior*. By Kerry Patterson et al. Published 2005, Ibid, ISBN: 10: 0071446524

Initiate your EMR discussion by sharing some facts about EMRs and the new U.S. healthcare realities. Start off with open-ended questions designed to invite staff responses. You might ask these key questions:

1 If the government succeeds in bringing 31 million uninsured Americans into the healthcare system by providing some sort of insurance, what would it mean for our practice? Could we handle an influx of new patients in our practice with our current paper-based clinical records approach?

2 If the trend of mandating quality outcome reporting continues and we can get incremental reimbursement, how can we capture the data and bill for improved outcomes? Is there a practical way to do this without an EMR?

3 How can we keep current staffing levels if we allow our practice revenue to diminish further? If EMRs can enhance practice revenue, how will that benefit everyone?

4 How could an EMR improve our workflow without changing overall staffing levels?

Any of these questions will initiate the larger discussion of exploring an EMR as a possible solution to one or more of these challenges every practice faces today. How would having an EMR affect workflow during a medication recall, or when new warnings have to be evaluated against every patient in the practice and require chart pulls and other tedious manual interventions? Would an EMR in any way expedite or simplify these situations? How could everyday workflow bottlenecks be expedited by an EMR? How might an EMR create new ones?

Choosing Your Research Point Person

When you reach consensus that EMR adoption is worthy of further investigation and discussion, the next step is to assign an EMR "Point Person" to gather and present information on EMRs at future meetings. Once your staff and colleagues begin to envision and ponder how deploying an EMR can solve larger problems, you are well on your way to a meaningful dialog.

Your office manager is a likely Point Person candidate. Assure whoever you make Point Person that you are available to help and provide access to resources they need. Most providers who have not yet automated their practices have only a vague idea of what an EMR is, what it can do for them and how to proceed. You are free to copy any charts from this book, which can help you document your thought process and decisions. The Scorecards at the end of chapters document the Crucial Decisions you make and list any Action Items requiring attention. They will help when it's time to write your Request For Proposal (RFP) after you have had EMR developers demonstrate their products. Chapter Scorecards and some charts and diagrams fare available at the MSP ESP Portal Web site, www.ehrselector.com.

Protect Your Anonymity When Researching EMRs

One key Internet EMR information caution: don't browse all over EMR developers' Web sites looking for EMR product information at this stage in your process, it will simply trigger an avalanche of premature sales follow-up contacts. Use only Internet sites that protect your privacy and do not disclose (or sell) your names to any EMR developers. The very first thing to read at any Internet site is its Privacy Statement. Check for use of Web-bugs too. Think ahead before registering at every EMR site Google directs you to. Uninvited and disruptive sales contacts are easier to avoid than to turnoff, once they have begun. If a site doesn't guarantee your anonymity, don't go there.

Next Step – Confidence & Consensus Building
The change to EMRs is coming but it doesn't have to be overly complicated. What's needed is a pragmatic approach based on impartial, reliable EMR information and most importantly, the will to improve your practice. Reassure your staff that making this transition will succeed if everyone works together. After all, the majority of the largest practices in the U.S. have already automated. Learn from the experience of these early adopters.

When EMR developers were asked, "What have physicians done to overcome adoption barriers?," the top responses included:
- Researched the topic to get up the learning curve and in some cases hired EMR consultants;
- Found ARRA and Stark funding source to finance EMR adoption;
- Educated their staff to build a consensus about the specialty-specific EMR functions required;
- Attended conferences where EMR developers were exhibiting systems for their specialty (see Appendix II for a suggested list);
- Used an EMR/EHR selector tool that matches practice needs against EMR features available in commercial products (see Appendix III).

Many affordable resources exist to help you in the EMR adoption process. By researching before you choose a product, you can shorten deployment time, avoid backtracking and enhance staff satisfaction with, and use of, the EMR deployed.

Single Step (Big-Bang) Vs. Multi-Step (Phased) Deployment
Once you decide to deploy an EMR you must also determine whether to deploy all EMR functionality in one step (a big-bang approach), or to adopt a multi-step (phased deployment) approach. The gating factors may include the amount of change your staff can accommodate and your budget constraints. If you decide that an integrated EMR and CPM (Computer Practice Management) system would be the best solution, you could deploy the EMR as step one and continue to use your existing CPM. When your staff has become acquainted with the EMR, switch over to the integrated CPM and retire your current CPM. Just because a product has many features doesn't mean that you need to deploy them all at once. The deployment sequence should be such that it doesn't overwhelm your staff but rather allows them to manage and become efficient with the changes as they are being introduced.

This is why many practices opt for a phased (stepped) approach rather than a big bang deployment, particularly for integrated EMR/CPM products. In some hospitals, deployment is a continuous process that spans 7 to 10 years.

Wrap Up

If you decide to adopt an EMR determine not to turn back. Think of it as a wagon train experience like the pioneers of old. When you hit a rough spot, remember the vision and reasons you made the decision to do this. No matter what the ultimate outcome of the political debate about healthcare reform, the right EMR is a tool that will empower your practice. Take the time to consider the issues and get it right the first time.

Deploying an EMR is no longer the venue of physician-computer geeks, it has become the province of mainstream medicine. Indeed, it is essential going forward to increasingly adopt evidenced-based, best practices. Chapter 1 has provided a broad overview of some good reasons to adopt EMR now. If you have decided to proceed, the remaining chapters will lead you, Crucial Decision-by-Crucial Decision, through the rest of the process.

There is no "one linear path" through all of the Crucial Decisions you must make. We cover Crucial Decisions in a particular sequence and logical order, yet some of those we cover later on may cause you to revisit earlier decisions that you have already made, based on new or additional information provided. Therefore, don't consider any Crucial Decision you make on the first pass through this book to be a final decision. Expect to make at least a second pass through the Crucial Decision process before casting your decisions in stone.

CHAPTER 2

How EMR Will Enhance Your Practice

Crucial Decision

What method will you use to build staff consensus to adopt an EMR in your practice?

This chapter also addresses the following questions:

- How can an EMR improve the patient experience?
- What are each stakeholder's EMR adoption goals?
- How do you determine if you have achieved your goals after EMR deployment?

EMR Adventures

Anne Roberts has a recurring pain in her abdomen that doesn't quite seem like indigestion. Her primary care physician, Dr. David Rodriguez, has referred her to Dr. Karen Bell, a gastroenterologist. She is trying to squeeze in her appointment at lunchtime before she has to return to the office for a client meeting at 2 P.M. When she arrives on time, only to find out she'll have to wait because Dr. Bell's office is backed up and the patient scheduled before her is sitting next to her in the waiting room, she immediately becomes anxious about the delay and her blood pressure rises.

Anne is handed a clipboard and a pen and told to fill out the forms with the same basic information that she has already given to all of her doctors, including Dr. Rodriguez. "Why couldn't Dr. Rodriguez share the information with Dr. Bell, when it was all on his new computer system that he was so proud of? Why do I have to fill this out all over again?" she wonders.

Anne questions why Dr. Bell cannot organize her practice more efficiently, like Dr. Rodriguez. Why is she behind schedule on this day of all days? If she kept people waiting this long, her business would lose clients. Is Dr. Bell a good doctor? She hopes Dr. Rodriguez knew what he was doing with this referral.

As Anne makes her way through the seemingly endless check boxes on the form, she thinks: "I've already answered most of these questions for my primary care physician, why can't these guys communicate with each other and just send the records over? Why can't a doctor visit be more like going to my bank, or seeing my accountant, or even my dry cleaner – each uses

---

Successfully Choosing Your EMR: 15 Crucial Decisions. By © Arthur Gasch and Betty Gasch. Published 2010 by Blackwell Publishing

a computer. When will doctors get out of the Stone Age and quit wasting patient time?"

Now finished with the 20-question part of the check-in, Anne pages through a magazine without much interest, every ten minutes consulting her watch. She wishes she had scheduled the appointment for a different day, but Anne had already put off scheduling the time twice this month and was becoming worried about her symptoms. Anne notices that her stomach is beginning to cramp and knows she has to stay for the visit.

Finally, the other patient is called in, 45 minutes late according to Anne's watch. Anne now realizes that lunch is out of the question due to the delay. As her stomach pain flares up, Anne fears it can't be heartburn, because she hasn't eaten – thanks to Dr. Bell's backup – and wonders if it's something more ominous, like an ulcer, or even cancer? "My time is just as precious as Dr. Bell's," she fumes. "Maybe she'd be more prompt if she had to pay me for all of my time that's being wasted," she thinks to herself. "Maybe I should ask her to deduct something from my bill!"

Finally, Anne is ushered into the exam room, where the nurse says, "Hi, how are you today?"

Anne replies, "Fine, except for these stomach pains." But the nurse can tell that something more is wrong. Anne seems frustrated and tense, like many of the other patients she greets each day. Guess that just goes with this job, she thinks to herself, as she starts to write down Anne's vital signs.

Improving the Patient Experience Using EMRs

Anne's long wait could have been shortened by improved office efficiency, something an EMR can certainly help to accomplish. But EMRs can do so much more. Our fictitious patient's frustration derives from the inefficient practice workflow that she is subjected to when she visits Dr. Bell's office. Anne perceives these inefficiencies as unnecessary, and thus, rude, which only heightens her sense of receiving poor treatment.

EMRs have the potential to change many aspects of the patient experience. As you begin to envision your EMR-enhanced practice, don't think about where you will fit computers into your existing space; rather, think about how to rework your current office area to accommodate the efficiencies that a computerized EMR will bring. Let's look at how an EMR might be used to benefit both your staff and your patients.

The patient's experience (the face-to-face part of it) begins in your waiting room, so start there and imagine your new office. One way to include your patients in making your office more efficient is to choose an EMR that supports patient entry (or transfer) of their own data from a Personal Health Record (PHR); or more likely, from the information they fill out and send over the Internet to your office the day prior to their visit.

Many patients today have computers with Internet connection. By using an instant medical history guided interview, information such the reason for your patient's visit, chief complaint, all drugs and dietary supplements they are taking, and so much more can be transmitted for your review prior to their coming to your office. The patient's medical insurance can be verified and their medical formulary loaded, long before they are greeted by your receptionist. This is all the data that your patients won't need to reenter when they arrive at your practice.

Another good reason to have the patient do their medical history interview at home, is that he or she has access to all of their medication and to their food supplements (including the doses). It will achieve a more complete chart and better idea of what your patients are really taking. You may be surprised at what they have added to their regimen without first checking with you!

Having your patients enter data at home is anywhere from one-third to one-fourth the expense of having it captured by a nurse or physician in the medical office setting.[1] Reduced cost at the same reimbursement levels means increased revenue to your practice. Editing patient-entered data is faster than entering it, and reduces potential for transcription errors.

For those patients without computers at home, a small kiosk area would allow patients to accomplish the same task after they have checked in with the receptionist. About two out of three patients that you see can accomplish this task without any staff assistance, and the other one-third can receive confidential assistance from a staff member.[2]

If your office situation allows, make your reception room a bit smaller and build in some kiosk alcoves. Alternately, open up one or two rooms – perhaps the areas where you previously stored your paper charts (once your active patients' paper charts are scanned in and moved to storage).

When your patient completes the computer-guided interview, the EMR can update the patient status White Board to alert the nurse to accompany the patient to the exam room and record the patient's vital signs and conduct any preliminary tests. By engaging your patients in the process, their wait time seems shorter and their data has already been gathered into the EMR, where it is ready for editing by the medical staff.

How Patients Can Become Even More Involved

Beyond the patient-centered topics already discussed, how else can you engage your patients in your office automation? What about allowing them to make their own appointment requests or to electronically request prescription refills? What about providing them with online educational materials customized to their specific health situations? Want to be really cutting-edge? Host a Personal Health Record (PHR) for your patients, and then import any data from it (with their permission) into your EMR. It will make your data exchange with patients task under 'Meaningful Use' requirements easier too.

---

[1] Data provided by Dr. Allen Wenner, MD, principal of Primetime Medical Software.

[2] Ibid

Get them involved in their own wellness program. Offer electronic consults, answering questions by secure e-mail and charge a small fee for that. All this and more is possible. Envision it, rethink your practice!

Enhance Your Patient Educational Resources

Don't overlook the possibility that your EMR probably includes patient education resources, either as a standard feature or an extra cost option. Many EMRs offer excellent educational tracts. If you want that and your EMR doesn't offer it, you can obtain these from third parties and run them on the same computer, in most cases. This is one way that an EMR helps to standardize your process around recognized best practices.

Educational materials can be quickly customized to specific patients by your staff, if needed. Patient handouts can be printed while your patient is still in the exam room and given to them there or held until the end of the visit for the patient to take home. The EMR can document that patient education occurred, listing the specific forms that were printed and passed on to the patient. In some cases, the EMR can then actually print the information.

Do you also want your EMR to make educational materials available to patients on your practice's Web portal? This can be very helpful when your office gets busy, as patient education is one part of the encounter that might be cut short if you are backed up or your patient is in a hurry to leave.

EMRs Are New Tools

These patient-centered scenarios underscore the need to begin thinking about the EMR as a new tool, and not just how to integrate it into your existing workflow and office layout. Rethink your exam rooms, your medication preparation and other office areas. In each case ask, "What does this new technology make possible that we could never have done before?" Don't ask, "How can this new EMR provide an electronic picture of my paper record, or fit into our present space?" These two questions are fundamentally different and will lead you down distinct paths to diverse outcomes.

Engaging Your Staff in Envisioning an EMR Solution

In envisioning an EMR-enhanced practice, your entire office staff will need to think outside-of-the-box from the way patient care has historically been delivered. Following are a few staff-oriented details to rethink, and they are only examples – let your imagine run for a bit.

What will you do with the space freed up by the removal of your old paper charts, or at least most of them? How will new technology integrate with your existing facility? The waiting room kiosk is an excellent transition example. Along with engaging your patients in a new way, an EMR with a kiosk may be a positive benefit for your administrative/clerical staff, helping to gain their support for adoption. Thinking beyond what's become the status-quo will encourage your staff in understanding what an EMR could mean to them.

The EMR visionary will need to set the tone initially and share his/her insight of EMRs, but it's a good idea to incorporate your entire office staff in imagining what each new office area could look like after deployment of your EMR and how your office workflow may change.

Hardware Choice Opportunities

Choices of what computer hardware you adopt will make a difference in how you envision your EMR-enhanced office. You have essentially three types of hardware to choose from: stationary PCs (desktop or tower), laptops and tablet PCs. PCs are useful on carts when wheeled into areas where they are needed. Laptops can be carried around, but not as conveniently as medically designed, tablet PCs. Tablets enable portability.

These all have different price implications, but cost (within reason) isn't the primary determinant. What hardware will best improve how your current practice functions is the crucial decision here. What works best to enhance staff workflow and interactions with patients is a much longer lasting and important consideration.

You will need to decide if you want one PC that moves with each provider from room to room or one PC located in each exam room – or a combination of both. Perhaps one caregiver wants it one way in his three exam rooms and a second caregiver a different way in her three exam rooms. That's OK. Nothing says that each person can't use a different type of computer. If one person wants to carry a tablet, get them a tablet. If another wants to push around a wheeled laptop because it provides a stable typing area, that's fine too. Hardware costs are always dropping and you pay for them once every 3-4 years. The time spent by caregivers and overall workflow efficiency is the real expense to focus on. We will cover the different hardware choices in detail in Chapter 5 and your staff may not know at this time how they would prefer to input data (or they may change their mind after interacting (later in your process) with various EMRs.

One caveat – experience shows that in your exam rooms, a desktop PC is a limiting choice because it's stationary and forces the physician or other caregiver to move to one place in the room, which is often not where a natural conversation with the patient occurs. It is often better to have the caregiver use a wireless, portable device (either a tablet or a laptop) and locate it near the patient so that the patient interaction remains as much like the pre-EMR encounter as possible; rather than a PC, such as is shown in Figure 2.1. This will allow you to keep your focus on your patient rather than on the EMR. Notice in the picture that the physician can remain engaged with the patient as he is making notes during the patient encounter. In a teaching setting, with residents and interns, the intern can capture the notes as part of the encounter.

The ability to have a portable EMR also gives physicians (who choose to) the opportunity to let patients see their chart. You will find that many patients are curious about your new EMR. In fact, you can use it to reinforce the quality of care you are providing by showing the patient the drug interaction screen, for example. If the patient has already used the computer to record medical information, he or she will be interested in watching as you edit and annotate the information entered. It also helps if you explain that the purpose of having the computer is to improve patient care, by catching medication interactions for example, particularly with over-the-counter vitamins or food supplements the patient may be taking, and doesn't think of as medication.

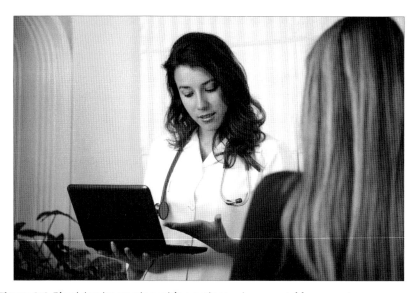

Figure 2.1 Physician interacting with a patient using a portable computer.

The EMR as Your Assistant

Think of your EMR as analogous to having a "silent assistant" in the room with you during the patient encounter. Information is flowing to and from the patient, to and from the physician, and into and out of the EMR application. Mostly, the EMR remains a silent listener as it receives data, but sometimes it will discreetly flash a message or other alert to catch your attention concerning a potential issue or to provide supplemental decision support information (if it offers that function), based on the symptoms or disease the patient has. It can also flag out-of-range values for vital signs, labs and other data.

Begin to think about how you want to interact with this new, silent partner. In most cases the physician/clinician will be operating the EMR during the exam using whatever type of interactions it supports; keyboarding, checking items on pick lists, speaking to the computer, using a stylus and writing on a screen form. We discuss this topic in detail in Chapter 5.

Developing Staff Consensus

In Chapter 1, we noted that the fourth most cited reason for not adopting an EMR was "lack of office staff support". Why is this?

One reason is that often staff members feel that an EMR is meant to replace them. In fact, the reduction of paper chart storage space required when your practice is automated has the effect of freeing up the potential for one or two new patient exam rooms. An EMR can facilitate increasing the number of patients that can be seen, along with practice revenue, resulting in more job security for your staff. The goal of an EMR, which should be made clear to your staff up front, is the more effective use of staff and expansion of the practice. Developing consensus on the decision to adopt an EMR should be easier once no one feels that their job is threatened.

Unless you are a solo practitioner, the consensus choice at the beginning of the EMR adoption process may be to procrastinate. The answer to procrastination is to inform your staff of the cost of not making a decision over the long term and the importance of efficiency (more on this in Chapter 9).

Who will accept the role of the EMR visionary, the person who lays out the benefits for the rest of the staff? The key is leadership. The visionary person has to be positive and have either direct or delegated authority in the practice in order to command the attention of the remaining office staff. It should probably be a physician or perhaps the practice manager as delegated by a physician.

A key to building staff consensus is not so much telling people they have to change what they are doing, but rather helping your staff envision how an EMR will enhance their activities and result in better patient care. We suggest you think of your staff as being in one of four groups (or roles):

1 An administrative/clerical role
2 A nursing or technician role
3 A physician or nurse practitioner/physician assistant role
4 An EMR technical support role (this is a new role that may come with EMR deployment)

Then together, develop a specific list of benefits and enhancements that each group can expect to realize by adopting an EMR (except for the EMR support role, which will be new). The more unanimous and committed to adopting an EMR all practice stakeholders are, the more likely it is that your EMR selection and adoption will be a success.

Building In-Office EMR Expectations and Goals

The new office EMR visionary builds staff consensus by involving all staff in listing their goals and expectations that the EMR can achieve inside the practice. These include two types of in-office goals:

• Practice level/patient-oriented goals;
• Individual stakeholder goals.

Encourage your entire staff to brainstorm EMR objectives and get them out on the table. Perhaps the goal of one physician is saving enough time so he can play golf again on Wednesday afternoons, while another physician wants to see enough gain in workflow so that the practice can begin to accept new patients again. Perhaps the practice manager wants fewer rejected bills from payers and the receptionist doesn't want to be interrupted all the time by patients calling to renew their prescriptions or asking questions about intake forms.

Don't judge anyone's goals, since that will make it seem unsafe to share and shut down the consensus process you are trying to facilitate. This is particularly true if the judgment is expressed by a physician or someone "higher up in the pecking order". This will instantly make it seem unsafe for those whose support you need to make the EMR succeed, to participate in and feel a part of the decision. If you shut people off repeatedly, watch out for resistance after YOUR system is deployed, you know – "that one YOU wanted but I knew would never work!" On the other hand, get your staff excited and involved in the process and they can make even a mediocre EMR a success.

One More Goal/Objective Level

It's good to add one more goal layer in addition to the above mentioned in-office level goals. The individual stakeholder goals will be those that affect each person in your office; the practice level EMR goals will be those that affect your entire practice (your patients, their safety, your mistakes, your malpractice insurance premiums). The third goal level focuses on the community; that is, how the EMR affects areas outside of your practice (the public health system, the CDC and quality of care in the U.S. in general). Here is how your practice-oriented goals differ from the community-oriented ones (although they certainly overlap).

Practice-oriented goals include items such as: reducing medication errors, verifying eligibility before the patient arrives for their appointment, being able to load a payor-specific prescription profile for the patient so that you aren't prescribing drugs that are off the patient's formulary.

Goals that transcend the practice include details such as knowing and following best practices or comparing your practice results with national benchmarks in order to improve care. You may want to be better able to exchange data with the CDC in an emergency situation or during disease pandemics.

As you and your staff review the benefits associated with EMR adoption and deployment, you probably will find common ground with each other and support for specific goals. Decide how well you must achieve whatever goals result from your discussions, in order to consider your EMR a success. Other questions you should generally consider:

- Who will be primary stakeholders in the EMR conversion process? Who will be secondary stakeholders? Be sure to include both in the overall process.
- Will those participating in adopting the EMR be equally invested in the financial results of automating the practice?
- Will you need an EMR consultant for your EMR planning? When will you need to integrate the consultant into the planning process?

Multi-Voting Can Be Useful

Whatever goals your practice stakeholders jointly agree to, embrace them all, but then rank them all. You are shooting for ranking goals as "Must Haves," then "Like to Haves," and finally, "Maybe Later." It would be highly unlikely that all goals could be achieved. How you put a specific goal into one or another category depends on many things and often a multi-voting approach is helpful.

Consider a practice of six people – two doctors, two nurses, one receptionist and one billing/office manager. Let's assume that there are 15 proposed goals on the table to be ranked. Give everyone seven votes, and let them choose the seven important goals for them personally, then tally the results. The goals that receive four or more votes go into the "Must Have" category. Those that receive two to four votes go into the would "Like to Have" category, and all other items go into the "Maybe Later" category.

The number of votes everyone has depends upon the number of goals on your list. Give everyone a number of votes equal to about one-third to one-half the number of items on the list. Set the category thresholds so that it takes about two-thirds majority to make an item a "Must Have", perhaps one-third to one-half for a "Like to Have", and below one-fourth to one-third are the items that go into the "Maybe Later" category. In this way everyone participates in determining how important various goals are, and the numbers will show you the level of consensus that exists for key goals. It will also surface any major divergence in support.

Splits most often occur when there are three or four alternatives and part of the staff supports each. In such cases all choices may get low votes, but for some EMR items, the goals may not be mutually exclusive. For example, there are four different input alternatives: handwriting recognition, speech recognition, document scanning and template/pick list. One physician may want speech recognition to be a "Must Have" since that is the only way he/she is willing to interact with the EMR, but (in the example above) the other physician and the nurses prefer template/pick list approaches, neither meets the criteria of getting two-thirds support. In cases like these, look for an EMR that supports both speech recognition and template/pick list (e.g. combine the two separate items into one combined item) and vote again (if necessary). It may be obvious that everyone supports an EMR that can accept both types of input.

This approach is just one effective way to build consensus. Incorporate any approach that allows everyone to participate, because that builds commitment for your EMR decision.

Measurement Approach

For the goals that are agreed to as "Must Haves," discuss with all stakeholders how to measure the degree to which you are achieving them after your EMR is deployed. Everyone needs to be on the same page regarding what the EMR needs to do for the practice in order for it to be considered a success. In setting up measurements, be aware that some EMR interaction types will make measuring some goals more difficult than others. This is discussed in Chapter 5. When you have finished that chapter, you may want to revisit the measures you have established for each of your goals. Common measures of EMR success might include:

- How many patients per day is the office seeing? With paper charts? With EMR?
- How much time does it take for each specific type of patient encounter (see Chapter 9)? With paper charts? With EMR?
- What is your lost patient chart percentage, or how long does it take to pull a chart for a patient? With paper charts? With EMR?
- Is Dr. Jones actually able to play golf on Wednesday, as he had hoped?
- What percentage of patients (that need them) receive patient educational materials? With paper charts? With EMR?
- What percentage of patients have you verified payor eligibility for before the patient arrives? With paper charts? With EMR?
- How many patients' formularies can be displayed on the chart when you are seeing the patient and ready to prescribe a medication? With paper charts? With EMR?
- What is the time taken by every person in the practice in interacting with the patient, pulling information before he/she arrives, etc.? With paper charts? With EMR?
- How long is the patient waiting to be seen – in the waiting room, the exam room, for an ECG or lab test or whatever? With paper charts? With EMR?
- How satisfied are your patients with the medication refill authorization process? With paper charts? With EMR?

Don't overlook patient quality improvements. What is the rate of visits to emergency rooms for your diabetic patients or CHF patients before and after EMR deployment? And so on.

You will think of more, this is in no way an exhaustive list. The point is to choose functions that will allow you to measure changes in your practice with "Must Have" goals. Also, while you are in the EMR evaluation process, share your "Must Have" and "Like to Have" goals with each EMR developer you are considering and ask his opinion about which of these his EMR can actually deliver, and how.

Negotiating the Trade-offs

Most people realize that they won't get everything they dream about in an EMR. Let everyone dream to begin with, but then start to talk about the trade-offs that may be involved.

Think through what trade-offs your practice is willing to make for the good of the office. If it takes you a minute or two extra to chart with a new EMR during the exam portion of the patient encounter, but it reduces your coder's time by 30 minutes a day and reduces rejected claims by 60 percent, increasing reimbursement by 15 percent and reducing days-receivables – is that an acceptable trade-off to the physician doing the charting? Should it be for the good of the office? Will it open up a bottleneck that now exists in your practice workflow?

If you spend extra minutes on each patient exam using an EMR so that when an FDA medication recall happens, your EMR addresses it quickly – is that a good trade-off? These are the kinds of concessions that need to be thought through. Appoint someone in the practice to be the de facto patient advocate in any staff discussions, because without one it is easy to overlook how the patient may view the changes you are discussing. Patient interests need to be represented in this process as well. If you have hired an EMR consultant, he/she may be a possible candidate for patient advocate (if they seem patient oriented). At the end of the goal setting/trade-off discussions, use the Scorecard at the end of this chapter to document what everyone agreed to and then post the results in a conspicuous place in the staff area of your office – as a reminder of the agreed-to areas of EMR adoption as your process begins.

A Word Concerning EMR Consultants

The choice of whether or not to use an EMR consultant is one that may become clear as your decision process unfolds. One indication that use of an EMR consultant may be wise is if you and your staff are having to learn an entirely new vocabulary in order to even begin the decision process. A good consultant will guide you in each phase of EMR adoption but will ultimately leave the final choice up to you and your staff – because they realize that you are the ones who will be interacting with this new tool on a daily basis. You can find EMR consultants using an Internet search and a list is also available at https://www.ehrselector.com/ehrselector/EMRToolkit/ASP/EHRconsultants. asp. In either case, ask for references and then ask their former clients for specific information. Ask them how available the consultant was to answer questions in between formal meetings, did it seem as if the consultant was favoring one EMR over others or did he/she simply guide the process, did the consultant have a wide source of reference information to help them up the EMR learning curve, etc. Prices consultants charge can vary greatly. It's wise to interview several to find the best overall value for the services you will require.

Wrap Up

Striving for patient-centered care in medicine is not new, but an EMR can either enhance or detract greatly from this goal. The use of an EMR by physicians/clinicians in an office setting will change the patient encounter, hopefully for the better. What you don't want to do is make notes while you're with your patient and then enter the data after the exam. Not only does that waste precious time, but it can cause the EMR exam data to be incomplete or missing significant details of work that was actually done in the exam, not to mention the potential for confusing patient observations. Charting later also defeats some of the advantages of having an EMR, like real-time decision support and medication interaction checking.

Think outside-of-the-box. The EMR is a new tool, not just a computer to automate the old way you have been doing things with paper. It's a paradigm shift, and the change it produces is not unlike the transition from the slide rule to the electronic calculator, or from listening to a patient's chest with your ear to using a stethoscope.

You can experiment with many different approaches before you make a decision as to how you want to proceed. Get a copy of this book for your entire office staff so that everyone can go through it, chapter-by-chapter and all be on the same page as you work the process together. Use a copy of the included Scorecard to document your initial goals, measures and benefits of adopting an EMR in your practice. You may want to post this Scorecard before any decisions have been reached in a conspicuous place where everyone will be reminded of what needs to be decided and can think through each question prior to your next meeting.

Once you have created and motivated your team and they have some idea of shared visions of the new, EMR-empowered practice, you are ready to wade into some of the configuration decisions. The first of these is covered in the next chapter.

Crucial Decision

What method will you use to build staff consensus to adopt an EMR in your practice?
Photocopy as needed or download Scorecard from www.ehrselector.com

List of problems associated with our patients and our workflow that we would like to see an EMR solve (think outside-the-box):
List of our agreed-upon initial goals/priorities for adopting an EMR as one of the following Must Have (MH), Like to Have (LH), Maybe Later (ML):
Our Goal:
Our Rationale:
Our Goal:
Our Rationale:
Our Goal:
Our Rationale:

This is just the beginning of your decision process. This Scorecard is to start everyone thinking about the possibilities and potential problems to be solved with an EMR. These goals and trade-off decisions will need to be revisited once you've read further. At this point, have some fun.

Crucial Decision

What method will you use to build staff consensus to adopt an EMR in your practice?
Photocopy as needed or download Scorecard from www.ehrselector.com

What trade-offs are we willing to make at this point in the process? Trade-off:
Our Rationale:
Trade-off:
Our Rationale:
What trade-offs are we NOT willing to make at this point in the process? NO Trade-off:
Our Rationale:
NO Trade-off:
Our Rationale:
What else do we need to think about at this point?

This is just the beginning of your decision process. This Scorecard is to start everyone thinking about the possibilities and potential problems to be solved with an EMR. These goals and trade-off decisions will need to be revisited once you've read further. At this point, have some fun.

CHAPTER 3

How EMR Will Impact Your CPM System

Crucial Decision
What level of EMR functionality will you deploy?

This chapter also addresses the following questions:

- Will your existing CPM be interfaced to a new EMR or remain separate?
- If an interfaced EMR/CPM, will it be one-directional or bidirectional?
- If bidirectional, who will modify your current CPM to "talk to" your new EMR?
- Will you replace your current CPM with a new integrated EMR/CPM solution?
- What is the growth path if you want to keep your existing CPM solution?

EMR Adventures

While in her private office, Dr. Karen Bell is visited by her office manager and receptionist. They look troubled, as they ask, "Do you have a few minutes to hear us out?" That doesn't sound good, but Dr. Bell does have a few minutes, so she replies, "Sure, what's on your minds?"

"Well," the business manager, Mary, begins, "I know you want to open up the practice to new patients as part of this new EMR we are all discussing, but I just don't see how we can do it with our current office staff."

"Neither do I," chimes in Linda, the receptionist.

"Do you see some problems that we haven't discussed?" Dr. Bell asks.

"Well, we are getting a lot of bills rejected once or twice," complains Mary. "And our coder says that I need to bill more conservatively because our charts aren't always complete and I'm afraid of what will occur if we are audited." There is a pause – "Yes, go on," encourages Dr. Bell.

Linda, the receptionist, speaks up, "I just can't handle any more patients. Between calling them to remind them of their appointments and handling all the calls from patients and pharmacies about prescription refills... and then there are the calls to verify insurance for patients we are seeing each day, and faxing and filling all the referral reports. I just don't have any time left, and I'm not doing the best job of greeting our patients when they arrive."

"If I am hearing you both, it sounds to me like there are a lot of activities you are performing currently that the new EMR we are considering isn't designed to address, is that right?"

Successfully Choosing Your EMR: 15 Crucial Decisions. By © Arthur Gasch and Betty Gasch. Published 2010 by Blackwell Publishing

"Yes, that's right," they both reply together.

"OK, then perhaps it's time to widen the discussion to not only adding an EMR, but perhaps replacing our old CPM with one new integrated system. How would that approach impact the issues you are concerned about?" responds Dr. Bell.

"I don't know, I didn't realize we could take that approach. I thought we were stuck with our existing CPM solution. I would have to give that some thought," answers Linda. "So would I," adds Mary.

Dr. Bell responds, "If we need to, we can look at replacing the CPM also. I've heard that some of the newer EMRs have CPM functionality integrated, and automatically manage things like notifying patients of coming appointments, proactively handling refill authorizations, directly sending scripts to the patient's pharmacy, calculating the E&M codes for billing purposes, and so on. Maybe we need to think about taking this approach."

"If some new system could do all that, maybe we could handle seeing more patients," say both Mary and Linda.

"Good, think about this for the rest of the week and bring up the topic at our Friday office meeting. I'll put it on the agenda so we can get everyone's thoughts. We'll brainstorm about how that might empower us to move forward," Dr. Bell says.

"That sounds great. We'll talk this over and present it on Friday. Thanks for your help. We'll let you get back to work now."

As this EMR Adventures illustrates, sometimes an EMR alone may not be enough to let your practice meet all of its goals based on how you envision the practice working after your EMR deployment. In addition to your EMR, many of the capabilities of your current CPM affect how smoothly your practice operates. Not only do you need to improve your office clinical charting with an EMR, you need to think about streamlining your overall practice workflow; the impact of an EMR or EMR/CPM system can be startling.

In order for Dr. Bell to meet her goal of opening up the practice to new patients again, she will need to figure out where her office bottlenecks are. Will simply deploying an EMR address these bottlenecks, or is a broader EMR+CPM integrated solution required?

Practice Workflow Optimization

If you can get your CPM and your EMR to work together effectively, you can minimize workflow problems such as patients forgetting appointments or arriving late, over-booking, payer verification, refill processing and more. You can pass flags from the EMR to the CPM to trigger billing for quality measures that have been performed, rather than doing it manually. Some EMRs capture all the clinical exam data automatically, indicate what E&M level you can bill at, and then the EMR communicates this data to the CPM automatically. This results in a reduction in the rate of rejected bills, and therefore helps you to be paid more promptly. Reduction of rejected billing is something that all physicians would like to achieve, but so far most have not realized this goal.

Improving workflow and billing success depends on the level of communication that exists between your CPM and EMR. EMRs that are added to an office with an already existing CPM will need to be "interfaced" to the CPM. Ideally, your office doesn't want to be the first to be interfaced to an EMR – it's better if an interface already exists and is working somewhere else. And the interface should be to the current CPM version, one that is still sold and supported. Interfacing to an older, now unsupported version of CPM software, is not a good situation. If it's to the newest version only, one newer than you have, that raises another decision. Why pay to upgrade to the newest version of your CPM, if your EMR has an integrated CPM that costs just a little more than your upgrade plus EMR? Why not get rid of the old CPM now and deploy the new, integrated solution offered by your EMR vendor?

Unless a working interface already exists from your EMR vendor to your CPM system, starting from scratch may actually work better than trying to get your current CPM to communicate with, or interface to, your new EMR. Some truly integrated EMR/CPM solutions have features such as patient reminder capabilities, automated phone calls, the ability to send e-mail, or even (snail) mail. They can also re-verify a patient's insurance the day before their appointment and even upload the patient's medication formulary and lab information to the EMR. These features and the enhanced workflow they enable may make it worthwhile to invest in an integrated system.

E&M and Billing Codes – Can EMR Talk To CPM?

All offices have to generate and transmit billing for services rendered. Doing this is not the sole province of your Computer Practice Management (CPM) system but also requires a good E&M module in your EMR and some communication between them. Given that X12 transmission standards are being upgraded to version 5010 by January 1, 2012 along with the delays in clarifying Meaningful Use requirements, any EMR you look at should be carefully considered for its ability to speak to your current CPM, just as your CPM needs to be carefully evaluated to determine if it can support ICD-10-CM by Oct. 1, 2013. This is crucial since there isn't a one-to-one correlation between ICD-9-CM and ICD-10-CM codes; in some cases the relationship is one-to-many.

Integrated Versus Interfaced Solution

The EMR/CPM decision depends on the quality of your current CPM and the quality of the CPM that is integrated with the EMR you are considering. If both are good or excellent quality CPMs (e.g. all CPM functionality being equal), then the clear choice is deploy the integrated product, don't upgrade your old CPM!

Why? Because an integrated application working from one code set (out of one, shared database) beats an interfaced application hands down. Integrated solutions work faster and offer more shared functionality, with full bidirectional data flow. It's just a better solution – one crafted from the beginning, not cobbled together by one party with which the other party didn't cooperate. But not all combined EMR/CPM solutions are one integrated solution – be careful! Just because one company offers both an EMR and CPM solution, doesn't mean that they are an integrated product. The EMR developer may be moving in that direction, but they may not be there yet. Here is a real-world example.

Henry Schein, the well-known medical equipment supplier, originally offered the interfaced approach. They understood the market trend and responded by acquiring two separate companies, MicroMD (which had an existing CPM solution), and Cliniflow (an Israeli company that had an existing EMR solution). They then renamed the Cliniflow EMR product, MicroMD EMR, but these two products were independently developed solutions, written by completely different developers (companies) and each used different database and code sets – that had been interfaced together. They sold this interfaced solution until July 2009. At that time, MicroMD CPM and MicroMD EMR were upgraded so that both products worked on the same platform, same code set and one integrated database. Henry Schein has now moved from an "interfaced solution" to an "integrated solution" with their EMR. That's typical in the current market.

CPM companies don't want to be displaced by EMR/CPM solutions developed by EMR companies, so they are buying EMR companies and doing the integration themselves. Likewise, EMR companies don't want to cripple their EMR solution by not being able to get data out of, or push data in to, another vendor's CPM solution, so they are writing CPM solutions themselves. And other companies, which are in neither of these segments (e.g. Henry Schein), are buying both an EMR and a CPM and integrating them to enter the market. So what does this mean to you?

The best case scenario is that the EMR and CPM are already integrated, and work well, and you purchase that integrated solution. The second best case is that one company, which made either solution, has purchased a competitor that offers the complementary solution, and is in the process of integrating them. In the meantime they are interfaced superficially. If the company is able to deliver what they are promising, then this will be a good choice AFTER the integrated version is announced, deployed, shaken-down and fixed. In the mean time, maybe you will want to keep your existing CPM and bank the money saved for the future upgrade.

A third alternative is to purchase an excellent EMR from one company which has a one-way (reads data from) interface to your current CPM vendor's product. The two companies aren't going to merge and there will never be an integrated solution, so buy an EMR that has a CPM (or is developing one) and bank the money until the new CPM is done and you are satisfied with its quality and performance. Then change.

The worst case is that the EMR and your existing CPM don't communicate. Don't be the group practice that finances the development of the EMR interface to your CPM system. Is your EMR vendor planning to introduce a CPM? If not, rethink deploying their EMR in favor of one that already has a CPM or is in the process of developing one.

Hallmarks of *interfaced* EMR/CPM solutions are that they were created at two different times, by different development teams, written perhaps in two different languages or using two different database, and two different user interfaces and menu structures. Interfaced solutions can have two independent technical support departments (which sometimes blame problems on the other developer).

Hallmarks of an *integrated* EMR/CPM are that it is one product, written in one language, using one database, presenting one consistent user interface. One caveat, be sure that any integrated solution will support the ICD-9-CM codes currently used and the ICD-10-CM codes that have to be accommodated by 2013 (at the latest). Not all systems are equally ICD-10-CM code ready. An integrated system has benefits, like a more consistent user interface across both products, making the integrated solution easier to learn than two separate solutions; it will offer enhanced functionality also.

Getting 220 EMRs to Speak with 198 CPMs

It will never happen, nor does it need to. Only a small subset of these suppliers have the brand identity and market momentum to grow and ultimately survive.

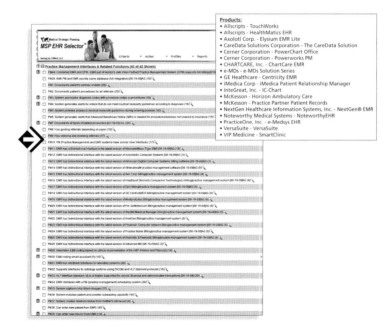

Figure 3.1 EMR Vendors EMR to CPM integration on the MSP EHR Selector

There are over 220 EMR developers and there are 198 Computerized Practice Management (CPM) system providers. Many of these CPMs have been interfaced to multiple EMR products, creating an enormous matrix of connectivity. Fortunately, there are only about forty CPM systems that have achieved substantial market share. There are dozens of developers on the MSP EHR Selector enable MSP to track these EMR/CPM interfaces by updating their information on the MSP EHR Selector Web site (www.ehrselector.com). Readers can access a current list of interfaced/integrated solutions at that site.

Figure 3.1 illustrates Practice Management Features/Interfaces from the MSP EHR Selector tool (www.ehrselector.com). By each CPM product there is a number in parentheses that indicates how many EMR products are interfaced to that specific CPM solution. In the case of Accumedics, for example, the number is 18 EMRs (see arrow in diagram).

In the case of more popular CPMs, the number is higher. After the number of developers, there is a magnifying glass symbol. When the magnifying glass is moused over, a drop-down list (as shown) is displayed, listing the specific EMR products that have been interfaced to some version of a particular CPM. Be advised that not all interfaces support the same functionality. The version of your CPM is also important, as the interface may not work well with all available CPM versions. Make sure that both the EMR and CPM versions are compatible. Even on the MSP EHR Selector, we don't list interface details. In addition, interfaces are being developed all the time and are hard to catalog in a book, which is a snapshot at one point in time only.

The number of EMR/CPM products that claim to interface to each other diminishes if you require the interface to be bidirectional and to be currently sold and supported versions only. Be sure to discuss this with your selected CPM developer. Ask your CPM developer about the communication and functionality support needed between your candidate EMR and the current software version of the CPM product. Check to make sure that the EMR that you are looking at can communicate with your current CPM in areas like appointment scheduling and patient reminders, formulary loading and patient eligibility, transfer of E&M codes and direct billing, and so on.

Avoiding Software Generation Changes

At some point EMR developers begin working on the next generation of their EMR application, as opposed to the next version of their existing generation. You need to know when this is going to happen and be cautious about adopting older generation and legacy EMR solutions. The EMR developer's next generation may have a very different evolutionary plan than their current one. New generations are likely to incorporate changes in programming language, operating systems, database systems, and other elements that are not necessarily backward compatible with existing EMR generations.

You should generally avoid a phased-in approach to deployment if your EMR developer has begun working on the next generation of their EMR application. If you are desiring a phased-in approach to EMR deployment, you would also be wise to consider only EMR developers that are committed to backward generation compatibility for current EMR products or whose EMR is in the early stages of its product life cycle.

If you opt for the phased-in approach, when it is time for you to deploy your second or third phase, if the EMR developer has moved on to a completely new system, you will be left with a difficult choice. Either you will be left with an obsolete EMR that will not have further development (and may not have aggressive fixes for bugs) or you will need to abandon your entire system and move to the latest new generation of the developer's EMR system. This forces your office staff to learn a new system all over again, something they are not likely to welcome. Be sure to get all verbal commitments of any timing of new generation development from your chosen EMR developer in writing, in your purchase contract.

Wrap Up

Your decision of either an integrated or an interfaced EMR/CPM comes down to a few key questions. What is the scope of the solution that you will have to deploy in order to achieve your practice goals? Can you afford to purchase an integrated EMR/CPM solution, or is that beyond your budget? If it's limited to simply deploying an EMR, then be sure to look for one that has an interface to your current CPM solution. If your goals require a broader, practice-wide approach, consider replacing your current CPM with a new integrated EMR/CPM solution that performs all the functions you need to achieve your practice improvement goals. Be sure to take into account how much change your office staff can accommodate at one time. Only if you have the budget, and the need, and a very flexible staff, should you consider deployment of one, integrated system all at once. This deployment tactic isn't called the "big bang approach" without reason. If you believe you need to replace everything, you can do it in two stages. Get an EMR that has both a CPM integrated with it, and one that also interfaces with your current CPM (which you will ultimately replace). You will always need to consider how your EMR and CPM are going to communicate with each other. Make sure all interfaced approaches you undertake are documented regarding their functionality, sustainability (as new software versions are introduced) and supportability.

Crucial Decision

Will you deploy an EMR or will you deploy an integrated EMR/CPM solution?
Photocopy as needed or download Scorecard from www.ehrselector.com

Based on our initial goals, budget, etc, we believe we want a:			
	Standalone EMR	No Direct Integration with Existing CPM System	
	EMR Interfaced to CPM	Bidirectional Interface to Your CPM Version or Later *The functions listed below can be used to determine whether interfaced EMR can receive from your current CPM*	
		Appt. & Scheduling	
		Loading Formulary	Verifies Patient Coverage Still in Effect and Loads Rx Formulary From 3rd-Party Payer
		Eligibility Verification	
		Appt. Reminders	Notifies Patient 1 Day Ahead of Appt.
		Transfer of E&M Levels	
		Direct Bill for PQRI	PQRI Measures Transferred & Billed
	EMR Integrated w/CPM	EMR & CPM From Same Vendor Using Same Database	
Our Rationale:			
Do we want to make any EMR + CPM changes in:			
	Two Stages		
	One "Big Bang" Stage		
Our Rationale:			

These choices are CRUCIAL to other decisions and you will probably return and reconsider these initial decisions. For example, if you choose integrated above, you have to choose the same EMR and CPM vendor. If both products don't match all your needs, this option won't be an alternative.

CHAPTER 4

Structured Data & Report Generation

Crucial Decision
Will a freeform or a structured clinical patient data approach serve you better today? What about 5 years from now?

This chapter also addresses the following questions:

- Do you want an unstructured data approach or a more highly structured EMR?
- If a more structured approach, do you want data to be structured at the billing code level or at the diagnostic code level?
- If more structured data, how can you get it without slowing down charting?

EMR Adventures

Because physicians using paper-based charts have no practical way of accessing the data in these documents, they may overlook the importance of being able to do this once they adopt and deploy an EMR, or undervalue the positive impact such information could have on their practices. They may also mistakenly believe that every type of EMR supports these functions, which is not true. The more structured the EMR, the better it does at providing data that allows physicians to evaluate their therapies and outcomes themselves – what worked and what didn't. In essence, an EMR can be a group's own decision support engine and analysis tool, if an EMR that collects the necessary data is chosen and the physicians take the time to query it once it is populated with data.

If you recall from Chapter 1, Dr. Rodriguez was in the early stages of working with the new EMR his practice had just adopted, but he was already seeing benefits (the medication feature helped him avoid a drug allergy mistake). Dr. Rodriguez's office has now had their EMR for six months and everyone is pretty comfortable working with it. Let's see how things are going.

As Dr. Rodriguez takes a quick break to grab a bite of lunch in his office, his associate, Dr. Goldstein, sticks his head in the door and asks, "David, did you see the latest info from the AAAAI[1] that just came in on the EMR? We already know of the dangers for our patients taking LABA[2] inhalers without

---

[1] American Academy of Allergy, Asthma and Immunology

[2] Long-Acting Beta Agonists

Successfully Choosing Your EMR: 15 Crucial Decisions. By © Arthur Gasch and Betty Gasch. Published 2010 by Blackwell Publishing, ISBN: 9781444332148

a steroid and the controversy of LABAs over the past few years, but the new info warns that too many patients stop taking their steroid inhaler because it is not of obvious benefit to them, while they continue with the LABA inhaler. The Academy is recommending that we contact all of our asthma patients to advise them to change to a combination steroid/LABA inhaler. The FDA might also issue a recommendation on this topic. Regardless, we need to contact our asthmatic patients."

"No, I didn't see that, but that's trouble, I wonder how many of our patients this affects? I think immediately of Sharon Tremain because I prescribed both type inhalers recently, but we need to know exactly who is on what and to do something about this soon, we have a lot of asthmatic patients of all ages."

"Yes we do," comments Dr. Goldstein entering the doorway. " I agree, we're going to need to get in touch with all affected patients quickly."

"I bet our EMR can help us with that," speculates Dr. Rodriguez. "It has a pretty powerful report generator. I'm sure we can create one for this situation. Let's take a look tonight when we're finished seeing patients."

"Sounds good. I mentioned the situation to Becky, maybe she can come up with something on how to do this," says Dr. Goldstein.

In a busy medical practice there are always surprises, but this is the first potential drug recall that had occurred since Goldstein and Rodriguez had deployed their EMR. Now it would be put to the test. They didn't specifically discuss drug recalls with the sales person who worked with them to fit the EMR system to their practice, so they weren't immediately sure how to handle the issue. To be continued...

Structured EMRs Bring Fundamental Paradigm Change

It's time to discuss how an EMR is different from a paper chart. Carefully reflect on each of these statements:

• The freeform structure of your paper-based chart doesn't exist in a structured EMR.
• There are generally no "pages" of information in a structured EMR, blobs not withstanding (blobs detailed shortly).
• Patient data is stored in related database tables that have specific field labels and values in a structured EMR.

Let's say this again in a different way, because it's very important.

• All of the clinical information that is written on one page of your current paper chart would be written into hundreds of different fields, in dozens of different database tables, in a structured EMR.

The converse is also true.

• The structured EMR is programmed to assemble data out of many different database tables and present it to you on a computer display in what looks like a "page," so you feel comfortable and think nothing has changed.

That's the paradigm change of structured EMRs. Consider the implications or you'll miss the value proposition of structured EMRs. Understanding this is critical to:

- Choosing the right type of EMR;
- Realizing what can and can't be achieved by a particular type of EMR;
- Learning to interact with your EMR efficiently; and so much more.

The EMR Value Proposition

If you can grasp the new structured EMR paradigm, you will begin to realize the many new possibilities EMRs bring, options not possible with paper charts. Think of an EMR as a librarian who looks up relevant information and works with you while you are conducting your patient exam, sort of an electronic intern. You probably would never think of your paper chart in that context.

- A paper chart could not self-organize a list of possible diagnoses and prune it as you entered data from the physical exam, but a structured EMR can.
- A paper chart can not select a list of medications that have been shown to be effective against the diagnosis you are considering, and then sort it by which prescriptions are on the payer-approved formulary and which are not, or by the price of the prescription, but a structured EMR can do that.
- A paper chart can't automatically correlate a prescription against a chronic disease your patient has, or an allergy, or the current liver or kidney lab profile, or the patient's gender and age, but the e-Prescription module of a structured EMR can do that for every patient.

Why an EMR is Not an Electronic Version of a Paper Chart

A structured EMR brings new information to you, which leads to a very practical question – what do you want on the EMR screen display? If you are still thinking of an EMR as an electronic version of a paper record, you will probably organize the EMR screen much as your paper-based chart is currently organized. But do you really want to do that?

There is no place on a paper chart for an EMR-generated diagnoses list, or a list of drugs on the patient's formulary. There is no place for a list of medication interactions, or a display of recent prescription compliance and refill history. There is no place for a list of lab and diagnostic tests that are indicated by the various diagnoses and diseases the patient has. Would any subset of such information be helpful to you in the exam room? If so, where do you want it on the screen? Can you control where it's displayed?

EMR – Have it Your Way

Make your EMR display better than your paper chart and have it fit your wants and needs. How big a display will you need for this extra information – 12", 15", 19", 23" or 25"? What is the smallest font you can comfortably read (from the distance you will view the EMR display)? How much control will the EMR give you over the information on the display? How can you restructure it to suit your needs? In Chapters 9 and 10 we are going to revisit these very questions and decisions, but keep them in the back of your mind for now because when you choose a particular type of EMR, some of these features are available, but others may not be. It all depends on what you specify.

Everything you see on an EMR screen is a "form" or a "report." You are seldom looking at unprocessed source data. Think of an EMR computer display as an interactive report (or form filled with data) that you can modify, as contrasted to a non-interactive printed report. Don't be fooled because the EMR displays a pseudo-page motif, remember that what you are seeing is a report (or form filled with data) extracted from a database. The screen display is the interactive report you deal with that accepts your input.

The more an EMR just automates your current paper motif, the less of the previously mentioned benefits it can provide for you. Think of the term EMR as an umbrella that covers a wide spectrum of products that organize clinical information about patients in very different ways, some structured and some more freeform.

How Structures Empowers EMR "Smarts"

Imagine an EMR as a database with only two possible types of fields – that's an over-simplification,[3] but go with it for a minute.

The first type of field has two parts, a field Label and a field Value. For example, Field Label=First Name and Field Value=Jane. Field Label=Last Name and Field Value=Doe. Field Label=oral temp and Field Value=101. Field Label=TempUnits and Field Value=degF. Field Label=laceration and Field Value=head. Field Label=country and Field Value=Brazil, and so on.

The second database field type is "blob." It consists of a Field Label such as HPI (History of Present Illness) and a Field Pointer to another location that contains a long string of totally unstructured text that contains, "The patient was surfing in Brazil, wiped out and hit her head on a coral reef and ingested sea water... had a severely lacerated and bruised head and within 8-hours a fever of 101 degrees, and so on."

How is Most of the Clinical Information Stored?

Creating an EMR mostly from these two different EMR field types, has very different implications for how you practice medicine. Using the second approach, which is more unstructured (like your current paper chart), you have no help in considering what tests are justified, considering treatment options, drugs and so on. If the entry is a blob from an EMR created by dictation and speech recognition (without natural language processing), you still don't have much help because while that EMR contains the data, it doesn't "understand" it, and therefore can't easily act on it independently.

---

[3] An over-simplification because there are also fields with types of "date," "integer," "logical or Boolean," and so on; but they all expect discrete values, so lumped them all together to make the distinction between the type of "blob," which you can think of as "paragraph" for example.

That's your situation if you purchase an EMR that uses (for example) speech recognition without Natural Language Processing (NLP), to eliminate (or reduce) transcription costs.

Suppose you could ask the EMR speech recognition program to scan for words like "temperature" or "cuts" or "accident." In spite of the fact that the patient Jane Doe has all of these problems, your search would fail because the speech recognition blob contained the words fever (not temperature), and lacerations (not cuts) and wiped out (not accident) – so you searched on the wrong terms. Unless you remember the vocabulary and exact words you used for a patient you saw 3 months ago, a search will be fruitless. Now multiply that by 500 active patient charts. Do you always use the same words in describing the same patient conditions? Do your colleagues use the same vocabulary you do? Using the speech recognition EMR approach without NLP, the record generated is legible, nicely typed, spelled correctly, but searches don't find all of the potential matches – e.g. it has weak data extraction and reporting capabilities. It does reduce transcription costs and if that is all you want from it, fine – but there is much it won't do for you that other, more structured EMRs will. How the computer stores physician observations determines how "smart" it is and its potential to help you with decision support tasks or quality measure documentation. It all comes down to what you want.

Front-End Vocabularies

The data structuring issue with the speech recognition approach could be overcome if there were a standardized "front-end" vocabulary of terms you had to construct the HPI from, when describing Jane Doe's problems. If the front-end vocabulary forced the terms "accident," "temperature," and "laceration," the HPI would have been less colorful, but the search conducted later and crafted from that same vocabulary would have succeeded in matching every term! Is that a good trade-off? It could also be overcome if there was some natural language processing that looked at the speech and actually structured it automatically to a standard nomenclature. In fact, there is such a system and it is described in Chapter 7.

In our vignette, Dr. Goldstein and Dr. Rodriguez would have a good chance to extract the data they are looking for from an EMR that stores highly structured data. They chose an EMR designed to collect patient data with high (very fine) granularity, e.g. with much clinical detail. In fact, each vital sign, each symptom (and all its modifiers), each drug, and more information, is captured by some highly-structured EMRs. This represents the high end of the data-structuring spectrum.

What Will It Be for Your Office?

This is a key decision your office faces – how much structure you want in your new EMR and the task and challenge of making that decision has implications.

Erring on the side of not enough data means that you won't have detail in reports or possibly won't satisfy the government's Meaningful Use requirements for ARRA reimbursement (that remains to be determined when the final criteria are announced). Erring on the side of too highly structured data will mean that you will be challenged to increase your productivity, and it may fall due to increased data entry times. You will need to find the right balance.

Unstructured Data in a Structured EMR

Even a highly-structured EMR may not have all data structured. Take lab results as an example. If (and only if) all labs return structured data (using LOINC or perhaps SNOMED syntax), will all lab results be automatically populated by your EMR as structured data. If results from even one lab are faxed to you, they will be scanned and stuck under an "Unstructured Documents" area as blob lab data – intelligible to you, but not to your EMR. In this case, only your visual inspection will determine if data reported is "out of normal range." Your EMR won't know to alert you in all cases.

Most practices with an EMR deal with many labs. These labs can include Quest (which can send all structured data, for an extra fee), LabCorp (which apparently cannot), various hospitals' labs (which may or may not be able to) and any national specialty labs. So you will have to look in two different areas of your electronic EMR, the Structured Lab section and the Unstructured Documents->Lab Results section, for data. Only when all labs report structured data will that go away, no matter what type of EMR you choose.

The same is true for Unstructured Documents in the "ECG Studies" section, where you will find a blob of information that might be labeled: "Ralph Johnson ECG 1-25-09." There is not much information about Ralph's ECG there, nothing about whether or not it's normal, or if abnormal, did it have an axis shift, ST-segment elevation or depression, an arrhythmia and so on.

However, if the same ECG has a direct interface to your structured EMR and the ECG sends over an ECG report labeled with (besides name and date): rhythm analysis, R-R interval measurement, ST-segment, and an interpretation, all of this data can be discretely stored and acted upon. The labeled data can be searched later and retrieved based on any of its indexed fields.

Intermediate Approaches

Some EMRs allow you to append values or labels to otherwise unstructured data. Suppose you have 50 pieces of paper: a variety of lab results, ECGs, pulmonary function results, etc. and none of them are structured or have direct interfaces to your EMR. Some document scanning systems will list the type of report on a menu: ECG, Lab Values, and so on. Once the user picks the correct report choice, the scanning system displays a set of information specific to the tests being scanned in. If they are lab tests, and the EMR is integrated with your CPM, or has a record of what was ordered for that patient, it may list the individual tests ordered. The user can then read the report and enter the values for each type of test.

That then brings structure to the unstructured data. Scanned in data goes into the EMR's unstructured document section, but the structured data is stored in database fields. You get a little of both with some scanning approaches; more structure than an unstructured document, but less than you would have if the device was directly interfaced, or the lab had reported data in a form (like "ELINCS") where the EMR could have stored the information for you.

Interfaces to Devices Directly Push Data Into the Database

The most structured method would be to have a direct interface from your EMR to your ECG machine (or whatever device you want to connect to). Having the data come in through a direct interface is better than scanning it in, not only because more details about the ECG are available from the direct interface, but because scanning takes staff time and is subject to problems handling the original ECG strips. Storing the ECG in a more structured format has obvious advantages.

This means you need to figure out what diagnostic devices you have and which (if any) are supported in each EMR by a direct interface. You will need to be very specific in checking with your EMR developer, as a direct interface to a Philips, GE, Siemens or other ECG machine is still somewhat proprietary, particularly if you have an older model.

Think of the implications for other external or diagnostic data as well. Can the images from radiology, endoscopy, ultrasound, cine films, X-rays, CT, MR and so on come to you in DICOM or some other structured format? If so, can your EMR accept and process them automatically, saving your staff from having to do a lot of manual sorting and scanning? Going electronic is not just having an electronic tool to do what you used to do with paper records, it is really an entirely-new paradigm for collecting, storing and displaying your patient records (which are now "database entries" for your patient).

Standards Create Structure-Ability

There are new standards for how structured lab data is reported. The best EMRs accept lab results reported as LOINC codes (via an ELINCS transaction). The matter was discussed at the Meaningful Use subcommittee meetings (2009), and it was suggested that LOINC reporting should be made part of the CLIA (Clinical Laboratory Improvement Amendments) for future lab certification. In the meantime you may pay extra for ELINCS reporting.

XML Used to Express Structure

In a more structured approach, data may be marked with Extensible Markup Language (XML) tags that identify each data element and its value, allowing the individual elements to be indexed and stored in the EMR's clinical database. Had the data on Ralph Johnson been tagged (via XML or any other way), the individual information like the rhythm, heart rate, R-R interval and so on, would be separately identifiable, as would comments on abnormalities in any ECG lead, all the patient demographics, the unverified interpretation and warnings. In fact, every piece of information the ECG machine could determine would have been indexed in your EMR (if tagged).

Drill Down Pre-Supposes Structure

Both structured and unstructured EMR approaches would be able to answer simple questions such as, "Did Ralph Johnson have an ECG, and if so, when?" However, if you ask both systems, "Did Ralph Johnson ever have an abnormal ECG with flat T-waves or one that showed arrhythmias in the rhythm strip?," only a structured EMR would be able to answer the question because those detailed combinations of attributes of Ralph's ECG don't exist as data in the scanned in (unstructured) ECG image.

Structuring Inferred from the Billing Level

Every patient encounter ultimately results in a bill, and that uses codes to indicate the patient's general problem or procedure performed. As a result, limited structure can be inferred from billing codes (CPT, ICD-9-CM, HCPCS (Healthcare Common Procedure Coding System) codes). Such codes are not detailed enough to be terribly useful. If the EMR has fields for the billing codes, it might capture the following information about patients who have Congestive Heart Failure (CHF), based on the ICD-9-CM and CPT codes:

- 391.8   Other acute rheumatic heart disease (includes congestive heart failure with active rheumatic fever)
- 398.9   Rheumatic heart failure (congestive)
- 402.01 Malignant hypertensive heart disease with congestive heart failure
- 402.11 Benign hypertensive heart disease with congestive heart failure
- 402.91 Unspecified hypertensive heart disease with congestive heart failure
- 404.01 Malignant hypertensive heart and renal disease with congestive heart failure
- 404.03 Malignant hypertensive heart and renal disease with congestive heart and renal failure
- 404.11 Benign hypertensive heart and renal disease with congestive heart failure
- 404.13 Benign hypertensive heart and renal disease with congestive heart and renal failure
- 404.91 Unspecified hypertensive heart and renal disease with congestive heart failure
- 404.93 Unspecified hypertensive heart and renal disease with congestive heart and renal failure

Billing level data structure provides only limited information about heart failure patients, certainly not the entire clinical story from which you may need to draw information. In many cases structuring data at the billing level is insufficient for tracking quality measures or other patient care purposes.

Structure at the Clinical Level

To obtain more structure, some EMRs use "front-end" vocabularies or terminologies. These fall into two groups – industry-standard, NCVHS-recognized nomenclatures/vocabularies, and vendor-proprietary vocabularies.

It would be extremely confusing if there were 220 different nomenclatures/vocabularies, one for each EMR vendor in the market and so there are two generally recognized and approved nomenclatures – SNOMED CT and MEDCIN. These two have very different origins and structures, but both have labels for diseases, findings, procedures, microorganisms, pharmaceuticals, treatments and orders, medications and so on. The point of using one of the two is that it allows a consistent way to index, store, retrieve, and aggregate clinical data[4] in an EMR's database.

It is the authors' opinions that MEDCIN is the superior solution, although some will disagree. Moreover, there are different implementations of MEDCIN and different user experiences in its various implementations, which are discussed more fully in Chapter 7. The basis for our preference is that it is nearly impossible in MEDCIN to index the same encounter to two different storage codes, a problem that can occur in SNOMED CT and which complicates subsequent data query and retrieval for reports. Only about a dozen EMR companies out of 220 have embedded MEDCIN in their products to date. About three times that number of EMR developers have embedded SNOMED CT, either as the front-end structure, or as a back-end structure against which their proprietary front-end vocabulary ultimately maps the data acquired. There can be significant differences in the time it takes to work with an EMR that uses SNOMED CT compared to some implementations of MEDCIN.

For Existing EMR Users

If you currently own a first or second-generation EMR with a vendor proprietary front-end nomenclature (vocabulary), you are probably wrestling with how in the world to migrate all of your EMR patient data (locked into that proprietary database structure) to whatever your second (or third) EMR system will be. If you were fortunate enough to have chosen an EMR based on MEDCIN or SNOMED CT (or RT), you have half a chance of succeeding. If you locked yourself into a vendor-proprietary approach, unless that vendor will map it into SNOMED CT for you, or there is a cross-walk (of field in their database to fields in MEDCIN or SNOMED CT), you are facing a daunting challenge. We discuss this in Chapter 8 – Interoperability Beyond the EMR. We would suggest however, that if your new EMR is one that supports either of the two recognized standard nomenclatures, your problem the next time may be significantly minimized or eliminated.

---

[4] Information taken from Wikipedia page on SNOMED, http://en.wikipedia.org/wiki/SNOMED_CT.

EMR Auto-Pruning of Front-End Vocabularies

Because front-end data trees associated with MEDCIN, and particularly SNOMED CT, are enormous, EMR developers have looked for ways to reduce the number of choices presented to physicians using EMRs with these front-ends. One fruitful approach has been dynamic pick list pruning. In this approach the EMR uses a mechanism to "watch" the data being entered and to "prune off" values (really secondary choices) from user pick lists that are no longer clinically relevant based on the context. This reduces the number of pick list choices, and thus expedites entry.

Knowing that the gender of a patient is female, allows the EMR to prune off items appropriate only to males, and vice versa. Also, once a medication is selected, inappropriate administration routes can be pruned off – for example a drug that is an ointment would not show a choice for intravenous infusion or injection. Amazingly, many EMRs do NOT make such eliminations and allow you to enter impossible routes of delivery without ever warning you.

Quality Reporting Requires Structure

Increasingly, the government is adding financial rewards to physicians who can demonstrate quality reports and the ability to generate these reports depends upon the level of structure the EMR enables.

The 2006 Tax Relief and Health Care Act (TRHCA) (P.L. 109-432) required the establishment of a physician quality reporting system, including an incentive payment for Eligible Professionals (EPs) who satisfactorily reported data on quality measures for covered services furnished to Medicare beneficiaries during the second half of 2007. Medicare named this program the Physician Quality Reporting Initiative, or PQRI for short. Increasingly, documentation (reports) are required to confirm compliance with PQRI and other quality standards and best care protocols (evidence-based medicine) for many patient populations.

For example, the Medicare Improvements for Patients and Providers Act of 2008 (MIPPA) (Pub. L. 110-275) made the PQRI program permanent, but only authorized incentive payments through 2010. EPs who meet the criteria for satisfactory submission of quality measures data for services furnished during the reporting period, January 1, 2009 - December 31, 2009, will earn an incentive payment of 2.0 percent of their total allowed charges for Physician Fee Schedule (PFS) covered professional services furnished during that same period (the 2009 calendar year).

There are standards for diabetics, children, smokers, CHF patients, ARDS (Acute Respiratory Distress Syndrome) patients, and patients taking particular medications. For a list of all of these standards, browse http://www.cms.hhs.gov/PQRI/Downloads/2009_PQRI_MeasuresList_030409.pdf on the Web. (Note: all of these are user-assertable criteria on the MSP EHR Selector, so you can determine which EMRs match the PQRI standards that you are interested in by going there.)

Is Electronic Patient Record a Valid Business Document?

An EMR should produce a valid business/medical record that prevents one caregiver from changing another caregiver's entries into the chart. Once an assertion is made (and the chart is signed off), only appended corrections should be made, which are noted along with the name of the caregiver who makes them. Again, this is not the case with every EMR available.

Some EMRs attribute all observations, by all caregivers to the one person (read physician) who actually signs the chart, (legally) implying that this physician made all of the data entries.

Avoid EMRs that allow one caregiver to change assertions made by another. Check out how EMRs that enforce "consistency" handle the correction of inconsistent data. The implications of that are enormous, and are discussed in Lawyer-Proofing Your EMR – Chapter 13.

Trying to "Structure" Freeform Data Entry

Being consistent in charting helps to make searching data more effective, particularly if you choose a freeform EMR approach. Several tools are available that can bring consistency to your charting in a freeform environment.

Abbreviated Text and Word Expanders

One is Shorthand-for-Windows (a text expander keyboard utility). Using a text expander tool can be extremely helpful because it allows you to enter abbreviations, and then the tool develops these into complete statements. For example, you might type "SOB" for Shortness-Of-Breath, which is replaced using programs like Shorthand-for-Windows with a statement such as, "The patient complains of being short of breath."

This can also work for diagnosis. If the diagnosis is COPD, the summary can be expanded to read, "Patient has Chronic Obstructive Pulmonary Disease." This approach allows you the speed of entering abbreviations or acronyms for medical terms but then develops it into a sentence-like phrase that is specific and that makes charts more readable. If the chart is then saved as a PDF (Portable Document Format) document and cataloged, an index to every key word is created and can later be searched, with data retrieved in context. This allows you to find and pull out more data, but it won't make creating quality report statistics a simple process.

We saw an interesting, home-made, freeform EMR demonstrated by a physician a couple of years ago. He had created his entire patient record using Shorthand-for-Windows, by predefining a series of terms for medical conditions as keyboard shortcuts. With just a few keystrokes, he quickly generated most sections of a chart, which had a natural flow to the observations entered. Admittedly, the data was freeform, but for $35 and some of his time, he had created an excellent medical charting tool. Even his medication orders were documented this way.

Of course, keyboard expander approaches to "structuring" freeform data are missing the critical drug-drug, drug-allergy, drug-disease state (e.g. asthma), drug-lab value, and drug-age/BMI checks of e-prescribing and Computerized Provider Order Entry (CPOE) modules, so they aren't a step forward in preventing drug errors, and would not meet e-prescription or CPOE requirements. Nor would this help you with any Meaningful Use outcome data necessary to receive government reimbursement. But a text expander like Shorthand-for-Windows, RapidKey or others could be used with any conventional EMR to enhance data entry speed, particularly in the subjective sections of the patient chart.

Whatever text expander program you choose, be sure that it is from a reputable company, and not a disguised malware program (explained in detail in Chapter 15). Avoid any program from an unknown company, particularly if it is free on the Internet. Text expander programs capture and monitor your keyboard use and need to be safe, as they are potential HIPAA breach points.

For safety, set your firewall to NOT allow such programs to communicate with the Internet (see Chapter 15). Also check that they do not launch other programs, such as browsers, that communicate through them indirectly. Make all updates to such programs manually, rather than allowing them to go out to the Internet on their own and automatically download updates. Figure 4.1 lists legitimate products that perform text expander functions.

Figure 4.1 Keyboard Expanders Available for Medical Documentation

Product	Source & URL	Comments/Support	Price
Shorthand for Windows	Healthcare Technologies	ShortCut, HTI's shorthand program lets you simply type in an abbreviation and the system will expand it to an entire word, phrase, sentence, paragraph, document, or macro.	$99
Abbreviate! for Windows 2000/XP	Sylvan Software www.sylvansoftware.com/expanders.htm	Abbreviate! is a useful utility that monitors all keystrokes as you work in your Windows-based programs. When you type one of the stored abbreviations, the abbreviation is replaced with the text you defined. Works with most software programs. Tech support included.	$79
Shortcut Word Expander for Medical Windows 95, 98, NT, 2000, XP & Vista 32-bit	Sylvan Software www.sylvansoftware.com/expanders.htm	ShortCut is an automated medical shorthand program (also know as a "medical shorthand," "speed typing," or "abbreviation expander"). Shortcut allows you to type in an abbreviation which can be expanded to a word, a phrase, a sentence, a paragraph, an entire document, or even a macro. It includes 30-day free support.	$86
Instant Text V Pro By Textware Solutions	Sylvan Software www.sylvansoftware.com/expanders.htm	An abbreviation expander offering: automatic glossary creation and sentence continuation. Instant Text allows you to use abbreviations for faster, easier, and accurate text entry. Abbreviation expanders have been around for over thirty years, but have required that you develop and memorize glossaries with hundreds of abbreviation codes for your frequent words and phrases. With products like Instant Text, this is not necessary.	$178

Scanning + Acrobat Convert Freeform Notes to Indexed Notes

If you are using a freeform approach, augmented with one of the above keyboard expanders (or not), you may want to employ Adobe's Acrobat Professional software to convert your typed pages into Portable Document Format (.pdf) files. These PDF files can then be indexed on every word using Acrobat's Catalog function. To avoid having to initiate the catalog update manually, you can set it to run as a scheduled task by the Windows operating system.

The PDF approach, when coupled with Optical Character Recognition (OCR), is useful for making unstructured scanned in data, granular at the word level, indexing it and making it searchable. Nuance makes Omnipage for that function, however it takes some doing to get Omnipage to work with most office supply store scanners in an automatic manner that can process documents easily.

An interesting alternative to the Nuance product is the Keyscan Keyboard/Scanner, a keyboard product that is also a document scanner, but one with a twist. Keyscan auto-triggers scanning as soon as a card or document is inserted, then automates the entire scanning process, doing the OCR conversion on the fly, and delivering a PDF document with words that can be indexed by Acrobat Pro's catalog feature. We detail this product in the next chapter under the scanning interface approach.

How User Interface Preference Infers Structure Level

Each of the major EMR interaction types have different data structuring granularities with some supporting more highly-structured data than others. Keep that in mind as you read about each type of EMR, as shown in Figure 4.2. Each user interface choice is discussed in detail in the next chapter but know that there have been some very interesting breakthroughs in speech recognition technology that now offer the possibility of structured data capture with what appears to clinicians using it, as simple dictation. This is detailed in Chapter 5.

Figure 4.2 Reporting Implications of Alternative EMR User Interfaces

Type of EMR System	Type of Data Structuring	Comment About Data Retrieval
Document Scanning as an image	Minimal structure	Each major section is a "blob" of unstructured information, which at best may be indexed by section or subsection.
Document Scanning w/OCR	Adds text that can be indexed, and can add barcodes also	If saved to Acrobat PDF format, can be indexed text, and can have 2D barcodes attached to index major document sections. See healthcare extensions of Adobe Acrobat discussed later.
Speech Recognition	Freeform, sentence structure	If converted to PDF and cataloged, words can be searched for, but synonyms remain a challenge. Training is an issue and in some cases working from more than one location is an issue as well.
Speech Recognition w/Natural Language Processing	Improved over SR without NLP	NLP helps to build the voice data into a finer structure. Look for EMRs that incorporate the new CliniTalk SR+NLP engine. Browse the Medicomp Systems (www.medicomp.com) Web site for more information on their OEMs using this new technology (see next chapter for details). Also see M*Modal (www.mmodal.com), a technology that allows physicians to dictate as they normally would and then captures an audio file from the spoken dictation, ultimately turning the dictation into a meaningful document.
Handwriting Recognition and Forms	As highly structured as the form is	Templates filled in by handwriting that is recognized are as good as those that are typed in. This is a popular alternative for EMRs implemented on handheld tablet PCs.
Typed in Data and Templates	Most highly structured data in general	If templates are well mapped to a structured database, provides the most highly organized & retrievable data.

And Now Back to... EMR Adventures

It's the end of the day and the last patient has been seen – time for Dr. Goldstein, Dr. Rodriguez and Becky Kelly, the practice's business manager, to put their heads together on the asthma medication recommendation problem. They all gather in Dr. Goldstein's office, Dr. Goldstein leads off the discussion. "How are we going to deal with this new recommendation?" he asks.

"Not a problem," Becky Kelly replies. "I've already dealt with it. I put together a list of our asthmatic patients who were on a LABA inhaler and a separate steroid inhaler and sent them all a notice that Dr. Rodriguez worked up. It advises them to call the office for a new prescription and for an appointment and follow-up instructions. In fact, we got our first call late this afternoon from a patient who received the notice as an e-mail."

"How in the world did you do that?" asked Dr. Goldstein in amazement.

"Well, if you want to know, I simply ran a longitudinal query against our EMR's clinical database, using its query tool. I picked "all patients" for the scope, and picked the RxNorm code for LABA inhalers and listed the first, last, full name, address, town, state, zip code, home phone and e-mail. I then submitted it. The EMR pulled 320 records out. I then sorted the records returned and split them into two groups – one we had e-mail addresses for and the other we only had mailing addresses for. I e-mailed the first group with the text Dr. Rodriguez worked up, and used our patient mailing program to type letters for those who didn't provide e-mail addresses. The e-mails have already gone, and the mail-merged letters should be finished printing in about half an hour. They can go out in the mail tomorrow."

"Unbelievable, you have been busy!" exclaimed Goldstein. "I thought this was going to be a huge problem! I remember the last time we had a drug recall, and what a pain it was to go through all those paper charts and figure out who was on Vioxx. It took us almost a week of overtime hours. This is really an improvement. You did an outstanding job, Becky," said Goldstein.

"Yeah, really great work Becky," chimed in Rodriguez. "We can all get home on time tonight and here I thought we were going to have to work late or over the weekend."

"Becky, I've noticed that you haven't been working late as often since we got the EMR," commented Rodriguez.

"You are right, and thanks for getting me the text of the cover letter so quickly, Dr. Rodriguez," said Becky.

This is a near best case scenario. A few EMRs would have allowed the report to be automatically merged with the letters and e-mails, rather than requiring a manual step. Others would have forced a much more fragmented and piecemeal approach. Some few would not even have supported the practice-wide, longitudinal search. In a few EMRs that store data as unstructured, free-formatted text statements (such as might be the case with a physician using a speech recognition system to list the drugs a patient is on), a query could still be run, but matching it to patient demographic and address information would be substantially more difficult. It certainly would not have gotten done that afternoon.

Wrap Up

This chapter has presented you with one of the most important decisions you will make in selecting your EMR – how structured your data will be. We have presented consequences of all of the various choices. Before you cast any decision in stone, read the next chapter that discusses different ways of interacting with your EMR. Once you have completed that chapter, you will probably be ready to decide both what type of EMR you want and how structured its data must be. This will substantially narrow the spectrum of EMR developers from which you can select. Here are the key ideas of this chapter:

- A structured EMR not only makes charts more legible, it makes patient care safer by reducing drug errors and may even provide real-time decision support. The future is towards structure, as it better supports billing, referral, quality and pay-for-performance incentives – which form much of the rationale for adopting EMR systems in the first place. If you are looking for an EMR that won't quickly become obsolete, favor a more structured approach, but don't settle for one that is poorly implemented and slows practice workflow.
- A structured EMR can help collect patient data that can inform providers about aspects of care and workflow that they have no other practical means of developing.
- Usually, but not always, charts created by structured EMRs do not contain observational contradictions, and may therefore provide a better legal document (see Chapter 13, Lawyer-Proofing Your EMR).
- If you choose a structured data approach, you will then have to also choose whether the data is structured at the billing level or at the clinical level (see details on this in Chapter 7, Standards, Vocabularies & Interoperability).
- EMRs with freeform or unstructured data are faster to interact with, and perhaps can be deployed more quickly. They may also have a shorter learning curve for staff, but also a shorter useful life. The trend in the industry is away from unstructured approaches, as they don't provide a good growth path to the future in many cases.
- EMRs with unstructured or partially structured data can allow conflicting statements about a patient, their systems and vital signs that would be very troublesome during audits, or if your records are ever involved in any litigation.

Now that we have explored structured versus unstructured data and reporting, let's look at how that impacts the type of user interactions you want to have in your EMR. That is the topic of the next chapter. Use the Scorecard provided to capture the group's decisions about data structuring. Be sure to update it if the next chapter changes any decisions you have made here.

Crucial Decision

Will a freeform approach or a structured clinical patient data approach serve you better today? What about 5 years from now? Photocopy as needed or download this Scorecard from www.ehrselector.com

Do we want a freeform, unstructured data approach, or are we willing to adopt a more highly structured EMR that offers more detailed reporting?
Our Decision (or preference at this point):
Our Rationale:

This is a Crucial Decision in which the choices are mutually exclusive. Remember, the more structure you want, the more specific the data entered must be, and that can take more time on every patient encounter, unless your EMR has a very well-designed user interface and outstanding, encounter-specific templates.

Crucial Decision

Will a freeform approach or a structured clinical patient data approach serve you better today? What about 5 years from now? Photocopy as needed or download this Scorecard from www.ehrselector.com

If we want a more structured approach, do we want data to be structured at the billing code level (ICD-9-CM, CPT and HCPCS codes) or at the diagnostic code level (MEDCIN or SNOMED CT)?

We would like to further explore the following products/approaches:	
	Text Expander Program
	PDF (with OCR)
	Keyspan keyboard scanner

Our Decision (or interest at this point):

This is a Crucial Decision in which the choices are mutually exclusive. Remember, the more structure you want, the more specific the data entered must be, and that can take more time on every patient encounter, unless your EMR has a very well-designed user interface and outstanding, encounter-specific templates.

Crucial Decision

Will a freeform approach or a structured clinical patient data approach serve you better today? What about 5 years from now? Photocopy as needed or download this Scorecard from www.ehrselector.com

<table>
<tr><td>

Our Rationale:

</td></tr>
<tr><td>

What else do we need to think about/act on now?

</td></tr>
</table>

This is a Crucial Decision in which the choices are mutually exclusive. Remember, the more structure you want, the more specific the data entered must be, and that can take more time on every patient encounter, unless your EMR has a very well-designed user interface and outstanding, encounter-specific templates.

CHAPTER 5
Interacting With Your EMR

> **Crucial Decision**
> **How does everyone prefer to interact with an EMR?**
>
> This chapter also addresses the following questions:
>
> - Should you request/allow patients to input data into the EMR?
> - What user interface options are available for data input with an EMR?
> - If people work different ways, can you get one EMR to satisfy everyone?
> - Which EMR developers support each of the methods of user interaction?
> - Where can you try out the interaction approaches before purchasing an EMR?

EMR Adventures

When Dr. Brian Goldstein first brought his idea of purchasing an EMR to the office staff, there was confusion surrounding how data had to be entered into it. Dr. Goldstein was the "techie" guy in the office so he had a number of different ways in which he would be comfortable entering data. But Brian was concerned about Dr. Roy Jones, the senior partner in this four-physician office. Roy wanted to retire in two or three more years and wasn't opposed to an EMR but didn't want to have to learn "techie" ways of interacting with it. Roy had made it very clear to Brian that he wasn't a typist and felt uncomfortable with keyboard entry for patient data. "I don't want to be pecking on a keyboard and looking like an idiot in front of my patients," Roy had told him. The business manager, Becky, the receptionist, Sue and Alice, the nurse, all had to enter data in a way that fit their needs as well. At an office meeting prior to their EMR adoption, the five individuals were discussing how they wanted to interact with their soon-to-be-purchased EMR. Let's listen in.

"I know we are going to have to figure out what kind of EMR we want," says Brian, "You all work in such different ways and one of the things we need to decide is how we can each be comfortable interacting with any EMR we eventually purchase."

"That's true," Roy replies. "I dictate my clinical notes now, and the transcriptionist types them up. I'm not a very good typist, but can I keep working this way when we get an EMR? When I saw an EMR at the last convention I attended, it was all screen templates and the sales guy typed information into it. I just can't work that way, I'm too old to learn to type."

Successfully Choosing Your EMR: 15 Crucial Decisions. By © Arthur Gasch and Betty Gasch. Published 2010 by Blackwell Publishing

"I prefer to type in any information that I gather," says Sue. "I'm a good typist and know the keyboard layout well and already do that for billing. That would be my preference – typing data in directly."

"I believe I would like to try the handwriting recognition approach. I have fairly legible handwriting, better than you doctors (a few chuckles), but I could type patient complaints and the vital signs into the EMR if I had to. I don't mind either method," adds Alice.

"I would prefer to use a pen-entry approach as well," says Brian. "Because I figured we would all have different needs in this area, I asked Becky to do some research on what exactly our options are in EMRs. Becky, can you give us an overview?"

"As I've been looking into things, I've found we can get one EMR that supports different data entry methods," says Becky. "I've come across EMRs that support voice input, so you can continue to dictate, Dr. Jones, and some of the same EMRs support handwriting recognition too – which seems to be what Dr. Goldstein and Alice are looking for. And most EMRs allow typing of information so your needs are met also, Sue. There are advantages and disadvantages to each approach that we will have to understand. Some EMRs let you enter data one way for the subjective parts of the encounter, and use a different way for other parts."

"That's great, I didn't know that one EMR could support different types of interactions," Alice replies.

"Neither did I," says Roy. "I guess there is something out there that would satisfy all our needs! We will have to get the rest of the staff in here soon so that they can begin to learn about possible choices."

Brian then asks, "What about our patients, will they be willing to enter some data into the EMR?"

"I didn't know we were going to have patients enter data at all," says Roy. "We don't ask them to do that now. How will they feel about that? Where will they do that – in the waiting room? There isn't much privacy there and who will help them if they have questions?"

"In researching EMRs, I've found several that offer patient kiosks and guided interviews where patients enter their own data. These replace the clipboards and questionnaires used in many paper-based practices," says Becky.

"Our clipboard forms have no branching logic and sometimes I wish I had more information on specific patient conditions that are checked off, but there is no supplemental information on the paper form, so I have to take time during the exam to capture this extra information," comments Roy. "Could we get that extra information if we used a computer-guided interview on a kiosk?"

"I wonder if the patients would be able to do this," says Alice. "Some have trouble just filling out the current paper forms. I am always getting questions about what some term means."

"A well-designed, kiosk-based computer-guided interview has Help Frames that can be silently displayed on the screen as needed, to clarify terms for example," replies Becky.

"I wonder if there are also audio messages that a patient wearing a headset could get?" asks Sue.

"I don't know – I could look into that," Becky replies, "but in either case wouldn't the process be more private and HIPAA compliant than the normal verbal exchange between the patient and you guys, which is audible not only to the patient, but many other patients sitting in the same reception area?"

"Probably!" says Alice. "Definitely!" adds Sue, "and we wouldn't be interrupted so often by patients asking questions about the paper forms."

"We would have to rearrange the seating in the waiting room, and put in a few alcoves for the patients to use in interacting with the kiosks," comments Brian. "It would be important to position the kiosk display so that there is no one behind the patient who can see the screens of questions and the answers the patient is entering. This can often be achieved by using cubicles or other devices to keep screen displays private."

"I've got an idea," says Roy. "Let's get the patients to do this at home, over the Internet, before they even arrive for their appointment. If done at home over a secure link, all HIPAA requirements would be met."

"Not all of our patients have Internet access," cautions Brian. "But many of our younger ones do," replies Roy. "Even many of the older ones do, if they live with the kids. And the Baby Boomers often do."

"Well, even if it works for 40% of our patients, it would reduce our office workload, and I'm all for that," says Sue. "So am I," adds Alice quickly.

"All right," says Roy. "but how many EMRs support this computer-guided interview approach?"

"Well, I pulled down a list from the EMR/EHR Selector we are using," says Becky, "and it lists McKesson's Practice Partner, GE/IDX, Epic, Eclipsys, Amazing Charts, Bond Technologies, Cerner, eClinicalWorks, e-MDs, Med3000, Medfusion, The MD Net (Medical Communications Systems), Medseek, NextGen, Praxis, Sage and SOAPware – and there may be more."

"That many! Well I guess this is a practical approach," comments Roy.

Different People, Different Interface Preferences

There are five major user interface options for EMRs (six if you include patient data entry approaches) and each has ramifications for how you practice medicine. Every care provider in your practice needs to decide how they would prefer to interact with an EMR. It may be possible to accommodate everyone's first choice, or it may not. If it is not, then you can decide what user interface best fits the majority of the staff preferences and try to convince the others to adopt it. Exploring different EMR approaches and allowing each person to express their preference will help boost staff acceptance and willingness to use the EMR.

In using an EMR, it is helpful (but not essential) if you can type. Those who find this an obstacle, often lean towards after-the-encounter dictation, particularly if they are already dictating notes. This however will circumvent many of the advantages of the EMR, such as real-time decision support and real-time drug checking benefits. Dictation will also leave you tied to your transcription service, but probably with reduced costs.

While it may seem simplest to interact as you do now with your paper charts, that may not be the best long-term approach to adopt. You may want to interact with different parts of the patient exam in different ways – using speech recognition and natural language processing in some parts and working with templates and pick lists in others, for example.

As explained in Chapter 4, you need to weigh the level of structure you want in an EMR (from highly-structured to unstructured) against the different types of user interfaces available to you. You also need to consider whether or not you will encourage your patients to enter some of their data into your EMR.

Patient Data Entry Modes

A kiosk-based, computer-guided patient interview is able to enhance the information that was previously gleaned from your patients using a clipboard and paper form. To assist your patients, each item on the electronic form can have a help frame so that they know what information you want from them. If properly implemented, kiosk help screens can head off the need for (most) patients to ask the receptionist about questions they don't understand.

John Bachman, MD has written a wonderful article entitled, *The Patient-Computer Interview: A Neglected Tool That Can Aid the Clinician.* In his article, Bachman points out, *"that a physician will interrupt a patient within 24 seconds after the patient begins speaking."* This physician behavior is removed from the equation when the patient is interacting with a computer-guided interview, because the computer doesn't interrupt the patient. As a result, physicians obtain more information than if they had interviewed the patient in person, sometimes surfacing very relevant information.[1]

When the patient is allowed to enter data (at home or in your office), it will take about two minutes of caregiver time to edit the information, according to data from Primetime Medical Software. But patient entry is excellent for including the subjective history of the patient in their record – it's their contribution to describing why they are making the visit. Primetime reports that 40% of patients can enter data from home, and that of the 60% who enter data in the physician's office, 40% can do so unassisted, while 20% will require staff assistance to enter their data.

At Home or In-Office Patient Data Entry

If you would like to include your patients in your new automated office, the first thing to determine is where the data entry into your EMR is going to start; in your office or in the patient's home – or both (see Figure 5.1). Could your waiting room be rearranged to have a private area with a computer screen and

---

[1] *The Patient-Computer Interview: A Neglected Tool That Can Aid the Clinician.* by John W. Bachman. Published January 2003 Vol. 78, No. 1, pp. 67-78, Mayo Clinic Proceedings

keyboard that arriving patients could use to check in, or to enter the reason for their visit, or other information? Having your patients enter data certainly makes the visit more interactive for them. Any data presented to patients will need to be structured, and will need to be reviewed by the staff as part of the medical exam.

The following list is a sampling of what can be entered by patients:

- Their (patient) demographics;
- Their (patient) insurance or other eligibility information;
- Their (patient) payment guarantee;
- Their (patient) information necessary for scheduling some pre-ordered tests;
- HEDIS standards information[2].

Having patients enter some of their own data is a novel idea to some medical practices, yet research shows that many patients (of all ages) like this approach. Some even have their own Personal Health Records (PHRs) on the Internet at sites like Google Health or Microsoft Health Vault, and may want to transfer their data into your EMR. Consider purchasing an EMR that includes an Internet-accessible patient portal and setting up your own PHR for patients.

Enhancing Patient Interactions – Using HIPAA-compliant Kiosks

If you decide to replace clipboards and pencils with computer-guided patient interviews, your patients can use a stylus or the keyboard up/down arrow and return keys to make the "yes/no" check marks on the kiosk screen form, just as they did previously on your paper form. Using electronic kiosks can expedite form completion and facilitate capture of more in-depth information about medical history or current complaints. Kiosks need to provide privacy.

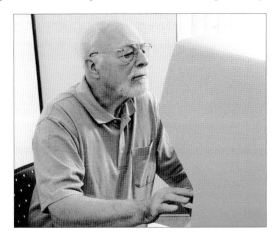

Figure 5.1 Kiosk in a Physician Office where patients can enter their information.

---

[2] The Healthcare Effectiveness Data and Information Set (HEDIS) is a widely used set of performance measures in the managed care industry, developed and maintained by the National Committee for Quality Assurance (NCQA).

Kiosk designs vary and support a wide range of displays, including the newer, all-in-one computer+display (see Figure 5.2), which are quite compact and available with screen sizes up to 25 inches. As patients age, larger screens running at medium resolutions (1024 x 768 or 1280 x 1024) provide larger, more visible characters for visually-impaired patients. To assure HIPAA compliance, kiosk design and placement must be such that screen displays are not visible to bystanders or other patients. Touch screens are helpful, and use of 3M privacy filters help to keep screen-displayed data private. Addition of a card reader (if your patients have machine-readable health plan ID cards), or a biometric ID (finger print) scanner are extra-cost items.

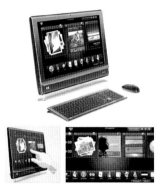

Figure 5.2 HP integrated CPU+display/IQ500 or IQ800 Series All-in-One Computers

Another alternative is to have the patient use a tablet PC, like the Motion C5 (shown in Figure 5.3). The disadvantage is that tablet PC displays are only about 12-14 inches diagonally and therefore the information is presented in a smaller character format that can be challenging for some patients to see. Also, they can weigh 3.5 pounds, which may be too heavy for some patients.

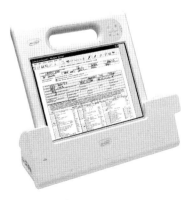

Figure 5.3 Motion Computing C5 Tablet PC

What About Cross-Contamination with Kiosks?

Possible cross-contamination is an issue amplified by using touch-screen PCs instead of a clipboard to capture information, but one that is easily addressed. Sealed keyboards are now available that can be sprayed with disinfectants. Others are available that have membranes over the keys. Keeping disinfectant sprays or wipes in each alcove is helpful, as patients can spray or wipe the keys before typing. That means you will need paper towels and a waste container in each area (see, EMRs are NOT totally paperless).

Selecting Staff EMR User Interface(s)

How your office staff interacts with an EMR is a very important issue if the adoption of your EMR is to be successful. The user interface determines how menus or other control structures appear, where they are located, how they sequence, what is included in the presentation menu, how "deep" the menus are, and so on.

The user interface has a lot to do with staff perception of how easy-to-use any EMR seems. If the user interface is well designed, then the EMR will seem fast and intuitive to use. If not, as you are searching around for functions you want, it may seem as if the EMR is slowing you down and killing your productivity. That's why this is a Crucial Decision.

Often, the first step to deciding what interface each person on your staff prefers is watching demos of EMR products so that each person is aware of the potential choices they have. Keep in mind the interplay between any user interface and the data structure decisions you have already explored.

Not all user interfaces will support highly structured data capture and different user interfaces can be employed to enter data into different parts of the EMR chart. For example, speech recognition could be used to enter subjective data, but templates with selection lists could be used to enter data into the objective sections of the chart. Many EMRs support more than one type of user interface, although they usually have a dominant, underlying user interface approach to which the others are limited use alternatives.

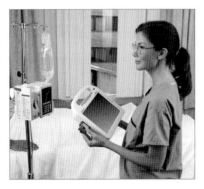 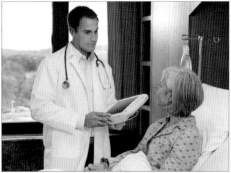

Figure 5.4 Newer (Panasonic) tablets offer enhanced features for medical use

Different Interface for Different Areas of Practice

An interface that works in the office EMR setting may not be the right choice for an EMR being used in an inpatient setting, or in the home care setting. Inpatient shifts run 8-12 hours, so if computers are battery operated, they will need to support features like "hot-swap" batteries (shown in Figure 5.4), that allow the computer to remain "on" while the batteries are removed and changed for recharged ones.

This may not be as much of an issue in an office setting, or in an inpatient setting if a cart-mounted, tablet PC is chosen. Hand-carried tablet PCs could be ideal for physicians making rounds (also shown in Figure 5.4) because the physician won't be using it for so long that battery discharge becomes a factor. If a physician brings his/her own PC, it is helpful if data is stored in an industry-standard format (such as HL7 CCD) and can be readily transferred to any EMR the hospital staff is already using. Alternatively, if the physician PC is supplied by the hospital, obtaining a CCD-formatted encounter summary to update the physician's own EMR patient chart, would be helpful. This is the topic of interoperability and standards, discussed in detail in Chapter 7.

Select an Interface That Enables Use

It's important to select the right type of EMR so that no care provider needs to make notes on paper while seeing a patient and then transcribe that data into the EMR after the exam. Not only does that make more work and waste time, but it could also lead to EMR exam data being incomplete. It also circumvents important patient alerts that the EMR provides during the exam. Choosing an input mode that is natural for caregivers is important to interacting effectively with an EMR.

EMRs are designed to support one or more of these five major user interaction approaches:
• Typing in data using a keyboard;
• Dictation with speech recognition without natural language processing;
• Dictation with speech recognition with natural language processing;
• Handwriting the information using handwriting recognition software;
• Scanning in data using a document scanner with barcodes or category sheets to index it.
Each approach has some strengths and weaknesses related to how the patient data captured can be retrieved and used after the patient encounter, as well as cost implications related to the expense of the patient encounter.

Cost Implications of Different Interaction Approaches

Let's discuss the costs first. Dr. Allen Wenner at Primetime Medical reports that handwriting is the slowest method (unless speeded up by highly structured, predefined presentation lists and forms). Handwriting occurs at about 30 words per minute and works well for users who can write in a way that the computer can repeatedly process without errors. If you want to know if this method will work for you, try it. If you are getting more than six errors that you have to go back and correct, this method probably isn't a good choice for routine clinical use. Handwriting recognition requires looking at the tablet (or electronic paper) you are using in order to stay within the handwriting area and to minimize mistakes (which will break eye contact with your patient).

The next fastest input method is typing. A good typist might obtain 60 words per minute routinely. Typing speeds can be dramatically enhanced by using keyboard expander software, which allow clinicians to enter an acronym (such as COPD) that the computer then expands to Chronic Obstructive Pulmonary Disease, at faster rates than the user could achieve by typing the phrase directly (see Figure 5.5).

An even faster method is dictation (on the front end) – people can speak at rates up to 180 words per minute. We cover this in detail shortly.

Pick lists that allow editing of data can occur at an equivalent rate of over 7,000 words per minute, depending upon the length of the data statements involved. There are different pick list approaches.

One approach is for the EMR to display the normal information for any condition being addressed and then the clinician includes what is pertinent to the current patient or excludes or brings up an abnormal list if the patient presents with an abnormal finding at the current time.

A second approach is for the EMR to show all of the possible abnormal findings for any condition being addressed and then the clinician includes what is pertinent to the current patient.

A third pick list method is for the EMR to enable the patient's prior office visit to populate the EMR screen and allow the clinician to address the specific previous abnormal complaints to determine if they are resolving. This third approach is the fastest data entry method and therefore the least expensive way of working – but still must be the method-of-choice for each user or it will not be an advantage in the long run.

Not all EMRs enable all three pick list approaches, but typically use only one. As shown in Figure 5.5, the speed for use of structured pick lists is much slower if the lists are not pre-populated with normal/abnormal findings or with information from the patient's previous visit.

Popularity of Various User Interaction Approaches

The adoption level information in Figure 5.5 is taken from the MSP/Andrew EMR Benchmark. No approach is correct or incorrect – it all depends on your purpose for adopting an EMR. Keep in mind that some EMRs support a primary approach and one or more secondary approaches. Dictation and speech recognition are common secondary approaches for data input.

Figure 5.5 Primary EMR Data Input Category by EMR Developer

Data Input Category	% Supporting	Relative Speed	Typical Charting Time
Structured Pick List	69%	up to 7,200 words/min.	RN 2 min. + MD 3 min.
Handwriting Recognition	20%	30 words/min.	up to 4 min.
Direct Typing by Caregiver	3%	60 words/min.	up to 8 min.
Dictation w/Speech Recognition	4%	180 words/min.	up to 3 min. + transcriptionist costs
Document Scanning	4%	N/A	N/A

MSP/Andrew EMR Benchmark/also data from Dr. Allen Wenner – Used with Permission

While it's apparent that a structured pick list is the predominant input approach offered by 69 percent of EMR developers, handwriting recognition is the second most popular approach by far. However, the actual success of handwriting recognition is a function of the accuracy of the recognition, which is user dependent.

Dictation or speech recognition is much less popular than one might imagine. Speech recognition usually does not create charts that support semantic interoperability, unless there is back-end natural language processing to structure the recognized speech. A breakthrough in back-end natural language processing for speech seems to have been achieved by the latest Medicomp CliniTalk voice structuring software (details follow in the speech recognition section).

Scanning is just as popular as dictation and speech recognition, but requires setup and does not provide information that inherently supports semantic interoperability.

Each of the various EMR input types are discussed individually in the next sections of this chapter.

Structured Pick List Approaches

Pick list approaches are by far the most widely deployed types of EMRs, probably because they result in clinical data being structured at either the billing or the clinical data levels.

The oldest, most common and more structured approach to EMR design is the use of pick lists in combination with practice and diagnostic-specific templates. For example, there may be a template for Congestive Heart Failure (CHF), others for diabetes and other conditions. If a patient has two conditions, often two separate templates are required, with some of the data duplicated on each template.

Figure 5.6 lists (in alphabetical order) some companies that support the pick list approach;

Figure 5.6 EMR Developers Supporting Traditional Pick List Approaches to EMR

EMR Product Name	EMR Developer	Guided Patient Interview?
AllMeds	AllMeds	
Enterprise EHR	Allscripts	
Professional EHR	Allscripts	
AmkaiCharts	Amkai	
BetterHealth record	BetterHealth Global	
Bond Clinician EMR (MediNotes)	Bond Technologies	Yes
ChartWare	ChartWare	
EpicCare Enterprise Clinical System	Epic Systems Corporation	Yes
Centricity (ICU and ED solutions)	GE Healthcare	Yes
HMS	Healthcare Management Systems	
ICU and OR interoperative EMR	iMDsoft	
InteGreat EHR	MED3000	Yes
SmartDoctor	Intelligent Medical Systems	
EncounterPro	Encounter Pro (was JMJ Technologies)	Yes
KeyChart	KeyMedical Software	
Mercure	Lakes Health Systems	
Emphasis Clinical Information Suite	M2 Information Systems	
MedcomSoft Record 2006	MedcomSoft	
MD.net EMR	Medical Communication Systems,	
ChartMaker	Medical Information Systems	
MedicWare EMR	MedicWare	
MediNotes	Eclipsys	Yes
MedtuityEMR	Medtuity	
Mountainside EMR	Mountainside Software	
NextGen EMR	NextGen	Yes
Physician's Workstation	Nightingale Informatix	
AHLTA	Northrop Grumman IT	
OmniMD	OmniMD	
Optimus EMR System	Optimus EMR	
Concerto Medical Applications Portal	Orion Health	
Amelior ED patient care system	Patient Care Technology Systems	
PatientNOW	PatientNOW	

Continued

Figure 5.6 EMR Developers Supporting Traditional Pick List Approaches to EMR

EMR Product Name	EMR Developer	Guided Patient Interview?
ICIP Suite – Xtenity Enterprise (ICU setting)	Philips Medical Systems	
	Picis	
ED PulseCheck (Ibex)	Picis	
Pulse Patient Relationship Management	Pulse Systems, Inc.	
Purkinje EMR	Purkinje	
RelWare's Clinical Application Solution	Reliance Software Systems	
SolComHealth	SolCom	
EMRge	SSIMED	
Systemedx EMR Navigator	Systemedx	
T-System EV	T-System, Inc.	
VersaForm EMR	VersaForm Systems Corporation	
VersaSuite	VersaSuite	
Wellogic Consult	Wellogic	

The organization of the EMR is often in a paper chart motif, with sections to address complaints, history of present illness, patient exam, etc. This is not necessarily the best organization because it imposes the limitations of the paper-based paradigm of practice on the EMR.

Strengths of the Structured Pick list Approach

- Pick lists allow EMR users to express clinical observations in a structured and content-determined manner, eliminating variations in the EMR.
- The structure can be mapped to a developer-proprietary or an industry-standard vocabulary or back-end clinical codification system. If indexed at the clinical level (using MEDCIN or SNOMED CT), the data will also be cross mapped to billing levels (ICD-9-CM, CPT) by most EMR systems.
- E&M work levels can be determined to guide billing. This can expedite and streamline back office operations, reduce claim rejections, shorten days-receivable and enhance cash flow.
- Pick lists empower a variety of structured reports on individual patients (multiple encounters), multiple patients (longitudinal patient reports) or on all providers (longitudinal provider reports). These reports help identify where practices are departing from evidence-based protocols or standards of care. Pick lists can trigger real-time decision support alerts if the EMR is one that supports this function.
- Structure doesn't have to come at the cost of having slower data entry on the front end, particularly if assertions for the current visit are pre-populated from previous visit results, so that only changes need to be edited.

Limitations of the Structured Pick List Approach

- Without pre-population of clinical findings, data structuring using pick lists can increase documentation time, particularly if the approach does not automatically delete the pick list choices that are not relevant.
- If you are interested in an EMR that takes this approach, determine if the EMR you are considering provides such pruning.

Handwriting Recognition Approaches

Handwriting recognition is the second most popular approach, possibly because handwriting recognition can result in highly-structured data. Many of these systems utilize tablet PCs programmed to display forms with check boxes and drop-down lists to provide structure to medical notes. EMR developers in offering handwriting recognition are listed in alphabetical order in Figure 5.7.

Figure 5.7 Sixteen EMR Developers Supporting Handwriting Approaches

EMR Developer Name	EMR Product Name	Guided Patient Interview?
AdvantaChart	AdvantaChart	
Amazing Charts	Amazing Charts	Yes
AutoMedicWorks	AutoMedicWorks	
Brunmed	Medscribbler Lite	
CPSI	CPSI System	
CureMD	CureMD EMR	
Database Constructs	Med-Center	
DavLong Business Solutions	MedInformatix	
Doc-U-Chart	Doc-U-Chart for the Tablet PC	
Integritas	STIX	
Kietra Corporation	Kietra XPR for Clinicians	
Meditab Software, Inc.	Intelligent Medical Software	
ObTech	ObGynPocketPro	
Poseidon Group	Navigator Web	
PracticeXpert	Xpert EMR	
QuadraMed	QuadraMed EMR	

Most handwriting approaches use tablet PCs. Several tablet hardware developers that have customized their products for the medical market include Fujitsu, Dell, Panasonic, Motion Computing and Hewlett-Packard. MSP has evaluated some of these tablets and found the most medically oriented platforms to be

Panasonic, Motion Computing (and its various OEMs) and HP (in that order). About two years ago, Intel, Motion Computing and other developers got together to design a next-generation portable, wireless, medical computing platform and came up with the Motion Computing C5.

Some of the advances it offers include:
- Light weight and an integrated handle for portability;
- Hot-swap batteries;
- Extended operating time compared to most laptop PCs;
- Biometric ID for user authentication;
- Integrated wireless networking;
- Integrated scanning for patient wristband and medication ID;
- The ability to switch easily from portrait to landscape display mode;
- two (or three more) noise-cancelling microphones built into the display for speech dictation without having to use a headset in a quiet location, that work no matter which display orientation the tablet is being used in.

All of these features substantially differentiate this product from previously available computing platforms. While the form factor is ideal, the C5 implementation had some issues. It didn't do well when it was dropped and evaluations at one large, West Coast health system found battery-operating time issues, and processor speed issues when the tablet was operating on batteries, particularly as they discharged. Another hospital on the East Coast had issues with lost data when the C5 was used in a wireless setting (but that problem might be due to a myriad of other issues). Nor is the new Motion platform without room for improvement, something that Panasonic picked up on.

At the 2009 HIMSS conference, Panasonic showed their H1 tablet (shown in Figure 5.4). It overcomes all of the Motion C5 limitations for medical applications by extending operating time, and adding improved shock mounting of the hard drive that allows it to meet military standard 810F (and IP54 test procedures). It has integrated GPS (ideal for home healthcare) and both an RFID and barcode scanner more conveniently located at the bottom of the tablet. The integrated mitt makes holding the H1 more comfortable and secure during charting, and the unit comes with a 3-year warranty. The H1 weighs 3.4 pounds. Unfortunately the Panasonic H1 is only available through dealers, which limits access in some areas of the country.

An alternative to either the C5 or the H1 is a mini-desktop computer from HP, the dc7900. It can be mated to the back of a flat panel display, and then mounted on a mobile cart that provides power to it via an integrated UPS (see Figure 14.6). The Infologic/JACO Ultra SL series cart (not shown in Figure 14.6) is also a good host for the HP dc7900 units. These products can be seen by visiting the Infologic and the Hewlett-Packard Web sites respectively. This approach includes a cart and means the platform is pushed around, rather than carried around by the caregiver.

Strengths of the Handwriting Recognition Approach

- Handwriting recognition is often the most natural way of interacting with an EMR and requires little special training to use. If you want to increase the speed of data entry, shortcuts are available that can be quickly learned.
- Handwriting recognition is able to support highly structured data approaches.
- Most users choose handheld tablet PCs if they like the handwriting approach. These PC tablets are also excellent for providing on-the-spot patient education displays that integrate text and graphic information.
- The graphic "pictures" are incorporated in the charting as well, such as circling an area on a torso where the patient indicates they are having pain, or have been bruised, lacerated and so on.

Limitations of the Handwriting Recognition Approach

- Accuracy of a user's basic handwriting can be enhanced by a variety of means, but the handwriting approach may prove challenging to some users depending on their handwriting quality.
- Some developers provide special writing areas where the characters can be scribed larger than in the final text and therefore more accurately recognized. Other developers provide QWERTY type keyboards at the bottom of the display, which allow users to choose letters by tapping keys, but this approach can be much slower than direct typing or dictating.
- For handwriting recognition you are pretty much locked into using a tablet PC approach, which is a more expensive hardware platform. However, because the tablet PC is carried around by clinicians, you only need one per user (not one per exam room as with the stationary PC). Tablet PC prices range from around $2,000 to as much as $3,000.

Dictation with Speech Recognition

Many physicians are used to dictating charts, so Speech Recognition (SR) could be a natural choice for them, but this approach generally results in poorly structured (freeform) data.

SR EMRs that store data can have that data converted and stored as Adobe PDF files. These files can then be indexed by making use of the Acrobat catalog function, however that doesn't automatically tag the results for "what" the data represents. This technique for structuring freeform (SR or scanned) data is detailed in Chapter 4.

So the SR user interface does not necessarily lead to structured records that support semantic interoperability with other EMRs (of specialists/consultants in other offices, for example) or for use by Electronic Health Records (EHRs). The SR approach also has trouble distinguishing between speaker variations in synonymous terms used to describe the same condition, myocardial infarction and MI for example. Nor does the SR approach generally allow data retrieval using phrases rather than individual words. However, the SR approach results in more structured data than many document scanning approaches.

SR offers the potential to reduce transcription costs if you use packages like Nuance's Dragon Naturally Speaking Medical, but we will shortly cover the limitations with this addition.

The use of medical context speech recognition is critical to achieving the level of accuracy that you expect in a SR-EMR approach. One way that speech recognition systems determine what homonym best fits a context is by processing words in groups of three. In such phrase triplets as, "condition is acute," a SR system has to determine whether the word spoken was "a cute" or "acute." You don't want to correct "a cute" to "acute" every time you use your SR-EMR and you can train the system by saying, "A cute" and then "acute" without the pause, but this is annoying. Some out-of-the-box speech recognition technologies do not have the necessary medical context for words like "acute."

Figure 5.8 Five EMR Developers Supporting SR w/wo Natural Language Processing

EMR Supplier	Product Name
Alma Information Systems	TexTALK MD
Assist Med	MediPort
Cyber Records	Medichart Express
HemiData	MD-Journal
Medicomp Systems	CliniTalk

Make sure that any speech recognition EMR you are looking at has covered all your other technological requirements. Make certain that it runs on robust hardware platforms, with plenty of CPU speed, a very fast front-side bus and lots of (2-3 Gbytes) memory. You can quickly lose patience if speech recognition is run on slow computers, on some tablet PCs, or on computers with too little memory or that have poor audio components and make too many mistakes during dictation. Try out any SR product you are considering on the hardware you will be using it on before you finalize your purchase.

Be aware that obtaining the accuracy you want may require you to wear a small headset and microphone. Some physicians are reluctant to dictate when they are in the room with a patient and therefore they either take notes manually and dictate after the fact, or they try to remember what the patient said and dictate after the fact. Both approaches lead to missed information or decreased accuracy.

There are now hybrid approaches that add documentation templates to pure SR, which allows SR to be useful for areas like history of present illness, normal and abnormal findings, diagnosis and planning. The hybrid approach uses pre-determined choices by simply speaking them rather than using point-and-click. SR can also be used to navigate in SR-enabled EMRs. SR also is useful for dictating communications to patients and for referral reports, particularly in some specialties like radiology, pathology, dermatology and others. You will need to decide if the SR approach, with its need for error correction, will work for you in your practice setting.

The EMR developers shown in Figure 5.8 use SR as their primary user interface. The issue of capturing unstructured/freeform data in a SR (or any) EMR is how to transform freeform entries into specific diagnostic codes and assertions, which can be later searched to build your patient and management reports. To impose structure, speech recognition systems adopt standardized document outlines (akin to templates) that include a number of elements, and can improve accuracy and decrease your dictation time.

These standard documents/templates can be provided by the EMR developer or created by someone in your office. Built into these standardized documents are macros, which are a succession of keystrokes and/or commands that are carried out by triggering a keyboard key or command. SR is well suited to use with macros to generate large amounts of text using only a few commands, as long as the text can be pre-dictated. This approach would be very useful in radiology, diagnostic test areas, or if your practice centers on one patient specialty type.

Natural Language Processing and Speech Recognition
Dictation that is processed by SR alone generally results in unstructured text; however, when it is also processed by a Natural Language Processing (NLP) back-end system, data captured can become fully structured. Until recently there have been very few SR products with NLP subsystems, but that is changing.

Two SR Approaches That Offer Structured Data
In 2009 Medicomp introduced the CliniTalk SR+NLP engine, which employs the underlying MEDCIN front-end vocabulary. This is an extremely interesting development. Watch for SR solutions from MEDCIN EMR partners to begin appearing in 2010.

CliniTalk is the first Speech Recognition (SR) product with practical Natural Language Processing (NLP) that allows dictation but stores assertions in a MEDCIN-structured data record. The clinician has simply to dictate the chief complaint (or other information) in his/her own words, and it is captured like any other SR product, in an apparently unstructured format. However, behind the scenes the data is being structured, and it is also compared to observations from any previous encounters. Results from past encounters are brought to the present screen, noted as normal or abnormal findings, and then easily modified as needed if the patient's condition has changed. There is an interesting demo of this system at http://CliniTalk.medicomp.com/wp-content/themes/medicomp/video/CliniTalk_Final_TECH_DEMO_WMV9_Widescreen_960x540.wmv.

A second company, M*Modal, takes a different approach to structuring. Once the physician has dictated in his/her typical manner, M*Modal employs speech technology that builds a draft document. The transcript that results is automatically structured and encoded according to the healthcare provider's documentation rules, using M*Modal software. For a more detailed explanation, visit the M*Modal Web site at www.mmodal.com.

Figure 5.9 illustrates the NLP technologies EMR developers have included in their SR-EMR.

Figure 5.9 EMR Developers Integrating with Which Speech Recognition Technology

Product Name	% Integrating
Microsoft OS (Not EMR specific, focused on voice command of OS)	65%
Dragon/Nuance (the major SR developer left in this approach)	40%
Dictaphone NLP (before being acquired by Nuance)	24%
Philips Speech Recognition (before being acquired by Nuance in 2008)	20%
IBM/Viavoice (essentially out of the market)	18%

There are only a few NLP engines from which an EMR developer desiring to SR-enable their system can choose. In 2006, Nuance (parent company Scansoft) purchased Dictaphone and took the Nuance name. In 2008, Nuance purchased Philips Speech Recognition. Microsoft has not offered any medical speech recognition products to the best of our knowledge. Unfortunately, several EMR developers that use this approach declined to complete the MSP/Andrew EMR Benchmark and therefore are not listed in the table.

Caveats to SR with NLP

In the way of final remarks about NLP, Dictaphone (now Nuance) claimed to have this technology before being acquired by Nuance but would never risk demonstrating it to the trade press. Philips Speech Recognition demonstrated their product to us yearly, but never offered an EMR with which it integrated.

If any EMR developer offers NLP to you in a released EMR, check it out very carefully before committing to it. The Dictaphone solution was Web-based and never proved to be commercially viable. Given the additional acquisitions, we don't believe that any Nuance product has yet achieved general NLP processing that is applicable to a broad cross-section of medical specialty needs.

Manual approaches to data structuring using SR-based EMR exist. Developers have the ability to automatically parse dictation to a specific field in charts with template structure, which assists in capturing data as structured. Some EMR developers charge extra for this feature and some use third parties to create these templates. It is worth your effort to carefully assess each SR system for this feature and compare costs among the developers. Being able to view and edit online is a feature that the majority of SR developers include, so you will likely end up with this feature, but you may pay more for it. Figure 5.10 shows how SR EMR developers characterize their EMRs.

Figure 5.10 Characteristics of Speech Recognition Approaches

Characteristic	Yes	Future	Not Supporting
Track and Display Status of Processing Dictation File	64%	14%	21%
Dictated Message Automatically Directed to Transcriptionist	82%	07%	11%
Transcriptionist Productivity Reports by Physician/Clinician	48%	24%	28%
Automatically Parse Dictation to Specific Fields	63%	28%	09%
Allows Clinician to View/Edit Online	85%	15%	N/A

Improving SR

SR is now available with digital USB (rather than analog) microphones. In some cases this can improve the quality of the signal compared to using an analog microphone and an older PC sound card. If you are having accuracy or speed of recognition problems, try switching to a newer, digital microphone.

Strengths of the SR Approach

- Patient charts are legible and highly comprehensible;
- Transcription costs can be reduced;
- Text from the medical chart can be easily re-used for letters to patients or to specialists;
- Charts can be stored electronically and concurrently accessed from several locations by multiple caregivers.

Limitations of the SR Approach

- We find SR approaches benefit from training by each individual who will be using them; without training these systems are less accurate. While the amount of training required has decreased with each new version, it is still required. Plan on 2-3 hours of training to improve recognition accuracy.
- Many physicians/clinicians prefer not to dictate notes in front of patients in the exam room. SR works best for specialists who do not dictate while the patient is present (radiologists and other imaging specialists, pathologists, and so on).
- Most who dictate ignore the screen due to the short delay before the text appears. Users often notice recognition errors when they pause, raising the question of when to correct these errors. Corrections in real-time using correction commands works fairly well, but disrupt patient interactions and take practice and SR software is prone to making the same mistakes, even when a phrase is repeated by the user. So you might want to leave this task to a transcriptionist. The reality with SR is that there will most likely be a continuing, albeit reduced, need for transcription.

- The speed and accuracy of SR is dependent upon the sound system hardware quality, processor time and available memory. Some laptop audio software is not adequate for speech recognition, even if the laptop has built-in dual microphones. Some tablets with SR lack enough speed in their processors to keep the screen information current while you are dictating.
- Speech profiles are generally stored a computer where your EMR is running. Recently, SR developers have begun offering the option of running on computers over the Internet, as an ASP application. If you routinely dictate from more than one office and use several computers, consider the application service provider approach.
- Without functioning NLP, SR data remains fairly unstructured, often stored as freeform text, making the data is difficult to query and quantify. Pure SR approaches do not provide full EMR functionality and should be considered EMR-lite approaches.

Document Scanning Approaches

Almost every practice that adopts an EMR will have some experience with scanning because it's a common way to get some of the information from existing patient paper records into your new EMR.

Document Scanning (DS) with Optical Character Recognition (OCR) approaches (like the SR approaches just described) are also easy to initially adopt and document scanners are fast and inexpensive. They have up to three major elements:

- The first element is the Document Scanner (DS), which converts the paper document to a picture.
- The second element is the Optical Character Recognition (OCR) engine, which converts any text elements of the scanned picture into a usable form (ASCII text). OCR engines are available from companies like OmniPage (current version 17) or Abbyy FineReader.
- The third element is an Editor/Classifier that allows scanned elements, whether pictorial or text, to be labeled and in some cases classified.

Only when pictures and data have been converted, labeled and indexed do they become searchable entities in your EMR. Otherwise, they remain pictures or patient "blobs of information" (see Chapter 4) that must be read by a human to be interpreted or acted upon.

Scanning approaches, like pure speech recognition approaches, are sometimes referred to as "EMR-lite" functionality, particularly when coupled with some e-pharmacy or Computerized Provider Order Entry (CPOE) capabilities. Some EMR-lites even throw in E&M coding modules. Because they are less expensive and easy-to-use and adopt, they are popular with practices looking to achieve or improve documentation clarity with some indexing of clinical data but not all of the functions of a full-featured EMR. EMR-Lite is detailed in Chapter 1.

Interestingly, scanning approaches result in some of the highest satisfaction levels, particularly for practices not looking to fully automate patient data capture or that don't need retrospective longitudinal analysis of patient records. However, scanning approaches differ significantly in their ability to structure and parse data into terms that can be retrospectively searched to document quality measures or to qualify for Pay-for-Performance incentives.

Indexing and barcodes provide a partial answer to structuring patient chart data, but require some level of effort and manual intervention by your office staff. Optical Character Recognition (OCR) technology has improved and some DS/OCR approaches use document tabs, barcodes or other codes or symbols applied to the source documents that act as markers to the OCR and Editor/Classifier software to separate the patient charts by encounter into the conventional sections (chief complaint & history of present illness, personal history, review of systems, etc.). However, generally they don't index or tag information below this level in each section.

The paper chart is separated into the different encounters by date of office visit. Each encounter could be arranged into indexable sections, as described above. Some use physical index sheet section separators, others use barcode tags applied to the first page of each section, others use pseudo-tags that the scanning operator picks as the documents are scanned. Tags are either manually attached, or automatically appended by the software, as the pages are scanned in. There can be tags at the beginning of the lab results, medication, patient complaints and history of present illness sections and so on. Some scanning approaches are more batch oriented and automated than others. The EMR software then uses the tags to arrange the scanned chart information. Some scanning systems require you to do the work first, others scan each page and ask you to do it on the fly.

Even if you choose some other type of EMR user interaction than document scanning, most EMRs will accept scanned documents (for existing patient records) as indexed images, but such images won't be easily searchable.

Scanning Hardware

There are many small and inexpensive scanners that are fast and capture one or both sides of a page. The price point is constantly dropping, and the speed and capabilities constantly increasing.

On a side note, one interesting product we have seen is a keyboard integrated with a document scanner (shown in Figure 5.11). We saw the Keyscan Model KS811 at the 2009 HIMSS conference, but it has been around for a while.

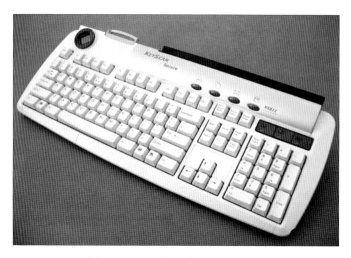

Figure 5.11 Keyscan Model KS-811 Keyboard/Scanner

There are two models. The model KS811 has an integrated fingerprint recognition scanner making it BioAPI-compliant and comes with a USB plug and OCR software that converts images into standard Adobe PDF format. The model KS810 has additional function keys on the upper left side of the keyboard where the fingerprint scanner is located.

It is useful in any medical practice, independent of the EMR user interface you choose, and fits well at the reception desk, as it is able to scan and process healthcare insurance cards, drivers licenses, patient reason-for-visit, HIPAA compliance and other forms. It could be equally helpful in the back office for billing and administrative functions. Keyboard with scanner lists for about $149, but can be found at medical conferences on special for as low as $99. There are undoubtedly quantity discounts as well.

EMR products that adopt the scanning approach provide a range of structured electronic charts. Some EMR developers use scanning to capture graphical and tabular report information to supplement a well-structured approach to charting. As discussed, structuring methods range from barcoding of existing records which are then scanned in and indexed, to scanning of handwritten charts with little or no structuring of the lab, prescriptions or other components.

Some EMR developers offer significant document scanning capabilities as a secondary EMR input modality, but chose to be listed in other categories in the MSP/Andrew EMR Benchmark. Figure 5.12 lists five EMR developers with scanning approaches.

Figure 5.12 Five EMR Developers Supporting Document Scanning Approaches

Product Name	EMR Developer Name
eDOMA for Healthcare	DOMA Technologies
eMedRec	Holt Data Systems
Optio Healthcare Quick Record Suite	Optio Software, Inc.
SRS Chart Manager	SRS Technologies
Wellness Connection	BlueWare, Inc

Be sure to inquire about paper record scanning and integration when investigating EMRs. This is an item that is often overlooked in vendor responses to RFPs because it makes the EMR quote higher, and EMR developers fear that the physician will reject the response without realizing that it contains chart scanning services while competitors' proposals omitted these expenses. Often they are correct. Be sure to put in your RFP that all EMR developers bid the document scanning item, and then you can compare apples to apples.

One more note on scanning. You will need to decide when you will scan in your existing patient records, once you have chosen an EMR to deploy. You may choose to scan in only your active patients or you may choose to scan in all of your patient records. Scanning in all records at one time makes them available in your EMR for scheduled patients as well as for unscheduled patient visits. Alternately, you may choose to scan in each patient record the day prior to their scheduled office visit. Neither approach is right or wrong.

Strengths of the Scanning Document Approach
• Scanning is an ideal way to enter and manage your paper data, from the patient charts that will need to be input once you choose an EMR system to the information that will continue to be sent in paper form.
• Scanning is an easy technology for offices to begin with, prior to going to a full EMR. Data can be scanned in by nonclinical personnel and then be brought online just prior to seeing each patient.
• It is also a common way of capturing and indexing results from medical devices like ECG machines, pulmonary function devices, stress testing and other devices that do not have a direct, electronic interface to an EMR. If the EMR scanner/EMR Lite incorporates the OCR element and or the Editor/Classifier element, searching for patient data downstream is made easier.

Limitations of Document Scanning Approaches
• Scanning of information requires time and, although many EMRs claim that they are able to receive scanned information, make certain that means that you can access, query and interact with any scanned-in data.
• Document scanning does not generally provide full EMR functionality, and does not result in highly structured records.

Multiple User Interaction Approaches

Figure 5.13 lists some EMR developers that support multiple EMR user interaction approaches in the same EMR. These are among the most versatile developers because they have adapted their EMR to support a variety of user input modalities. Each, however, has a core input foundation to which the other input types have been grafted on. Be sure to determine the core approach and understand its limitations.

Figure 5.13 Twenty-Three EMR Developers Supporting Multiple or Other Approaches to EMR Input

EMR Developer Name	EMR Product Name	Guided Patient Interview?
MDI Achieve	Achieve Matrix	
AdvancedMD	AdvancedEMR	
AutomationMed	EKiosk	
Daw Systems	ScriptSure	
Eclipsys Corporation	Sunrise	
Health Care Software	INTERACTANT	
Health Probe	Health Probes Professional	
Ingenious Med	IMBILLS	
LanVision dba Streamline Health	accessANYware	
LoginClinic	Login EMR	
McKesson	Horizon Ambulatory Care	
MedAZ	MedAZ	
Medical Office Online	Medical Office Online	
Medsphere	OpenVista	
Allscripts	Allscripts Homecare	
Momentum Healthware	Momentum Healthware Care Management	
MRVIEW	Document Scan. Service	
Point and Click Solutions	OpenChart	
Practice Partner/McKesson	Practice Partner	Yes
PracticeHWY.com	eIVF	
Software Performance Specialists, Inc	Easychart	
Spring Medical Systems	SpringCharts EMR	
VantageMed	ChartKeeper Express	

It's important to determine for which size practice an EMR was developed, as this will affect its pricing and functionality.

EMR Product Demonstrations

If you are not certain which data entry approach is best, consider EMRs that support more than one method. We have listed each EMR developer in one category that best describes their system (based on their instruction), but several EMRs offer multi-category data entry functionality.

The Big Picture

When you want to assess EMRs that support standards and interoperability, a national medical conference is a good place to go; particularly if it has an Integrating the Healthcare Enterprise (IHE) demonstration. Unfortunately, very few of the 220 EMR developers attend any single medical conference. HIMSS, the largest healthcare I.T. meeting, only attracts 50 to 60 EMR developers. There aren't enough physician prospects attending HIMSS to make it profitable for smaller EMR developers to exhibit at HIMSS. Thus, HIMSS EMR exhibitors tend to be the bigger and most expensive suppliers. See Appendix II for a list of conferences to consider. The smaller the medical specialty, the fewer EMR developers that support it, and the fewer that attend the conventions.

Make Appointments

If you want an in-depth EMR demonstration at a conference you plan to attend, schedule an appointment with that EMR developer in advance. Be aware that you may be seeing developmental (non-released) software with fictitious patient data. The EMR being shown may have all the new features that an EMR developer is working on, none of which may be actually deployed yet. A conference exhibit floor is not a clinical setting. If the EMR you are considering is hosted on the World Wide Web over the Internet (as an ASP product), the conference demo you are shown could be running from a Web server located in the developer's booth, rather than over the Internet. This arrangement makes their keyboard response times somewhat faster than you would experience in your office when you are connected to a distant Web server.

Another way to compare EMR characteristics without the expense and bother of traveling to a conference, is at the MSP EHR Selector Web portal. But here you will only see a subset of EMR developers that are willing to have their product information vetted and are comfortable with side-by-side comparisons of their product features. Usually this group is between 25 and 45 EMR developers, but will grow after "Meaningful Use" is clarified.

A more comprehensive source of information (on over one hundred EMR developers) is the MSP/Andrew EMR Benchmark™. MSP is expanding the MSP EHR Selector to include some of the results from this Benchmark.

Patient Interactions With Your EMR

You and your staff aren't the only people who will be interacting with your new EMR, so will your patients – at least if you want to achieve Meaningful Use and receive reimbursement. According to Paul Tang, e-copies of the patient's health record will be a requirement in 2011 and on-demand patient access to their full medical records will be required by 2013.[3] Access can be provided by Web portals or in-office kiosks, or ultimately over the Nationwide Health Information Network (NHIN), if it's operational by then.

In-office kiosks are our first choice to provide patient access because the patient has to show up in person and that eases the challenge with remote, electronic patient authentication, security and audit trail issues. We advise foregoing Web portals for a year or two until you are more experienced with managing a basic EMR system. Consider planning some space for patient kiosks. This may require rethinking your overall office layout or at least your patient waiting room layout.

In-office kiosks are also excellent tools for providing patient educational materials, something that is highly valued and associated with quality by patients. How comprehensive, complete and specific are the patient education materials you are providing to your patients now? Is there room for improvement? What education/instructional materials are you providing to patients today to help them understand:

• Their disease?
• Your treatment and procedures?
• What they need to do when they get home?

Is this education material customized in any way to the individual patient? Is it available electronically (via the Internet or a patient portal supported by your EMR)? Patients want to know about their care in all healthcare settings.

Learn a lesson from hospitals where more than 77% of patients indicated that communication about their care was more important to them than accommodations and billing issues.[4] EMRs that provide printed patient instructions and that can also host patient access from home to personalized education materials and personalized care instructions, have an advantage in attracting (and continuing to satisfy) patients.

A good EMR should provide comprehensive, clearly-written patient education materials that document the care and therapies you provide. Printed instructions help patients remember verbal instructions and thus avoid complications from not understanding or following instructions properly. The EMR should chart all educational materials provided.

---

[3] *Is the Bar Still Too High?* By David Raths. Published September 2009, Healthcare Informatics p. 38

[4] *A Better Hospital Experience.* By Hurt D. Grote, et al. Published Nov. 2007 by The Mckinsey Quarterly

Wrap Up

This chapter focused on the pros and cons of each user interaction approach available in your specialty and practice setting. Any choice you make will substantially narrow the number of EMR developers available to you. Consider the trend towards adopting approaches that provide more structured data. If you choose an EMR that is structured at the clinical (rather than the billing) level, the number of EMRs will shrink further (see Chapter 7 – Vocabularies, Standards & Interoperability).

Note on the Scorecard which of the data entry approaches each person in your office prefers and how you are going to provide your patients with electronic copies of their chart summaries. Photocopy the Scorecard as needed. Additional copies are available at the www.ehrselector.com Web portal.

Crucial Decision

How does everyone in your office prefer to interact with an EMR? Should the EMR be accessible to patients to enter their own data? Photocopy as needed or download Scorecard from www.ehrselector.com

If we decide that we do want our patients to be able to enter data, do we want them to use the Internet or enter data in the office – or both?	
	Internet
	In-office
	Both approaches
Our Decision (or preference at this point):	
Our Rationale:	
If we want our patients to be able to enter data over the Internet, what do we need to do to our Internet to ensure HIPAA privacy?	
If we want patients to enter data in-office, how will we rearrange our patient waiting area to ensure HIPAA privacy?	
What hardware do we need to add in order for patients to enter data?	
	Tablet PCs
	Keyboards/Computer Displays

This is a Crucial Decision in which some choices eliminate others. Check with EMR developers to determine their core input approach but realize that many offer multiple modes of entering data.

Our Decision (or preference at this point):
Our Rationale:
Any other items we need to decide/explore related to our patients being able to enter data? (desks, dividers, kiosk walls, any educational material wanted, etc.)
Selecting your user interface: Photocopy this page as needed and each person should determine the method(s) of interacting with an EMR they think they prefer at this stage.

	Structured Pick List
	Handwriting Recognition
	Direct Typing by Caregiver
	Dictation w/o Speech recognition
	Dictation w/Speech recognition

Multiple Interface Approaches (list below):
Our Decision(s) (or preference at this point):

This is a Crucial Decision in which some choices eliminate others. Check with EMR developers to determine their core input approach but realize that many offer multiple modes of entering data.

Our Rationale:

We are leaning towards using the following methods to enter our paper chart patient information as well as our ongoing information received in paper form:

	Scanning ability only
	Scanning ability w/OCR
	Scanning ability w/Editor/Classifier
	Scanning ability w interface to:

		ECG
		Stress test equipment
		Pulmonary function

Other Equipment (list below):

Our Decision(s) (or preference at this point):

Our Rationale:

Anything else we need to think through/explore at this point in the process:

This is a Crucial Decision in which some choices eliminate others. Check with EMR developers to determine their core input approach but realize that many offer multiple modes of entering data.

CHAPTER 6

Where to Deploy Your EMR

Crucial Decision
Do you want an in-office or a Web-based EMR deployment?

This chapter also addresses the following questions:

- With an in-office EMR, do you want a software-only or a turnkey solution?
- Do you want an EMR as a capital asset, or an ASP SaaS (Web-based) EMR?
- What special issues do either of the above deployment decisions impose?

The Fork in the EMR Deployment Road

The choice you make for this Crucial Decision will take you in two very different directions – in your office or as a service over the Web. Each approach will impact how easily the EMR you want can be customized (see Chapter 9), what sort of Crisis Planning & Mitigation (see Chapter 15) and security planning (see Chapter 16) is required, and your purchasing contract or licensing agreement (see Chapter 18). We suggest that you read all of these chapters and consider the pros and cons of each approach before you settle on one or the other.

EMR Adventures

Dr. Karen Bell, along with her business manager, Mary, and her receptionist, Linda, are having another meeting to discuss their options for an EMR. They finally made the choice to replace both their EMR and their CPM (see Chapter 3), but now they have another important decision to make. As the meeting starts, Dr. Bell says, "When it comes to the decision of whether we want the EMR to be located physically here in our office or on the Web, I am very much in favor of locating it right here in the office. I just can't see letting our medical records be stored by someone who I don't know and have no idea if they are secure or even HIPAA compliant – HIPAA compliance is becoming stricter under the Obama Administration."

"I see why you stress that," says Mary. "But I have no idea who will take care of the day-to-day running of a system or the maintenance associated with it, let alone what security software is good for protecting our data – programs like firewalls and anti-virus, and there is something I think called malware? How can we possibly figure all of that out?"

Successfully Choosing Your EMR: 15 Crucial Decisions. By © Arthur Gasch and Betty Gasch.
Published 2010 by Blackwell Publishing

"Don't look at me," adds Linda. "I think we should at least look at the Web approach because I believe the EMR developer takes care of all those programs. But if we go with the in-office EMR I think we can get help from Riverview Hospital's I.T. department."

"Yes," agrees Dr. Bell. "We will look at all options but I also know that with the Web approach, when the developer makes changes to the software, we all change along with them – even if we are pleased with the EMR the way it is. We change if they change. Nevertheless, we need to explore and list all the pros and cons of both the in-office approach and the Web approach. Then we can determine which makes the most sense all around."

This is not an unusual scenario for small physician practices. The differences of these two approaches need to be carefully considered and after exploring the already mentioned, additional chapters, you will be able to make an informed decision.

If you are currently maintaining your Computer Practice Management (CPM) system yourself, your EMR may be handled the same way. If not, perhaps whoever manages your CPM would also be willing to handle your EMR, if you ultimately decide to deploy an in-office solution. The Stark Safe Harbor legislation opens up the possibility that your practice can obtain technical support services from your hospital I.T. department, without it being considered a kickback. That can be a real help for smaller practices that lack in-office I.T. expertise. Talk with any hospitals where you have admitting privileges about what level of services they might be willing to provide and at what cost. About one-third of hospitals may be willing to provide some level of support.

In-Office Network Requirements

No matter where you locate your EMR server software (whether in a location in your office or someplace across the Internet), you will need to connect the computers accessing it to a wired Local Area Network (LAN) or a Wireless Local Area Network (WLAN) deployed in your office. A local area network is simply a group of interconnected computers, almost always using Ethernet.

That raises the question about what network approach and protocols you will need. In deploying either an in-office or one implemented across the Web as a Software as a Service (SaaS) Application Service Provider (ASP) EMR, you will need a firewall in your office to protect you from hackers. If you decide to locate the EMR in your office, you will also have to install and maintain additional computer equipment (the file server, backup equipment and other utility and security software). Except for the firewall, the additional software is not required in the SaaS ASP EMR deployment, as these should be handled for you on the Web server side by your ASP provider. This is all detailed in Chapter 16 (Protecting Your Patient Data).

If you choose the in-office approach, you must also decide if you want the EMR developer to provide just the software application or the software already loaded on computer hardware, as a turnkey EMR solution. Let's explore the in-office, turnkey decision implications.

Implications of a Turnkey Solution

The turnkey solution determines who provides the computer and networking hardware your EMR application will run on; does it come from your EMR software developer or does it come from independent hardware vendor(s)? There are benefits to purchasing and receiving support from one developer, but only if the developer can provide good support. Most EMR developers are smaller companies and do not make hardware, therefore there is no real profit in their supplying and taking on support of your hardware for them. As a result, most EMR developers don't offer the turnkey option.

Those that do offer turnkey solutions are among the largest suppliers, and you can be sure that you will pay a premium for such systems. At the 2009 HIMSS conference, eClinicalWorks announced that it had a partnership with Sam's Club that allowed physicians to order an eClinicalWorks EMR over the Internet from Sam's Club, and have it delivered on the specified computer hardware as a turnkey, integrated solution.

Advantages and Disadvantages Summary

There are advantages and disadvantages of selecting an EMR from a developer that can offer a turnkey solution. Turnkey EMRs are more expensive and out of the price range of most smaller group practices. They may also keep your practice from realizing savings on hardware and network components, on less expensive and more robust security components, and to some extent on assistance that might be available from local providers like your hospital I.T. personnel or a trusted independent service person (such as the person currently maintaining your CPM system).

Few EMR developers offer integration of their software with hardware. eClinicalWorks is one EMR company that offers hardware, through a special arrangement with Walmart/Sam's Club. The eClinicalworks system is only available on-line and not available in local Sam's Club stores.

Figure 6.1 details the advantages and the disadvantages of the components of this solution.

Figure 6.1 Advantages/Disadvantages to Turnkey EMR (EMR/CPM) Solutions

Item to Be Considered	Advantages of Turnkey	Disadvantages of Turnkey	Cost Implication for Deployment & Comments
EMR/CPM Application Software	One vendor to call, one sales agreement covers everything.	EMR and CPM may not be available from one source.	The more loaded the EMR solution, the greater the maintenance fees. You will be paying for a service contract on all components whether you need them or not.
CPU Hardware	Difficult for component suppliers to blame each other when something isn't working.	Available at lower cost from 3rd party than from any EMR developer.	EMR developers mark up hardware being supplied, raising the hardware cost of deployment. It contributes to their profit margin as well. May not support the most robust and current solutions.
Network Hardware	Practice doesn't pay until entire solution works.	Must work with your Internet access method. Generally two vendors will be involved in any case.	Vendor-supplied security may be less robust and more expensive than commercial security utilities.
Security & Utility Applications	Practice is ultimately responsible if security tools prove inadequate, although developer may also be responsible.	Security utilities from developer may not be adequate to assure complete HIPAA compliance. Any software (or hardware) you add may be cited as interfering with the system they support.	The MSP/Andrew EMR Benchmark found poor EMR testing of available security products – a weak link in all deployments.
Periodic Maintenance		Fewer EMR developers can provide this and those that do are among the costliest.	Maintenance may be contracted to a 3rd party anyway, and not performed by EMR developer. If so, it will be marked up twice (once by the developer and a second time by the actual service organization).

Comparison of In-Office and Web-based SaaS EMR Solutions

The implications of in-office versus remote, Web-based ASP approaches are summarized in Figure 6.2. We'll cover the details after this summary.

Figure 6.2 In-office Versus Application Service Provider EMRs Pros and Cons

Item to Be Considered	Web-based ASP Approach	In-Office, Client/ Server Approach	Comments, Strengths and Weaknesses
Total Hardware Costs	Less, only requires Web browser at each office workstation, but requires higher operating and site prep costs.	More, requires an office server and workstations with individual operating systems that must be network compatible.	Computers can have different Operating System (OS) versions, which will complicate support and networking issues. Since some processing is done on the client workstation, in-office hardware may need to be more capable, costing more.
Technical Support Required	Less, since only the browser is part of the EMR. Practice should plan to use the same brand and version of browser to minimize browser variation issues. Software updates done by ASP.	More, the entire server will need to be supported, as well as all workstations and the network, network policies, backup, software updating.	In both, individual workstations need to be secure, without viruses/ malware. But servers and networks are more complex to support, secure, and administer than workstations with browsers.

All browsers are not the same and each can render code in different ways. Test any ASP EMR with the specific browsers you'll use and be aware that there may be quirks when new browsers are bundled with new computers and OS, which can cause existing EMRs to malfunction. |
| Server Reliability & Redundancy | Depends on the Internet Service Provider (ISP) that is running the EMR application. Practice may still need emergency power backup, or can relocate to other locations with power and wireless Internet. | The server is in your office and your practice fully supports it, including all backups (on-site and off) and all site hardening (like emergency power). | Servers should have access to emergency power, which means a standby generator on-site, which many medical buildings lack. Determine whether you can add one and the costs. Backup power to support one medical practice can cost $4,000 to $6,000 for the generator and transfer switch, plus installation. They require access to natural gas (no gasoline) for their power. |

Continued

Item to Be Considered	Web-based ASP Approach	In-Office, Client/ Server Approach	Comments, Strengths and Weaknesses
Contract Period & Termination	Easier – a practice can usually terminate with minimal notice to ASP and without penalty.	Often a minimal contract period and more notice required to terminate.	Since the ASP owns and controls its software, simply providing a service to the group practice, termination is usually easier, faster and less expensive in the ASP approach.
Network Internet Contingency Issues	Internet connection, speed, and robustness are critical. If the Internet fails, your practice can be paralyzed. Internet access costs (an ongoing operating expense) will definitely be higher -- you'll pay for two Internet access connections, not just one.	Here, the robustness of the Internet is less of an issue, as it is used primarily for submitting bills, obtaining remote test results, and sending secure e-mail, none of which will shut down your practice if they are interrupted.	With the ASP model, you will need to have a backup and independent path to the Internet. The point is to have two independent connections, one used for daily operations and the other for emergency situations. What if an auto accident takes out a telephone pole that carries your Internet cable connection? How long can you afford to shut down your practice while the phone/power company gets around to restoring your service?
Physical Security	Need to secure only individual workstations (since there is no on-site server). Wherever data is located, on any device, it must be secure.	More complex: must secure all workstations and servers. Wherever data is located, on any device, it must be secure.	Security includes physical and electronic data security. Office should have an alarm system, with both copper and wireless (cell) connections to a monitoring center. All patient data should be encrypted and all applications that access it should require both password and biometric IDs.
Billing & Maintenance Issues	Usually an on-going charge based upon the number of "seats" or physicians using or concurrent users or patient encounters logged per month.	Usually, license is purchased, and later upgrades are provided by payment of an on-going maintenance fee ranging from 15-25 percent of the initial license cost annually.	ASP approaches lend themselves to expensing the EMR as an operating cost. In-office EMRs tend to have the initial price as a capital asset (that is depreciated) and the maintenance fee as an operating expense applied in the year it is incurred. Front-end costs are minimized with the ASP approach.

Continued

Item to Be Considered	Web-based ASP Approach	In-Office, Client/Server Approach	Comments, Strengths and Weaknesses
Patient Data Access & Portability	Every client's data is migrated forward to whatever format the most current version of the EMR software supports, which is superior, but carries some risk.	Individual practices may have to run different versions with different data formats, which is undesirable.	Patient data is more likely to incorporate standards like CCR or CCD and be written in industry standard data structures. Nearly all EMR developers store data in proprietary formats, so look for EMRs that can both export and import patient data in CCD-structured formats, regardless of deployment model.
Software Customization Implications	Little chance to customize basic functionality, as all clients run the same applications. Individual templates for certain practice specialties may be available, but that's it.	Customization possible (at a cost), but custom features in the current version may not be carried forward in future versions or compatible with them.	Choose a system built upon a workflow management system that lets you customize workflow without depending on the developer. Customization should include modification or creation of new screen layouts and templates without programming or making the EMR application non-standard, thus harder and more expensive to support.
User Interface	Some compromises due to the limitations of browsers and server-side code. Make sure you like their interface, too.	No limitations because the application has full access to your computer's resources.	In approaches that use Web browsers, browser applications run inside of a "sandbox" on the computer, which protects other computer programs from code running in the browser.

Whew! A lot of things to consider, probably some new terms too. Let's start the detailed discussion by focusing on the Internet EMR approach.

Web-based SaaS ASP Considerations

Before we launch into the details of this approach, let's define two terms. ASP and SaaS. Software-as-a-Service (SaaS) refers to the EMR software that enables your office to become automated. Application Service Provider (ASP) is the place on the Web that provides the SaaS.

One of the advantages to the Application Service Provider (ASP) approach is that you do not need to purchase (or maintain) the server or the network that your EMR application will run on. You still need the latest virus/malware protection and to operate behind a firewall though. This makes managing your office network and computers much simpler, a blessing if you are not comfortable with computer technology.

In the ASP Software-as-a-Service (SaaS) model, Internet connection is essential because your SaaS EMR is located on the Web and requires a connection to the Internet. This makes the Internet a single point of failure that can take out your entire practice at once. Without the Internet connection, you are out of business until it's restored.

If you use two methods to connect to the Internet that share the same infrastructure, both can be rendered inoperable at the same time (perhaps an auto hitting a telephone pole). It's safer to have one wired and one wireless connection to the Internet, which makes losing both connections at the same time unlikely. Most practices don't go to the trouble of establishing a second Internet connection path, betting that they won't need it.

This approach may be right 99.9 percent of the time, but if you ever do need a second connection, you will find that having it installed can take a week or more in good times, and longer if the provider is engaged in fixing problems with many subscribers who are also without service. Storms in Seattle took out phone and Internet service for two weeks in some areas in 2008, and because crews were working three shifts to repair existing lines there was no capacity to install new service. Of course, conditions in each area of the country vary so you must assess the potential impact of losing Internet connection if you are deploying an ASP EMR approach.

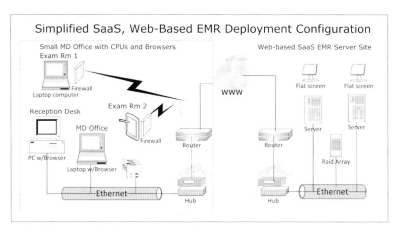

Figure 6.3 Diagram of Software-as-a-Service Information Flow

Figure 6.3 shows a typical (but simplified) diagram of a Web-based, Software-as-a-Service (SaaS), EMR deployment. On the left side of this diagram is your office. The cloud in the middle is the Internet. On the right side is your distant, Web-based, SaaS EMR Application Service Provider (ASP).

Your office is called the "client side," while the Web-based location is the EMR "server." The way your Web-based EMR works is that the server sends your Web browser (at your office, the client side), a screen to display. You interact with that screen by either clicking on a control or entering data. When you are finished, you submit it and the information is sent back to the server (via the Internet) and processed there. The result might be another screen sent over to your browser, or perhaps a report, if you requested data or output.

The clinical charting process is reduced to a series of such exchanges; a send from the server, a send back from your browser (two trips across the Internet), with data stored on the Web server, in a database server or other file storage modality. This means that the ASP has your patient records.

You will want to know two things for sure. Who is the ASP – is it the EMR developer or a third party the developer has hired to host the application? And if you want an electronic version of all your patient records (because perhaps you want to move to another EMR provider), how do you get your patient records back (and in what format)?

ASP Not Necessarily EMR Developer

Many physicians envision this approach as a two-party arrangement between themselves and their EMR developer. But not all EMR developers have their own data centers, some contract to have their EMR application hosted at a different site on the Web. In this arrangement, the Application Service Provider (ASP) is a separate site on the Web that is maintained by a different company, the Internet Service Provider (ISP), which is hosting the Web-based EMR application. In the worst case scenario, there are three different companies involved in the Web-based SaaS model:

• Your ISP (connects you to the Internet);
• Your EMR developer's ASP (runs their application for them as a Web service);
• Your EMR developer (developed the EMR application that is running).

This is important because if the ASP is not the EMR developer, there is a contract between these two parties. In the absence of terms to the contrary, the ASP is the one who physically has your patient records, and unless your licensing agreement says otherwise, you have no contract with that entity concerning your data rights, should the EMR developer default in their contract with the ASP or go bankrupt, or whatever.

You definitely don't want to get caught in the middle of a dispute between your EMR supplier and their ASP. While this may be deemed unlikely by your EMR developer, who will seek to dismiss it, such contingency planning is an important part of deploying the Web-based ASP EMR model.

Some EMR developers do act as their own ASP, making this a true two-party affair. As an example, Siemens in Malvern, PA is a large application service provider, hosting EMR and other Information Technology (I.T.) services for themselves, many U.S. hospitals, the U.S. government and others. The site is part of the U.S. security network. Many different applications are hosted there. If you have a Siemens Soarian EMR, running from Malvern, then Siemens would be your Application Service Provider (ASP).

The major issue for an ASP deployment is making Internet access more secure and less vulnerable to outside attack and evaluating how well the ASP has accomplished this for their server, so that interruptions don't occur at either end of the Internet.

Web-based EMR Responsiveness

At a medical conference, a Web-based EMR being demonstrated at a booth may run well and quickly because the server may be only a few feet away (in a closet at the booth location and out of sight), but the actual server that you would use in your office may be located halfway across the U.S. This reality could greatly impact the response time from your office location; you may find it to be vastly slower. It is a good idea to test response times before you commit to this type of EMR. Have any demonstrations carried out in your office over your Internet connection during the hours and days that you operate your office. That is the best test.

Internet data packets can slow down as they pass through each router on their journey over the Internet. The journey across the Internet is a distinct "route" that any message (data packet) takes as it "hops" from router-to-router. Disruptions like a virus spreading across the Internet, or floods, storms, snow, ice, tornados and hurricanes can also change Internet response time. Internet response changes are quite variable and will manifest in your EMR as a delay in having your next screen come up after you submit a form. In an office-based system, that delay would not exist.

Your computer uses a command to track the route your information is taking. It's called "TraceRt" (short for trace-route) and it displays listings like the ones in the next few figures. To perform this function, open a DOS window (Start>Run>Cmd). That will give you a black screen like the ones you see in the next few figures. To run the actual tracert, type in the address of the EMR server on the Web – one easy way to get this is to ask for it from your EMR developer.

MSP has two Web sites, one is two miles away and the other is in Texas. Figure 6.4 shows the route taken to go two miles from our New Jersey office to our Web site also in New Jersey. The hop number (left column), shows that it took 14 hops to reach this two-miles-away destination. In the process the message went into and back out of New York because of the way the Internet routed it. The fourth column (Figure 6.4) shows how long the message took to be processed on each leg of its journey. The entire journey consumes only 17 milliseconds to reach the destination (shown by the last number of the last hop and that's the round-trip time).

```
Tracing route to www.medsp.com [64.59.193.40]
over a maximum of 30 hops:

 1    <1 ms    <1 ms    <1 ms  Wireless_Broadband_Router.home [192.168.1.1]
 2     8 ms     4 ms     4 ms  L100.VFTTP-11.NWRKNJ.verizon-gni.net [72.76.24.1]
 3     6 ms     4 ms     4 ms  P3-2.LCR-01.NWRKNJ.verizon-gni.net [130.81.38.192]
 4     5 ms     4 ms     4 ms  130.81.29.188
 5    10 ms     9 ms     9 ms  130.81.17.6
 6    12 ms     9 ms    24 ms  0.ge-2-2-0.BR3.NYC4.ALTER.NET [152.63.3.130]
 7     9 ms    12 ms    12 ms  204.255.173.54
 8    13 ms    19 ms    17 ms  vlan99.csw4.NewYork1.Level3.net [4.68.16.254]
 9    10 ms    12 ms    12 ms  ae-61-61.ebr1.NewYork1.Level3.net [4.69.134.65]
10    20 ms    17 ms    19 ms  ae-2-2.ebr1.Newark1.Level3.net [4.69.132.98]
11    12 ms    12 ms    12 ms  ae-12-51.car2.Newark1.Level3.net [4.68.99.6]
12    13 ms    12 ms    12 ms  ge-10-2.car1.Newark6.Level3.net [4.68.145.234]
13    13 ms    14 ms    12 ms  64.9.35.246
14    13 ms    14 ms    17 ms  www.medsp.com [64.59.193.40]

Trace complete.
```

Figure 6.4 Hops From Lincroft, NJ to Shrewsbury, NJ – Two Miles Distance

However your Web-based EMR server is not likely to be two miles from your office and the response time in that case could be longer. To give you an idea of how much longer, we did another from our office in Lincroft, NJ to another of our Web servers in Texas.

```
Tracing route to www.ehrselector.com [72.32.12..146]
over a maximum of 30 hops:

 1    <1 ms    <1 ms    <1 ms  Wireless_Broadband_Router.home [192.168.1.1]
 2     4 ms     4 ms     4 ms  L100.VFTTP-11.NWRKNJ.verizon-gni.net [72.76.24.1]
 3     6 ms     4 ms     4 ms  P3-2.LCR-01.NWRKNJ.verizon-gni.net [130.81.38.192]
 4     8 ms     7 ms     4 ms  130.81.29.188
 5    13 ms     9 ms     9 ms  130.81.17.6
 6     8 ms     9 ms    39 ms  so-6-0-0-0.PEER-RTR1.NY111.verizon-gni.net [130.81.17.129]
 7     9 ms    12 ms     9 ms  so-0-3-1.mpr2.lga5.us.above.net [64.125.13.33]
 8    18 ms    17 ms    19 ms  so-0-2-0.mpr2.jca2.us.above.net [64.125.26.105]
 9    55 ms    54 ms    54 ms  so-1-0-0.mpr4.iah1.us.above.net [64.125.28.50]
10    55 ms    54 ms    54 ms  so-1-1-0.mpr2.jfw2.us.above.net [64.125.26.133]
11    73 ms    54 ms    54 ms  xe-1-1-0.er2.dfw2.us.above.net [64.125.26.214]
12    55 ms    79 ms    54 ms  xe-1-0-0.er1.dfw2.us.above.net [64.125.27.77]
13    55 ms    54 ms    54 ms  209.133.126.42
14    55 ms    54 ms    54 ms  vlan901.core1.jfw1.rackspace.com [72.3.128.21]
15    55 ms    54 ms    76 ms  aggr4a.dfw1.rackspace.net [72.3.129.15]
16    54 ms    54 ms    54 ms  72.32.121.146

Trace complete.
```

Figure 6.5 Hops From Lincroft, NJ to Texas, 1,600 Miles

The results are shown in Figure 6.5. This time it took 16 hops to reach Texas from NJ (1,600 miles away), but the response time (shown in column 4), was still only 54 milliseconds, or about three times longer than the two-mile trip. Again, this is a round-trip number.

In addition to the round trip travel time, the total trip time will include any computer processing time required on the Web server in Texas to perform whatever function we are sending it. In the EMR case, where it is serving many other group practices, that processing delay might be another couple of seconds or longer on a busy day.

Each trip across the Internet is different, so the response times can be different too, depending upon when they are transmitted. Doing a second tracert to Texas a few hours later generated Figure 6.6. Notice this time that it took one less hop to reach Texas, and the total time was 54 milliseconds (msec) – only slightly different. So the time it takes for a message to reach Texas is probably about as good as it gets.

```
C:\Documents and Settings\Arthur Gasch>tracert ehrselector.com

Tracing route to ehrselector.com [72.32.121.146]
over a maximum of 30 hops:

 1    <1 ms    <1 ms    <1 ms  Wireless_Broadband_Router.home [192.168.1.1]
 2     8 ms     4 ms     4 ms  L100.VFTTP-11.NWRKNJ.verizon-gni.net [72.76.24.1]
 3     5 ms     4 ms     4 ms  P3-2.LCR-01.NWRKNJ.verizon-gni.net [130.81.38.192]
 4     5 ms     4 ms     4 ms  130.81.29.188
 5     7 ms     7 ms     7 ms  0.so-5-0-0.XL1.EWR6.ALTER.NET [152.63.19.177]
 6    10 ms     9 ms     9 ms  0.ge-4-1-0.XL3.NYC4.ALTER.NET [152.63.3.101]
 7     9 ms     9 ms     9 ms  GigabitEthernet6-0-0.GW1.NYC4.ALTER.NET [152.63.20.49]
 8     7 ms     7 ms     7 ms  teliasonera-test.alter.net [157.130.255.206]
 9     8 ms     9 ms     9 ms  nyk-bb2-link.telia.net [80.91.248.153]
10   187 ms   189 ms   129 ms  chi-bb1-link.telia.net [80.91.248.196]
11    95 ms    92 ms    94 ms  dls-bb1-link.telia.net [80.91.248.209]
12    55 ms    54 ms    57 ms  rackspace-ic-127247-dls-bb1.c.telia.net [213.248.88.174]
13    55 ms    57 ms    57 ms  vlan901.core1.dfw1.rackspace.com [72.3.128.21]
14    55 ms    57 ms    54 ms  aggr4a.dfw1.rackspace.net [72.3.129.15]
15    55 ms    57 ms    54 ms  72.32.121.146

Trace complete.
```

Figure 6.6 Hops From Lincroft, NJ to Texas, 1,600 Miles – Second Attempt

These scenarios point out the need to test any Web-based EMR from your office and not from a demo at a medical conference, because in such cases you have no idea whether that result is typical of what you will experience in your office. Nor will the loading on the CPU in a EMR developer's booth be anything like the loading on a live system serving thousands of clients simultaneously.

Make a point of specifying what the maximum acceptable response must be in your licensing agreement, and what remedy the EMR developer is committed to make if the actual response time exceeds the maximum one specified in the agreement. A Web-based EMR may be the right decision if you are a small office, but be sure to read Chapter 15 on Crisis Planning & Mitigation and make provisions for a second Internet connection in case your primary connection fails. And put all of the terms and conditions you want in your licensing agreement with your EMR developer (see Chapter 18 – Negotiating The Agreement). This is another area that highlights the wisdom of EMR-specific legal advice.

In-Office, Client-Server EMR Deployment Model

Now what about your other choice, the in-office EMR deployment? The in-office EMR deployment avoids all of the previously addressed Internet and security obstacles but it poses the following additional challenges for your practice. Refer to Figure 6.7. Here is a short list of items for considerations.

*   More Hardware Deployment – You have to deploy, configure and maintain more computer hardware (including a file server with a server operating system, perhaps a backup server or repository) than you would in the Web-based approach.
*   More Security Concerns – You have to deploy, configure and maintain more security software, because there are extra components on your network (such as the file server and the backup hardware). Managing access rights and security defenses on a server is more intense than managing policies on Web browsers alone.

- Manage Your Backup Plan – You have to do your own server backups and have them secured on and off site (out of your office). Overlook this at your own risk; servers fail and hard drives crash occasionally, and when these problems occur, a system backup may be all that you have from which to retrieve your electronic records. Redundancy is your friend if your EMR system is going to be located in your office.
- Handle Maintenance Releases – You have to do periodic updates of all system components and you have to determine when it is safe to do them. Any operating system is constantly being patched (code used to repair problems with the original software), and new versions of browsers are released each year. Wireless infrastructure is also being patched. Usually after hours is a good time to do updates, which means someone will be putting in hours that they aren't now. Who will that person be?
- Create a Secure Server Location – You may have to do some office modification to make space for your EMR server. Since computers are smaller today, space isn't as much of a problem as it once was, but it still is a security problem. You will want your server(s) to be locked away from everyone but the system administrator(s).
- Find a System Administrator – Depending upon your own computer skill level, you may need someone you trust, who knows a lot more about hardware and software than you do, in order to manage an in-office deployment. The Stark Safe Harbor legislation now makes it possible for you to contract with your hospital I.T. personnel to perform this service for you, if you know that the personnel are trustworthy.
- Use Leasing to Avoid Capital Expenses – You may be forced to purchase the system and the maintenance agreement, rather than being able to pay a fixed fee per month (or per patient encounter) to deploy the system. Of course, you can use a third-party leasing organization and take the monthly payments as an expense, since you will not technically own the EMR until the last lease payment is made. This is also an advantage because you can bundle the hardware, the initial software and even the yearly maintenance agreement into the lease for a fixed period of time. This may be a good idea in today's economic climate.

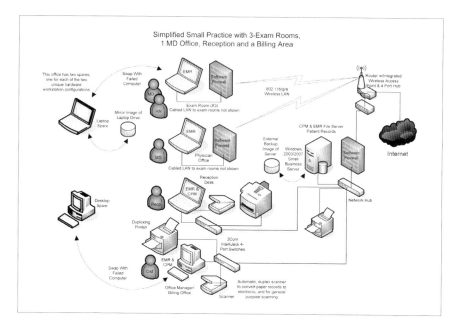

Figure 6.7 Simplified Diagram of 1-Office, 2-Physician Practice

Now let's consider advantages to in-office EMR, like the simplistic one depicted in Figure 6.7. This is not a workable design (see Chapter 14 – Configuration & Deployment). It is missing essential security components.

- Improved Response Time – The response time you experience when working with your EMR is likely to be faster, depending only on the EMR processing time. Some in-office EMRs seem substantially more responsive than their Web-based competition.

- You Control Your Patient Records – You store and manage your own electronic patient records, no second or third party has control of them or can limit your access to them. This means if the EMR developer is acquired or fails, your records are secure, and potentially (if you have chosen the right EMR), they can be written in some open standard format that will allow them to be read into whoever supplies your replacement EMR.

- No Forced Upgrades – When a new version of software comes out, you aren't automatically forced to upgrade to it. If you are comfortable with your current version, you can wait and let some other practice be the guinea-pig that tests the upgrade.

- No Duplicate Internet Costs – Continuous access to the Internet may not be required in a simple, in-office deployment, and having one connection to the Internet may be sufficient. This avoids the monthly cost of a second (backup) Internet connection – a saving of from $50 to $150 per month.

- Choice of Workflow-Enhanced EMR – You have more choices of EMRs that are built upon workflow engines with the in-office approach. This may be very important if you desire to optimize office workflow as part of the justification for adopting EMR.

- More Choices – Overall, there are more developers that offer in-office EMRs than offer Web-based ones, although that is changing. Many EMR developers that in the past only offered in-office solutions, are now also developing Web-based, SaaS EMR approaches.

Any in-office EMR server will take up some of your office space. You can probably place it where your CPM server is (if you have one). If not, you will have some new space freed up in your record room, which may be repurposed after deployment and initial paper chart scanning. You will not need a lot of space – as little as 100 sq. ft. or so (enough for two computers and their keyboards, mouses, and UPSs). The LCD monitor can be shared if need be, so in a pinch, these could all fit on one 48-60″ wide desktop (or in even less space if you are using a rack-mounted blade server approach – detailed in Chapter 14).

With an in-office EMR, your patient and other data is stored on the in-office server(s), which provides both control and risk compared to the ASP deployment approach. With this approach, you appoint yourself as the trustee for all your patient data, and therefore, it becomes solely your responsibility to insure its integrity, prevent its loss, encrypt it, keep copies off-site, create a secure environment for the data that is safe from hackers and viruses and other data predators. Someone must learn about and take responsibility for all these issues and it probably shouldn't be a clinician. These are tasks that you delegate to a skilled professional who performs them on a regular and scheduled basis, unless you are very accomplished with computers and are willing to devote the time it takes to manage these tasks.

This raises another point – discuss who will provide such services to your practice with your EMR developer before you commit to their system. What network of qualified service professionals is the developer aligned with in your area of the U.S.? Do they know of any organizations that might be able to take this on? If not, your hospital I.T. group may be willing to handle these services for you. Who is taking care of your practice management system now? Are they qualified? Contracting from outside your office is good because you don't incur full-time expense.

Understand, however, that whoever performs these tasks becomes a key part of your practice, even if you are just buying a slice of their time. Be certain that whoever you employ to maintain and update your in-office EMR is someone you can talk to and trust, as they will have access to all your patient data. In essence, you are putting your entire practice into their hands.

Two Alternatives (So Far)

Let's summarize. The in-office configuration has an (EMR) application server and a (patient data) file server (both may be running on one computer (referred to as "the server"). This approach also uses client workstations that access files from that server. This is called the client server model and it can have some variations. Each workstation is connected to the one in-office server over a Local Area Network (LAN), which is simply a computer network covering a small physical area, like your office, that can connect either wired or wirelessly.

The alternative, Web-based, remote ASP (SaaS) server uses individual Web browsers on computers in the physician office that are connected to the Internet through an office "gateway" (computer or router). The EMR application runs on the remote ASP server somewhere on the Internet (out there in the "clouds," so to speak). It communicates with the Web browsers on each of the caregiver workstations in your office. The patient files created are not kept and maintained in your office, but in the storage of the Internet ASP server. The remote Internet ASP server talks to Web browsers in your office. Apart from your browsers, no local EMR applications are running on any of the caregiver computers in this model; although there may be CPM or other applications running on these computers.

So far, we have discussed two configurations, but there is a third that blends them both together. This EMR application can run on the client workstations, but the patient data files can be kept on the server.

The ASP Blended Model

The third alternative is the in-office, Web server based blended with a remote Web server. Let's call this the ASP "blended" model. Think of it as a combination of the two previous models, with the difference being that the in-office server is a Web server, not a file server. Indeed, in this model, you are running your own, internal Web server, just for your office personnel.

The in-office Web browser connects over your Local Area Network (LAN) to your in-office Web server. The in-office Web server then connects over the Internet to the remote, ASP Web server (somewhere out there in the clouds). This model therefore has two distinct Web servers – one running in your office, connected to a second over the Internet.

This approach takes the most hardware, costs the most, requires local maintenance, just like the client/server model – so why would you want to do this? One reason is that it offers a fail-safe (crippled) operation mode and is tolerant of Internet outages, which can take down your whole office in the pure, ASP Web server model previously discussed. Another good reason is that with the blended model, your office is more independent because you are really running off of equipment in your own office 99% of the time. If your ASP is disconnected you just keep running off the Web server in your office!

In fact, the remote site is a support site for your local Web server. It can take backups of each record as it is closed and stored back on the in-office Web server, so that you always, automatically, have off-premises backup copies of all patient records. If there is ever a fire, flood, or other on-site disaster, that off-site backup is worth its weight in gold. In essence, your patient records are maintained on both Web servers, locally in your office and across the Internet on the remote Web server.

About the only other difference you will notice from inside your office is that your staff uses their computer's Web browser to work with the EMR, and not a standard computer application.

The blended Web server in-your-office approach is a great alternative to either of the two previously described models. After Internet outages, the two servers simply resync their files, so that patient records updated in your office during the outage, are sent over the Internet to the remote server to get it "back in sync."

The down side is cost and complexity. The cost for the in-office server could add $3,000-$4,000 in hardware cost, and it doesn't eliminate the monthly operating Internet charges, although it does reduce them because you no longer need a second (redundant) Internet connection like you would in the pure remote ASP Web server model. That can save $100/month alone.

If this approach appeals to you, check with EMR developers that offer this model, they may be able to do some of the administration and maintenance on the in-office server for you, from their side over the Internet. That may make the maintenance of the in-office Web server less complicated or painful.

Just remember to close the remote administration ports when you don't need to have them open. These are an invitation to hackers. If you are lax, or a hacker is clever, all your patient records are at risk. If there is a breach, the question will arise as to where the breach occurred. If it is on your in-office Web server, your EMR company is off the hook for any damages involved. This suggests you will need a skilled I.T. person to manage your in-office Web server components.

Assuming the proper I.T. support, this is our configuration of choice. If an in-office client/server approach appeals to you (e.g. the server keeps the files and the client computers run the EMR application) or a thin client/server approach is appealing (e.g. the server hosts the EMR application for every thin client, and also hosts the patient files), then why not go a step further and choose an EMR that uses a Web server and run it in your office? If you decide on this approach, be sure to read Chapter 16 – Protecting Your Patient Data – carefully. (Thin client refers to computers limited to only essential applications with the main function of processing keyboard input.)

One final thought. The majority of EMRs are client/server approaches, but that is changing. More are becoming remote, Web-based ASP (SaaS) applications. Of these, only a few offer the dual Web server (in your office and remote) blended configuration, so make sure the EMR meets all your medical and other needs first, and then look at how it is implemented – rather than doing it the other way around. No choice on configuration outweighs the basic functionality of the EMR application. If that isn't right, don't implement the EMR.

Wrap Up

No matter which deployment approach you take, you will have to interact with a computer, so the questions are what type and where to put them. No matter which approach you choose, you will also need some computers in your office. Be sure to refer to (reread if necessary) Chapter 5 – Interacting With Your EMR, as it contains a discussion on structured data that is important to your EMR decision and should be addressed with any EMR developer you are considering.

Also refer to Chapter 15 (Crisis Planning and Mitigation) that covers options for power loss, Internet loss and hardware failures – the three most common problems that will shut down any EMR.

If you find computer maintenance issues intimidating and you can find Web server ASP EMR solutions that meet ALL of your medical application needs, then lean toward one of the ASP approaches. If you have a trusted I.T. person, even a part-time one, the in-office solution offers you more EMR options and control. And, as we stated above, the blended model is a great choice and takes some elements from both the other two models.

Crucial Decision

Do you want an in-office (client-server) or a Web-based (Software-as-a-Service) EMR deployment? If the latter, do you prefer an in-office Web server plus a remote Web server ASP blended approach? Photocopy as needed or download Scorecard from www.ehrselector.com

Our Decision:	
Our Rationale:	
	In-office C/S or Thin C/S (Capital Asset that is depreciated)
	Remote, ASP Web server (license fee is operating expense, limited up-front investment for computers with browsers only)
	Blended, in-office LAN Web server + remote Web server (more up-front invest for in-office hardware, plus ongoing operating expense for ASP fees)

Type of Deployment: Turnkey from one vendor, or separately from multiple component vendors?

	Turnkey with hardware (one package includes everything supported by the EMR developer directly or through business partners)
	Purchase components and Integrate

What special issues does above choice impose on our practice staffing?

	Add I.T. person to staff
	Contract I.T. with hospital

Remember that choices to other Crucial Decisions may force you to return and reconsider these decisions. Future chapters that cover other topics may impact this initial decision.

Crucial Decision

Do you want an in-office (client-server) or a Web-based (Software-as-a-Service) EMR deployment? If the latter, do you prefer an in-office Web server plus a remote Web server ASP blended approach? Photocopy as needed or download Scorecard from www.ehrselector.com

	Contract I.T. w/outside company
	Service contract with EMR developer

Other I.T. Strategy, Describe:

Our Rationale:

Action Item(s):

Remember that choices to other Crucial Decisions may force you to return and reconsider these decisions. Future chapters that cover other topics may impact this initial decision.

CHAPTER 7

Vocabularies, Standards & Interoperability

Crucial Decision

What level of data structuring will meet your needs today, as well as 5 years from now?

This chapter also addresses the following questions:

- If you choose to structure information capture to the clinical level, how will you decide among SNOMED CT, MEDCIN and proprietary EMRs?
- If you choose an EMR that is structured to the billing level, especially ICD-9-CM now, how can you assure it will work with ICD-10-CM by Oct 1, 2013?
- What are CCR, CDA and CCD summary document standards, and how do they help you achieve interoperability?
- Do you want to populate your new EMR with paper chart summaries from active patients, and if so, how?

EMR Adventures

Dr. Alex Glass, an ophthalmologist, along with the physician assistant, Scott, and the office manager, Lynn, are discussing the need to replace their current EMR-Lite with an EMR that offers in-depth decision support. Dr. Glass and Scott want to add some structure to their patient data so that they can search the information, as both are writing articles for scientific journals. Unfortunately, the EMR developer that supports their current EMR-Lite, does not offer this level of data structuring.

Dr. Glass starts the conversation by saying, "I am concerned about how we will move all of our patient information from our current EMR-Lite into any full EMR that we choose."

Scott replies, "I understand the problem. I spoke with one EMR vendor the other day who said that the two EMR products cannot 'talk' to one another, as he described it. This could be a real pain."

Lynn adds, "I think there are some standards being developed for this very reason, but I don't believe that they will help us in our current situation. I know you two are looking at clinical data structuring for writing up your research, but on the billing side, there will shortly be a change from ICD-9 to ICD-10. When that happens, how will we move billing data to the new standard?"

Successfully Choosing Your EMR: 15 Crucial Decisions. By © Arthur Gasch and Betty Gasch. Published 2010 by Blackwell Publishing

"That's right," adds Scott. "Data capture is important but we also need to think about having an EMR that would be ICD-10 ready. Do you know much about this Lynn – you seem to have done the most research on the topic."

"I know it is important to be ICD-10 ready by 2013, but whether an EMR that has structured data incorporated in it, or is CCHIT certified, also means that they are ICD-10 ready is beyond me. I really am not sure," offers Lynn.

"We better check all of this out carefully," cautions Scott. "We don't want to end up with an EMR that falls short of our expectations."

"Oh, I am already doing research," says Dr. Glass. "I am talking to our service technician who takes care of the CPM system and who also services an internal medicine practice and a pediatric practice. He gave me the name of an EMR that both those practices like, and the EMR supports structured data."

"Yeah, but do they support ophthalmology as a specialty, do they support ICD-10 or exchange of information structures like the Continuity of Care Document and other basic important features?" inquires Lynn.

"You sound like my mother," interjects Dr. Glass. "This is a well-known EMR vendor, the product is expensive, it is CCHIT certified, I'm sure we'll be fine."

Clinical Information Capture vs. Charting Speed... and the Winner is?

There is a trade-off between capturing data with fine detail and the time it takes to chart information that has highly-structured data that uses standard vocabularies, empowers interoperability between systems; as emphasized by the NCVHS committee clarifying Meaningful Use criteria. Conversely, the finer the granularity of the information you chart, the more data you will have to input, and depending on the user interface, the longer it may take you to enter it. The challenge is where to draw the line between data granularity and increased charting time to capture it.

EMR Direction is Towards More Granular Data

The government, quality organizations and others are clearly charting a course towards collecting data with finer granularity (more detail). These groups are not mandating it directly, but the quality and outcome reports that are increasingly being required, emphasize the use of an EMR to generate the reports needed.

Some federal, state and local government agencies interested in receiving EMR data for benchmarking and other reasons include the Centers for Disease Control (CDC), CMS (Medicare/Medicaid), the American Health Quality Association (AHQA), public health agencies and others. Rather than build a separate infrastructure to gather the information they want, they are trying to leverage the data structure of EMRs by standardizing the way that EMRs code and store patient exam data. The problem is that EMRs have been developed independently, don't all share a common vocabulary and are stored in different ways by different EMRs. Many pre-date the development of EMR standards.

When longitudinal searches across the entire practice and all patients are necessary, more structure is better than less structure (or no structure at all). If capturing structured data is your choice, the next issue for you to consider is whether or not to collect data based on standardized vocabularies (like MEDCIN or SNOMED CT), or to use a proprietary vocabulary list embedded (and maintained) by your specific EMR developer.

Whenever data needs to pass to and be acted on by another EMR or caregiver, the adoption of a more structured approach using a standard vocabulary is helpful because it better supports semantic interoperability (explained shortly). This is why the approach is being encouraged. As a provider, you are free to choose whatever methodology you want, but the reimbursement of deployment costs is likely to be tied to the more structured approaches.

Standardized Medical Terminology (Vocabularies)

In order to enter assertions about your patient into the EMR database in a structured way, you have to have a vocabulary that the EMR can use. This is called a front-end vocabulary. Not all front-end vocabularies are standardized, some EMRs use proprietary (vendor home-grown) vocabularies and lists, because it's less expensive to used them than it is to license MEDCIN.

Standardized front-end vocabularies and structured data support a variety of reporting for PQRI and HEDIS quality and outcome measures that CMS (Medicare/Medicaid) is currently adding 2 percent incremental reimbursement when quality measures are performed and billing codes are properly modified. If you are going to do PQRI or HEDIS reporting, select EMRs that can report quality measure billing code modifiers to your CPM so that incremental billing for complying with quality standards measurements is both captured and billed to CMS. This avoids the need to manually bill them.

To achieve automatic billing for quality measures performed, you will need an interface from your EMR to your CPM. Put this on your EMR requirements list and research your CPM vendor to see if such functionality is supported. If an interface is not available, a manual process will be necessary before the bonus payment can be collected. Whom will that impact in your office?

The DBMSs Underlying EMRs

A Database Management System (DBMS) is a set of software programs that control the organization, storage, management and retrieval of data in a database. Of the 220+ EMR developers we track, there are almost as many different internal data structures as there are EMR developers. Most EMRs use traditional relational or newer, object-oriented Database Management Systems (DBMS), as shown in Figure 7.1. However, even if two EMR developers use the same DBMS, they may structure the front-end vocabulary schema (field definitions) somewhat differently.

SNOMED CT and MEDCIN (detailed shortly) bring some semblance of consistency to the organization of terminology (for those EMRs based upon them), however there are many EMR developers that don't use either SNOMED CT or MEDCIN, and have chosen instead to build their own, proprietary EMR vocabularies/data structures. This is why exchanging clinical data among different EMRs with different data structures, can be such a challenge.

Figure 7.1 Databases Used by EMR Developers for Their EMRs

Name of Database System	% of EMR Developers Using
SQL Server (Microsoft)	54%
Oracle	10%
MySQL	8%
Sybase Adaptive Server Anywhere	6%
Access (Microsoft)	3%
DB2	3%
Sybase Adaptive Server Enterprise	2%
M/Mumps/Cache	2%
4th Dimension	1%
FoxPro/Visual FoxPro (Microsoft)	1%
Domino (IBM/Lotus)	1%
Other	9%

Standard Nomenclatures

There are two internationally-recognized health terminologies (also called nomenclatures or front-end vocabularies) at the present time – SNOMED CT and MEDCIN.

SNOMED CT (Systematized Nomenclature of Medicine – Clinical Terms) is a comprehensive clinical terminology, originally created by the College of American Pathologists (CAP) and, as of April 2007, owned, maintained, and distributed by the International Health Terminology Standards Development Organization (IHTSDO), a non-profit association in Denmark. The CAP continues to support SNOMED CT operations under contract to the IHTSDO and provides SNOMED-related products and services as a licensee of the terminology.

The government doesn't give MEDCIN much press because Medicomp (its parent company) continued to develop its product after the government bought the rights to SNOMED CT and put it into the public domain. MEDCIN, not blessed with taxpayer money, has to continue charging for enhancing its nomenclature. Both of these products are well-structured and publicly described, and thus can represent patient encounters at clinical (rather than billing) data levels inside EMRs. Both enhance granularity and support semantic interoperability efforts, as mentioned previously, but one is somewhat easier to use than the other.

SNOMED, MEDCIN and CCHIT

MEDCIN (Medicomp Systems) and SNOMED CT (College of Pathologists/public domain) are often talked about in the same context, but they are really two different, but related, products – rather like tigers and panthers – both members of the cat family but different beasts. EMR developers can embed SNOMED CT for free. MEDCIN charges a significant licensing fee to EMR developers, which ultimately is amortized over all of the EMR developer's clients. Beyond the public/private differences, the two approaches are also very diverse.

Interface Terminologies & Clinical Reference Classification Systems

MEDCIN was designed to work as an "interface terminology," sometimes referred to as a front-end vocabulary. "Interface" means it is designed for you to interact with it as part of the graphical user interface of the EMR products that embed it. "Terminology" means that it accepts physician-observations about the patient and uses the terms defined to store them in the EMR database.

In contrast, SNOMED CT is a clinical reference classification system. It can also be part of the user interface, but more commonly it is on the back-end of the EMR, and provides a clinical classification descriptive system for patient conditions, drugs received, and so on. SNOMED CT strives to use the language the physician speaks (or captures) at the point of care; rather, as a clinical "classification system," it uses modifiers to build concepts about the patient and their medical conditions. Difficulty can arise if EMR developers attempt to use SNOMED CT as an "interface terminology" in real-time as it is simply too large and complex to easily accomplish that.

Charting the Asthmatic Patient

An example will illustrate the differences. Consider the disease asthma. Figure 7.2 shows the SNOMED CT links for this concept. Note the SNOMED CT approach is more deeply organized around data structuring first, and not optimized for capturing or expediting patient care in an office exam room or hospital clinical setting. Perhaps this is a result of the origins of SNOMED being rooted in pathology, a discipline that does not often interact face-to-face with patients. For clinical researchers, radiologists, pathologists and other disciplines of medicine that do not deal with patients directly, SNOMED is a viable approach.

However, when SNOMED CT concepts are coded into an EMR, many descriptors have to be entered for the disease asthma in order to fill out all of the relationships in Figure 7.2. The more descriptors required, the more impact on physician productivity, which can lead to user dissatisfaction. Compare the SNOMED CT structure shown in Figure 7.2, to the MEDCIN structure returned for the asthma, shown in Figure 7.3.

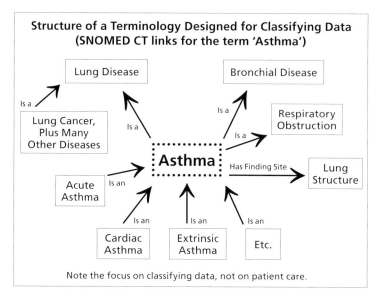

Figure 7.2 SNOMED CT Structure for Asthma

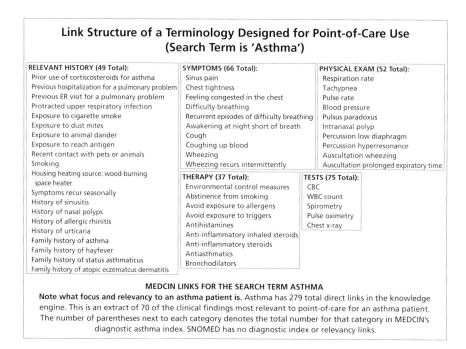

Figure 7.3 MEDCIN Conceptual Structure for Asthma

In the MEDCIN approach, the focus is clearly organized around patient care rather than raw information structuring. MEDCIN links show information that is clinically relevant to the patient encounter at the point and time of care, when the patient is in the exam room, in front of the physician. The MEDCIN approach is not so focused on creating clinical pathology descriptions or classifications. We believe this is a significant point of divergence between these two products that may play a more important role as the government moves towards prevention and management of chronic patient conditions.

From the over 260,000 clinical concepts with 68 million links focused on symptoms, history, physical examination, tests, diagnoses and therapy in MEDCIN, the MEDCIN knowledge engine selects those relevant to asthma, as shown. It also notes how frequently asthma occurs in patients, since many of these items can be found in other disease conditions as well. In this case there were 279 direct links for asthma in the MEDCIN knowledgebase.

How this information will be organized by any specific EMR depends on that EMR, but MEDCIN returns a set of selections for the EMR to work from. These basic selection boxes are shown in Figure 7.4 which shows six types of linkages that MEDCIN returns:

- Symptoms;
- Tests;
- History;
- Diagnosis;
- Physical; and
- Therapies.

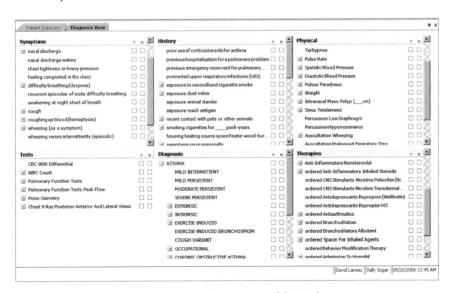

Figure 7.4 MEDCIN Decision Presentations Returned for Asthma

All of these are clinically oriented, not disease-classification oriented. Look at the length of each list and the items they contain. The list presented is a subset of the total list of symptoms, covering just those associated with asthma. Thus, MEDCIN prunes the number of choices available to you. If the patient has a co-morbidity of diabetes, items from that disease (concept) will be included also.

User-Interface vs. Information Reference Layers

Another way to differentiate SNOMED CT and MEDCIN is to conceive of them as two layers of data structuring; a top layer associated with the user interface technology and a bottom layer associated with clinical reference and classification information stored defined by a clinical standard. In this regard they are quite complementary. This is depicted in Figure 7.5.

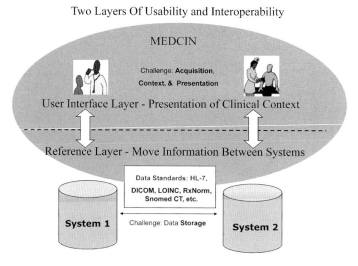

Figure 7.5 Front-End and Back-End Data Layers

You will want to consider which of these two approaches to clinical data structuring is the most user-friendly for your specialty and which requires the entry of fewer observations, or has observations most relevant to the data you need. The more data you are required to enter, the slower the capturing of the clinical observations will go and the longer the exam will take. You can evaluate this during a demonstration of an EMR that uses SNOMED CT and contrasting it with one that uses the MEDCIN front-end interface terminology. You can then determine the real impact of each approach for yourself. A list of EMR developers supporting both approaches is included in Figure 7.4 at the end of this chapter. Figure 7.6 is a select list of EMR vendors that embed MEDCIN in particular.

Figure 7.6 EMR Products with Embedded MEDCIN Knowledge Engines*

EMR Product	EMR Product	Implementation	MSP EHR Selector
Allscripts	Enterprise EHR	Blended Web/In-Office	Yes
AthenaHealth	AthenaClinicals	Web-based, SaaS Model	No
Eclipsys	Peak Practice EMR	In-Office/Hospital	Yes
EHS	Care Revolution	In-Office	Yes
Epic Systems	EpicCare	In-Office/Hospital	No
Impaq Medical	PhastNote	In-Office/Hospital	No
Med3000	InteGreat IC-Encounters	Web-based	Yes
Microsoft	Amalga HIS	Web-based	No
Northrup/DOD	AHLTA Global EMR	Enterprise	No
Pulse Systems	Patient Relationship	In-Office	Yes
Sage Software	Intergy EMR	In-Office or Web-based	Yes
SSI Med. Corp.	SSIMed EMRge	Blended Web/In-Office	Previously

*Note: In Figure 7.6, Epic uses the MEDCIN terminology without the MEDCIN knowledge engine and has developed their own mechanism for terminology integration. MED3000 was previously InteGreat. Don't confuse Microsoft Amalga HIS (using MEDCIN) with the older Amalga UIS that used Microsoft's old Azzyxi product and not MEDCIN. For a more complete list of EMRs that use either MEDCIN, SNOMED CT or have adopted their own, proprietary front-end terminology, see Figure 7.14 at the end of this chapter.

NCVHS Standard Nomenclatures

MEDCIN has been recognized by NCVHS as a core Patient Medical Record Index (PMRI) terminology standard. SNOMED CT and MEDCIN are both accepted into the Unified Medical Language System (UMLS) Metathesaurus. Here is a description of the Metathesaurus, taken from the U.S. National Library of Congress, National Institutes of Health at http://www.nlm.nih.gov/pubs/factsheets/umlsmeta.html.

"The Metathesaurus reflects and preserves the meanings, concept names, and relationships from its source vocabularies. When two different source vocabularies use the same name for differing concepts, the Metathesaurus represents both of the meanings and indicates which meaning is present in which source vocabulary. When the same concept appears in different hierarchical contexts in different source vocabularies, the Metathesaurus includes all the hierarchies. When conflicting relationships between two concepts appear in different source vocabularies, both views are included in the Metathesaurus. Although specific concept names or relationships from some source vocabularies may be idiosyncratic and lack face validity, they are still included in the Metathesaurus."

Proprietary (EMR Developer) Interface Terminologies

Let's contrast SNOMED CT and MEDCIN with proprietary front-end vocabularies created by specific EMR developers. If you don't choose either MEDCIN and SNOMED CT, the remaining alternative to structured data is getting an EMR with a vendor-proprietary interface vocabulary designed by the EMR developer. Some EMR developers reject SNOMED CT and also don't want to burden their EMR with the incremental costs for MEDCIN licensing fees – so they invent their own front-end terminology. You must decide if this is a viable and safe approach to structuring patient data at the clinical level.

For MEDCIN to fail, its base of support would have to shrink dramatically, since currently 14 or more EMR developers are using it. The number of EMR developers using SNOMED CT is even larger, with at least 35 EMR developers using it (in 2008). What's the situation with an individual EMR developer that has their own interface vocabulary – if that EMR developer fails, does the interface vocabulary fail with it? Who would maintain it going forward?

Unless you require that all EMR application software source code, including the reference terminology, be placed in escrow and donated to users in the event of a vendor failure (bankruptcy, etc.), you will have no access to the data structure schemas should the vendor who developed it - fail. Even if you do, sorting through these clinical structures and maintaining them is impractical for any small to medium-sized practices. Consider this when buying EMRs with vendor-developed, proprietary reference terminologies.

Structured Speech Recognition Solutions

Lest you think that all structured-data approaches are associated with Pick List/ Template-based EMRs, consider what Natural Language Processing (NLP) can do for dictated text and speech-recognized words, by organizing these words into proper clinical concepts. So far, the ultimate goal of speech recognition – organizing dictated information into clinically-structured text – does not appear to have been achieved by Nuance (or Dictaphone before it). Nuance is seriously pursuing this goal by acquiring Dictaphone and Dragon, and ultimately Philips' Speech Recognition group. To our knowledge practical NLP still eludes Nuance. However, it now appears to have been achieved by Medicomp, the same company that developed the MEDCIN interface terminology.

CliniTalk™

Medicomp demonstrated a new product called CliniTalk at TEPR and the 2009 HIMSS conferences. Dr. Caroline Samuels, a practicing physician and EMR consultant, saw CliniTalk at TEPR and was highly impressed by it. We saw it at HIMSS 2009 and were equally impressed. We believe that it will become commercially available by 2010, but how widely available it becomes will depend on how many speech recognition-based EMRs are willing to add the substantial licensing fees Medicomp will charge, to their EMR cost basis.

When CliniTalk does become available, it will empower physicians looking for a speech recognition approach to EMR, to be able to simply dictate a history of present illness, and end up with both the character-recognized and neatly-typed narrative, and with the structure data and concepts needed for quality reporting and Continuity of Care (CCD) Document interoperability (described shortly) – both automatically created by the EMR software that embeds CliniTalk. That is a major breakthrough because it provides structured data from freeform clinical dictation, something many physicians have been seeking. Physicians who prefer to dictate their information should watch CliniTalk development closely to determine which EMR developers pick up licenses from MEDCIN.

Audio File Formats

There are no standards for audio files use in speech recognition or embedded in EMRs, but there are many different audio file formats. These are important if you have selected dictation with speech recognition approaches for your input method, as they determine the flexibility of the EMR in handling dictation from various audio sources. They can also be important if medical tests include audio components, such as heart sound tests, and can be essential for capturing statements from patients or others in certain types of injuries, where litigation can be expected.

Audio formats supported by EMRs (from the most to least common) include: .WAV, .MP3, .WMA, .WFM, .DOX, .AIF, .DCT, and .QSM. If your patient documentation requires audio capture, try to choose one of the first three or four listed above. If the audio is only for documentation, but not speech recognition, using Adobe (PDF) document with a sound track is simple and effective, as you can dictate directly using the PC sound recorder. This may be useful if you are a pathologist, radiologist or cardiologist and want to dictate an interpretation of patient tests in legible, but non-structured, format for the referring physician.

While dictation and speech recognition may not be your preferred user interface, they may serve you well for obtaining a fast summary of each patient's paper records (albeit one that is unstructured), before moving their paper chart from your office to whatever offsite storage you use for archival purposes. While this works, using scanning or some means of generating a more structured record is recommended.

Terminologies vs. Billing Classification Codes

Billing classifications and clinical terminologies serve different purposes, but are complementary. Billing classification systems include: ICD-9-CM, ICD-10-CM, HCPCS and ICD-10-PCS. Some EMRs don't structure data at the clinical level, but rather stop at cross referencing it to ICD-9-CM and CPT codes (billing levels). These systems are for billing output and are not suitable

for primary documentation in an EMR, except to group data for some low granularity reports. Some EMRs try to use billing classifications for one or more of the following purposes:
- To determine quality or safety levels;
- To provide consumer outcome and cost data;
- To enhance clinical decision making;
- To pass information for continuity of care reporting;
- To support clinical research and epidemiological studies;
- To track public health risks;
- To track abuse in billing for unneeded services;
- To benchmark clinical or financial performance.

These are tasks that billing classification systems were never really designed to do. Moreover, ICD-9-CM is essentially a dead code, due to be retired on Oct. 1, 2013, when it will be replaced by ICD-10-CM coding. The rest of the world has already adopted their version of ICD-10 coding. This means that EMRs and CPMs will need to be able to support these newer codes, and track/document the clinical work required to bill against them; a capability that should be specified in your purchasing or licensing agreement. Learn more about ICD-10-CM at the AHIMA Web site – http://www.ahima.org/icd10/.

Mapping Between Terminologies and Classifications Needed

When billing codes are combined with front-end vocabularies or terminologies (like SNOMED-CT or MEDCIN) in an EMR system, an enhanced level of structure for data exchange is created. Work is needed to map SNOMED-CT and MEDCIN to ICD-10-CM/PCS and ICD-10-CM. This will have several business advantages and also make data somewhat more comparable.

Which EMRs are ICD-10-CM Ready?

The pending migration to ICD-10-CM coding raises an important issue beyond structuring clinical data. For example, which of today's EMRs are ICD-10-CM ready? How will records saved in ICD-9-CM structures be used once ICD-10-CM structures are implemented? This mapping needs to be bidirectional (one map from ICD-9-CM to ICD-10-CM, and a second from ICD-10-CM to ICD-9-CM). The ICD-10-CM codes also need to be mapped to SNOMED CT and MEDCIN, where possible.

   In talking with EMR developers, we find they vary in their readiness to integrate ICD-10-CM codes. One way of evaluating this readiness is to allow any EMR developer you are considering to take you through an ICD-10-CM demonstration. If they haven't progressed to the point of being able to show ICD-10-CM, then get a firm delivery commitment (and an exit clause to your EMR sales contract or licensing agreement if it isn't met). While actual billing is a CPM function, the best EMRs offer an E&M and coding module that is driven by the procedures performed. Tight communication between your EMR and your CPM is an important objective if your EMR is to deploy smoothly and enhance practice workflow.

We suggest therefore that you include administrative/billing staff on EMR selection teams making any site visits. Find out what ICD-10-CM issues or insights practices that have already installed an EMR have. See what is being promised by vendors about the adoption date for ICD-10-CM.

ViPS, a General Dynamics Information Technology company, demonstrated its ICD-10-CM WorkBench at 2009 HIMSS. They are one of several companies that are already introducing tools to help group practice CPM systems make the transition to ICD-10-CM.

AHIMA is offering tools and courses to provide a smooth transition. Check with these companies and organizations to determine what transition tools will be available to your practice.

Use of Standards

Whenever possible, favor EMRs that support standards, as this ultimately facilitates the potential for data exchange. Standards exist for imaging, laboratory, drugs and document exchange, and information exchanged must support such standards to be in a format the receiving computer can understand and automatically process. The degree to which that has been accomplished for lab, pharmacy and radiology is shown in Figure 7.7.

Figure 7.7 Support for Accepting Data from Various Sources (Format Unspecified)

Data Import From	Supported in Current EMR	Planned Enhancement
Laboratory Systems	88%	11%
Pharmacy Systems	74%	19%
Radiology Systems	58%	33%

The support of standards by EMRs is rapidly increasing, so you may find more EMRs support LOINC, RxNorm and DICOM than shown in the table above, depending on when you read this book.

Drug Nomenclature Standardization

With Meaningful Use requiring some drug interaction tests and alerts, it's important that EMR solutions use standardized prescribing terminologies. RxNorm is one such nomenclature for drugs. One of the reasons RxNorm was created was to include drug information in CCDs that are highly-structured.

"RxNorm is a standardized nomenclature for clinical drugs, created by the National Library of Medicine. In RxNorm, the name of a clinical drug combines its ingredients, strengths, and form. The form is the physical form in the drug specified in a prescription or order. With few exceptions (for packs), the RxNorm clinical drug name does not indicate the size of a package of drug units. RxNorm's standard names for clinical drugs are connected to the varying names of drugs present in many different controlled vocabularies, including those of commercially available drug

information sources. These connections are intended to facilitate interoperability among the computerized systems that record or process data dealing with clinical drugs...

The RxNorm model of a prescribable drug specifies the ingredient, strength, and dose form, adequately represents most prescriptions for medicines. However, some important medicines are not sufficiently or appropriately characterized by those three components alone, such as medicines that are dispensed in "Packs," like – Z-Pak, Medrol Dose Pack, and various oral contraceptive packages.

RxNorm's standard names for clinical drugs and drug delivery devices are contained in the Unified Medical Language System (UMLS) Metathesaurus. Since the Drug Listing Act of 1972 drug products are identified and reported using a unique, three-segment number, called the National Drug Code (NDC), which is a universal product identifier for human drugs. The NDC Number is a unique 10-digit, 3-segment number that identifies the labeler's, product, and trade package size."[1]

RxNorm harmonizes the same therapy when expressed in different ways. RxNorm is a collection of drug concepts, which can have multiple names derived from multiple sources but share a single RxCUI (identifier). It helps answer questions like, "Are the following four therapies equivalent?"

Ciprofloxacin 100mg/50mL IV Infusion

Ciprofloxacin 400mg/200mL IV Infusion

Ciprofloxacin Lactate 0.2% in Saline

Ciprofloxacin IV solution 2 MG/ML

RxNorm provides one code for therapies that are equivalent. For example, all names in a single concept RxCUI = 392151 are equivalent and could mean any of the following:

AMOXICILLIN 200 Mg ORAL TABLET

Amoxicillin 200 Mg Oral Tablet

Amoxicillin trihydrate 200mg tablet

Amoxicillin trihydrate 200mg tablet (product)

Since these are the same drug and dosage, an EMR can have and fire rules based on RxNorm codes when it detects overdoses (or underdoses) of a drug, even if the drug is expressed in different ways in the chart, based on their shared RxNorm RxCUI code (in this case 392151).

Middleware vs. EMR-Proprietary Drug Databases

Once you have decided between standardized or proprietary medical terminology systems, you must then decide between third-party middleware or proprietary drug formularies. There are a number of third-party middleware drug knowledge formularies available, including:

• Gold;

• Multum & First Databank (Cerner);

• Express Scripts Drug Digest Check Interactions;

• Micromedex Healthcare Series;

[1] *RxNorm Overview.* PowerPoint presentation by John Kilbourne MD (e-mail: kilbourj@mail.nih.nlm.gov). Presented October 2005, associated with the National Library of Medicine

- Drug-Reax Interactive Drug Interactions;
- Lexi-Comp;
- MedScape for WebMD Multi-Drug Interaction Checker; and
- Medi-Span (Wolters-Kluwer Health).

In fact, one drug knowledgebase can contain several individual databases. The Medi-Span Knowledgebase includes these separate drug databases:

- Adverse Drug Effects Database™
- AHFS Supplemental File
- Allergen Picklist File™
- Drug Dosing & Administration Database™
- Drug Image Database™ v2.0/Drug Imprint Database™ v2.0
- Drug Indications Database™
- Drug Lab Conflict Database™
- Drug Therapy Monitoring System™ (DTMS) v2.1
- DTMS Consumer Monographs
- Duplicate Therapy Database™
- Healthcare Common Procedure Coding System Codes (HCPCS) Database
- Integrated A to Z Drug Facts™ Module
- Integrated MedFacts Module™ (IMM)
- Master Parameters Database™
- Medi-Span Electronic Drug File™ (MED-File)
- Medical Conditions Master Database™
- Medication Order Management Database™ (MOMD)
- Parameters to Monitor Database™
- Payment Allowance Limit-Part B (PAL-B) v2.0
- Precautions Database™
- Rx Norm Cross-Reference File
- Standard Drug Identifiers Database

Medi-Span also offers the following toolsets.

- Drug Image and Imprint™ API
- Drug Information Bridge™
- Integrated Drug Facts and Comparisons™ API
- Integrated MedFacts Module™ API
- Trissel's IV-Chek™ API

If you choose an EMR that uses Medi-Span, in order to understand its full functionality, be sure to check which of these databases is included by your EMR developer. Unless you are practicing in a specialty with a very limited set of medications (used repeatedly), it's wise to favor an EMR that has embedded a drug database from one of the sources listed above, rather than an EMR developer that has engineered their own, proprietary drug database.

Even if your specialty doesn't use many drugs, your patients may be taking a wide variety of drugs for other conditions they have, or may be taking a wide range of over-the-counter health supplements that are potentially interactive with the medications you are familiar with and routinely prescribe.

No matter which approach you adopt, the "currency" of prescription information is important. This leads to the question, how often is the drug database updated? Figure 7.8 shows our research results.

Figure 7.8 Frequency of Drug Updates by EMR Developers

Time of Update	% EMR Vendors
Provided with each new EMR version release	69%
Daily to Weekly	3%
Monthly or Quarterly	10%
No Update Info Supplied	18%

No one likes to think the worst will happen, but there is going to be consolidation in the EMR market, there is not room for 220+ different EMR developers. Perhaps 150 or more of these EMR developers will fail in the next 5 years, as the government raises the entry bar with CCHIT-certification and now achieving Meaningful Use certification.

If your EMR vendor is acquired by another EMR developer, what support will there be for any EMR-proprietary drug database in the future? The acquiring company may want to switch you to their own, go-ahead EMR product that may utilize a third-party, middleware prescription database. Where would that leave you?

EMR systems that are large enough to cost-effectively imbed standardized vocabularies, patient history interviews, and drug interaction databases, are more expensive than those that don't. Even EMR developers with a small installed base, which use middleware drug databases, will have more expensive products than those that use proprietary drug databases, so don't always go for the least expensive product that meets your other needs. Look for EMRs that incorporate drug databases and support RxNorm (for formulary) nomenclatures and National Council for Prescription Drug Programs (NCPDP) for pharmacy.

Lab Data Interoperability Standards – ELINCS 2 & LOINC

Next, consider standardizing lab ordering and results reporting. There are simply a lot of labs in the United States. The nation's ~5,000 hospitals have almost 8,700 labs, and there are almost 12,000 other clinical and commercial labs, plus the labs in 108,734 physician offices (see http://www.cms.hhs.gov/CLIA/downloads/factype.pdf). These labs each use individual lab instruments or any of the 30+ different lab information systems, none of which employs the same data structures. To address this issue, the EHR Lab Interoperability and Connectivity Specification (ELINCS) was developed in California. It has subsequently been embraced by HL7, as a way of exchanging lab data.

ELINCS uses Logical Observation Identifiers Names and Codes (LOINC) as the identifiers for 95% of the most frequently performed tests[2].

The standard was developed with input from the Certification Commission for Health Information Technology (CCHIT); Connecting for Health (Markle Foundation); eHealth Initiative (eHI); Centers for Medicare and Medicaid Services (CMS); Integrating the Healthcare Enterprise (IHE); Public Health Information Network (CDC/PHIN); and Health Level Seven (HL7) groups, which explains its wide support. Many hospitals in California as well as national labs (Quest (12/09), LabCorp and Ameripath) use this standard, which was adopted by HL7 in 2008 and is part of the 2008 CCHIT certification. Some vendors whose EMRs support the standard include: Allscripts, e-MDs, GE Medical Systems, Misys, and NextGen.

Suppose you want your medication CPOE prescription system to check lab values for renal and hepatic functions to determine if the dose being prescribed (which is within normal range for a healthy patient) would constitute an overdose for a particular patient because of their depressed renal function. You could look this up manually (if you remember to do so for every patient), or you could expect your EMR to do it – if you choose the right EMR.

In order for the EMR to meet your expectations, it would need to accomplish that task automatically (without your intervention). For that to happen the computer needs to understand what lab values (XML tags) to read and what values for those tags would indicate a problem. If the data from the lab is reported as LOINC data, the value checking, flagging (or alert) functions could be written in a universal way, and would work for any lab that reports its data in LOINC format. That is the goal – to have data in a standardized format and write routines that access that format to process its data. EMR developers do not have the time or budget to write interfaces for each lab system and whatever report format it generates, so they support standards like LOINC.

However, just because lab values are reported using LOINC, doesn't mean your EMR can process them. But if lab values aren't reported in LOINC, if the lab data is just typed/printed as ASCII characters (untagged) text, the EMR by itself, has no way of identifying what values go with what tests. Figure 7.9 shows some of the data formats and the degree to which they are supported by EMR vendors collectively.

There is growing support for data standards.[3] LOINC provides human-readable data and computer-actionable data, as do certain types of XML-tagged data. In some cases, with national labs, you must request reports using LOINC

[2] *The Development of a Highly Constrained Health Level 7 Implementation Guide to Facilitate Electronic Laboratory Reporting to Ambulatory Electronic Health Record Systems.* By Walter V. Sujansky. Published May/June 2009 issue of the Journal of the American Medical Informatics Association, Vol. 16, No. 3, p. 287

[3] Health Information Technology Standards Panel (HITSP) has revised its standard IS-06 as of June 30, 2009 to accommodate changes for Meaningful Use. A draft of that standard, version 1.1.1 is available at http://www.hitsp.org.

formatting, and there is an extra charge for this. Hopefully, that will cease in the future, and LOINC will be the standard format for reporting all lab data, from national labs, as well as from various hospital labs device vendors.

Figure 7.9 EMR Import Data Into Patient Record by Supported Format

Document Format	% Current Support	% Future Support
RS232/422 ASCI	66%	16%
IEEE-1073 (MIB)	65%	6%
HL7 – Ver 2 Messaging	62%	10%
Laboratory – LOINC reporting	59%	13%
NCPDP (Medications)	58%	14%
XML Tagged Data	39%	32%
HL7 – Ver 3 For Clinical Documents	38%	35%
Other (Not Specified)	65%	4%

Image Data Standards (DICOM)

The standard for electronic images is DICOM (Digital Imaging and Communications in Medicine). This is a NEMA (National Equipment Manufacturer's Association) standard supported by the American College of Radiology (ACR). It covers the distribution and viewing of medical CT scans, MRIs, and ultrasound images. It is one of the first and oldest standards, dating back to 1985. Over the years, compliance to the standard has improved, as illustrated by the semi-annual Integrating the Healthcare Enterprise (IHE) demonstrations at the Healthcare Information and Management Systems Society (HIMSS) and the Radiological Society of North America (RSNA) conferences. Initially intended for images in radiology and cardiology, the format has become more generalized and is now available for a wide variety of medical images. You definitely want an EMR that can send and receive images in DICOM format.

Image Formats Supported by Scanning

EMRs in emergency departments and immediate care centers and pathology don't always have pictures in DICOM format, so it's useful to know what other image formats your EMR can provide, in case you are trying to document domestic abuse, track wound care or for many other purposes.

In fact, most of the common image formats are supported. These include JPG, TIF, BMP, GIF, PDF and fax. If you often include images in your EMR charting, be sure to check with your vendor to confirm what formats are supported. Another alternative for handling images is to "print" any captured image to a PDF file using Adobe Acrobat or any of the other programs that create PDF files. Once embedded in the PDF file, the image becomes a .PDF format, which many EMRs can handle.

Adobe PDF Used as Medical Document Wrapper

Adobe Acrobat (currently in version 10) is in no sense a medical standard, but is increasingly being used to package and convey medical record content because it has desirable attributes:
- It is widely available from more than one company;
- It maintains the format of the source information it displays, including embedded graphics and audio files;
- It generally results in a file that is smaller in size than the sum of the sizes of the individual items it contains;
- It can be password-protected with strong encryption;
- Documents scanned-in can be automatically converted into PDF format (see Nuance's PDF Converter 6 Professional for example);
- It is as easy to generate as printing a document. The open office organization now supports creation of PDF as a standard feature, without the need for Acrobat as a separate package, as does Abbyy, in both its PDF Converter and Fine Reader products. Fine Reader is a combination of document scanning and PDF creation, so it includes an OCR component. Nuance also includes OCR and PDF creation in its Paperport products. PDF documents support authentication and signature by their creators;
- PDF can be indexed and cataloged by every word (at least by the professional versions of Acrobat) and that catalog may be searched for a match on any word, with the resulting documents retrieved and opened in context to the occurrence of the search term. These features, plus secure document delivery, allow you to bundle and send documents in something Adobe calls a "PDF package." These are both password-protected and encrypted with Acrobat's tools;
- PDF incorporates "forms," standard documents with variable fields that can include information like patient name, ID and signature fields. Once completed, the entire form or just the variable data can be encrypted and transmitted to a repository and archived, providing an excellent audit trail for patient execution of HIPAA, living wills and other declarations.

PDF: A Vehicle for Providing Patient Access to Their Charts
While PDF is not a medical standard, it is a very useful and versatile documentation format. In preparing for EMR adoption, remember that Meaningful Use requirements may necessitate you to provide patient encounter summaries for their PHR, which includes lab results, the problem list, medication lists and data on allergies. Printing chart pages to a PDF document may be just the vehicle to

accomplish this. Get the patient to sign a form indicating they have received the PDF, and archive a copy showing their signature.

PDF's multi-media capabilities of recording/containing voice, plus plug-ins for DICOM and other medical formats, make it extremely useful in your office and an excellent adjunct to what your EMR can do. Any document you can print or scan or listen to, can be made into a PDF document in short order. If all PDFs are indexed by word, and placed in a searchable, PDF repository (catalog), they can also be readily searched on a word-by-word basis for drug names, diagnosis, or other terms or phrases.

Medical Use of Adobe PDF Format – DICOM Plugins

PDF is a very flexible format for medical data for the following reasons:
- It maintains document formatting;
- It can be locked with a password to prevent editing;
- It can be encrypted so that content is not seen unless viewer has the password used to encrypt it;
- It can be searched and indexed into catalogs by Adobe Acrobat or third-party PDF processing engines;
- Many medical reference texts are stored in PDF format, and the reader for that format is available free from the Adobe Web site;
- Some government agencies, like the FDA and DOC, now accept required submissions in PDF format.

Adobe PDF is the worldwide standard for faithfully representing paper documents and is part of all the standards that underpin healthcare. The DICOM 3.0 standard makes full provisions for encapsulating Adobe PDF files within a DICOM wrapper, allowing them to be archived to PACS (Picture Archiving and Communication systems) and transmitted with the same network protocols used by MR, CT, ultrasound, and other medical imaging devices.

Standards for Messaging & Documenting Care

Given the availability of standardized sets for drugs, lab results and diagnostic imaging, and EMRs that capture structured data for individual patient encounters, there is a need to assemble these components into an overall standard document. The need is for the document (and the data it wrapped) to have the ability to be exchanged among various stakeholders such as the physician and patient, two physicians, the physician and a hospital, nursing home, immediate care center or emergency department, etc.

The standard for the way electronic medical records store information (not the information itself) has three objectives:
- First, EMRs should be able to read documents and information stored in other, pre-existing formats, allowing information capture at the human level. An example would be importing a document in Adobe Acrobat (.pdf). People are able to read Portable Document Format (PDF) documents, as well as HL7 Version 2 messages.

- Second, EMRs should be able to wrap and unwrap, (assemble and disassemble, process and store) data in documents using standardized "envelopes." For example, if an HL7 CDA document contained an embedded DICOM image file, that file could be extracted intact and acted upon by the EMR. It should be able to be stored, printed, and transmitted as a medical image. People can't read an image in DICOM format directly, but they can read a picture created from a DICOM data file (a DICOM image) and interpret that. Thus, some formats can be read by both humans and computers, others by a computer that processes the data to create a human-readable record (or image).
- Third, the envelope needs a file format definition and a network communications protocol.

How medical data can be read is fundamental to what decision support is available at the point of care. Since decision support depends on the computer being able to know what data it has, if standard formats are not used, no decision support will be available, the information can only be stored and retrieved as a blob.

Simplified, Conceptual Data Flow Sequence

For structured medical data to flow from one place to another in a way that can be acted on by a computer at the receiving end, there is a sequence of steps that must be followed. Here's a simplified version that ignores some of the steps, such as obtaining consent from the medical data owner for the medical information to be sent, authentication of the sender and receiver, creation of an audit trail, positive patient identification, encryption, actual data collection and transmission, that all are present in real HIPAA-compliant exchanges of electronic health information. Here are the simplified steps:

- The request for data is made (using a HIPAA or other standard transaction message request), and it is acknowledged by the sender;
- The sending system collects data (hopefully in standard formats, LOINC, RxNorm, DICOM and so on) for the patient indicated. This is roughly equivalent to a clerk searching files to find content about an individual patient from an office file or wherever else they might exist;
- The data found is put into a file folder, and the sequence written on the outside of the folder; which is in turn put into a standard envelope (CDA or CCD wrapper);
- The wrapper (electronic envelope) is securely sent to the requesting party. This is roughly equivalent to personally taking the envelope to the post office, registering it, and requesting a return receipt when it's delivered;
- The receiver then reads the contents, unpacks the sections and processes them as appropriate. This is roughly equivalent to opening the envelope and reading the list of items it contains, then opening the folder and retrieving the actual contents and acting on them.

Standard Documents and Semantic Interoperability

"(Semantic Interoperability is) the ability of communicating entities to share unambiguous meaning. In other words, the sender must be able to reliably transmit all sufficient and necessary information; the receiver must be able to correctly interpret its interlocutor; and both must be aware of, and agree upon, each other's behaviors for given interactions."[4]

We add, that this refers to the sender's computer and the recipient's computers, as well. EHRs that achieve this have been called "intelligent" EMRs, by Dr. Peter Elkin, Mt. Sinai Medical Center, and provide a platform for achieving automated, best-practices, rules-based quality monitoring.[5] The government has funded research through NIST, (the National Institute of Science and Technology) to help realize semantic interoperability in medical software record systems. In their report entitled *High Confidence Medical Devices, Software, and Systems and Medical Device Plug-and-Play Interoperability, 2007*, the HCMDSS-MDPnP Joint Workshop issued the following abstract of that work.

"NIST researchers are collaborating with medical device experts to facilitate the development and adoption of standards for medical device communications throughout the healthcare enterprise as well as integrating it into the electronic health record. NIST researchers have developed a tool and corresponding electronic representation of an international standard's information model that provides several important capabilities leading toward device semantic interoperability.

We describe our XML schema (structure of the datasets) and tool developed which is built upon the medical device communication standard ISO/IEEE 11073. Central to this approach is a capability of the tool to develop and produce implementation conformance statements (ICSs). Users execute the tool to produce statements disclosing details of a specific implementation and specifying features provided by a particular medical device. Device ICSs can subsequently be compared and utilized across device interfaces to help overcome the semantic interoperability problem that is so prevalent today and has prevented proliferation of plug-and-play interoperable (EMR) solutions."[6]

In a nutshell, this means making the exchange of medical data unambiguous and actionable by the receiving EMR's computer without human intervention. The idea is to transmit data in formats that allow the receiving EMR application to act independently on the data being exchanged. That action may be as simple as asserting the data values into the appropriate fields in the receiving computer's EMR database; or more complex, such as creating user alerts, building decision support information triggered by the context of the exchanged data, or whatever. In the latest CCHIT standards, there are requirements for EMRs to support the Continuity of Care Document (CCD)

---

[4] Wikipedia definition at http://en.wikipedia.org/wiki/Semantic_interoperability.

[5] *iEHRs await federal action.* By B. Robinson. Published Nov. 2008 by Government Health IT

[6] *High Confidence Medical Devices, Software, and Systems and Medical Device Plug-and-Play Interoperability.* NIST documented workshop held June 25-27 2007. ISBN: 978-0-7695-3081-8), http://rtg.cis.upenn.edu/hcmdss07/index.php3

structured standards. As CCHIT requirements expanded, some EMRs didn't comply with newer requirements and dropped off the certified systems list. For ARRA reimbursement, pick EMRs with current certification.

Standardizing Medical Documents

An important aspect of selecting any EMR is understanding which (if any) standards it supports, and whether the EMR has achieved EMR import, export, or both (import/export) functionality. Structuring EMR data into some sort of standardized format has been pursued by several different groups, each with their own vested interests and objectives. Two of the standards organizations that have written specifications are HL7 and ASTM.

These specifications, for the most part, don't specify the format of the contents, they are more about the format of the file folder and envelope that will be used to deliver the information. HIPAA has provided some standard requests to initiate various types of data exchanges. HL7 and ASTM (with their wrappers) provide the envelopes. The standardized nomenclatures and data formats previously discussed, provide the actual data inside the wrappers.

CCR Backgrounder

The Continuity of Care Record (CCR) was a standard specification developed jointly by ASTM International, the Massachusetts Medical Society (MMS), the Healthcare Information and Management Systems Society (HIMSS), the American Academy of Family Physicians (AAFP), and the American Academy of Pediatrics. It documents individual episode(s) of care, providing a picture of the patient's status at a point in time when each episode occurred.

The goal of CCR was the improvement of the continuity of patient care coupled with at least a minimal standard of information transportability among healthcare providers; there was also a goal of reducing medical errors and preventing duplication of tests ordered. The CCR included various sections for such items as: patient and provider information, insurance information, the reason for a referral, the patient's health status (allergies, medications, vital signs, diagnoses, etc.), recent procedures and care provided, and the patient care plan.

CDA Backgrounder

The first CDA approach grew out of the legacy healthcare Information Technology (I.T.) vendors of large hospital diagnostic, medical and billing systems, which supported the Health Level 7 (HL7) standards development efforts. This resulted in the CDA (Clinical Document Architecture) specification based upon HL7's Version 3 RIM (Reference Information Model) concepts.

The goal of CDA is storing or moving clinical documents (lab results, X-ray readings, patient history, physical report, etc.) between medical systems. To accomplish this, the CDA standard utilized XML documents, which consist of a schema that defines what data fields the document has. Then a data document is made up of a combination of XML "tags" for the data field, and the data for that field. This CDA initially contained information of a single patient encounter.

An EMR for a particular patient would have many CDA documents, each detailing various encounters of the patient with a particular provider written as standard HL7 metadata and XML-tagged content. Because the format was ASCII[7] (plain text) that was XML-structured, it was easy to read by the computer receiving the CDA (also readable by a caregiver, although in a format that would be tedious and inefficient).

Several major providers initially adopted the CDA standard, including Mayo Clinic, and other providers, as well as EMR developers such as Allscripts, Epic, Eclipsys, GE Healthcare, McKesson, MediNotes, NextGen, Nuance, Siemens and more.

Standards Harmonization

Until about 5 years ago, both HL7-CDA and ASTM CCR proceeded on parallel development tracks. In many ways, CCR and CDA covered the same provider groups and EMR developers were faced with the decision of which to support, or the problem of supporting both at the same time. Two standards, two different groups of EMR stakeholders, independent of each other – the epitome of the American way. Fortunately, the two groups began moving intentionally towards a point of intersection.

CCR+CDA=CCD

In the end, logic prevailed and the CCR and the CDA groups worked together to harmonize their standards. In 2007, the two standards organizations collaborated via a memorandum of understanding on one newer, standard format – the Continuity of Care Document (CCD).

This work is supported by many organizations that are stakeholders, including ASTM[8], HL7[9], ADA[10], IEEE[11], College of Pathologists (SNOMED CT), ASC[12], NCPDP[13], OMG[14] and others. The work thus has wide support.

CCD Moves Ahead

Currently, the CCD is being phased into EMR certification standards written by CCHIT. The CCD was partially adopted in the 2008 CCHIT standards and

---

[7] ASCII – American Standard Code for Information Interchange

[8] American Society for Testing Materials

[9] Health Level 7 Group

[10] American Dental Association

[11] Institute for Electrical and Electronic Engineers

[12] Accredited Standards Committee

[13] National Council for Prescription Drug Program

[14] Object Management Group

2009 certification began to require codification of CCD sections – problems, medications and allergies, discrete data (individual field) import and export, and standardized IHE transport methods (ITI-XDS). By the end of 2009, this will allow semantic interoperability of the most requested sections of clinical data for physicians purchasing 2009 CCHIT-certified EMRs.

The CCD defines the organization of a particular type (name) of document, such as History and Physical (H/P). It also has a list of the sections that exist in that document, such as social history, current medications, and so on; rather like a book having a list of the chapters that it contains. The content, however, can be provided by other standards. The lab content, for example, may be expressed as LOINC data.

One strength of a CCD document is that it can be read, "understood" and acted on by another EMR application. That EMR application can answer questions like, what type of document it is, how many sections it has, the names of the sections, and so on. No person has to read that standardized document to answer such questions, the computer (EMR) can figure it out directly because of its structured nature and the use of XML tagged data.

XML Tagged Data

The code expression of the standards documents is XML (eXtensible Markup Language). XML's purpose is to aid information systems in sharing structured data, especially via the Internet. XML uses visually familiar (ASCII) characters, making an XML document readable by humans and, because XML also has the notion of a structure to the information it contains (a schema), it uses "tags" to identify "content." The tag is associated with data – the value of a patient's body temperature, for example. Since this is all expressed in an understandable character set (like this book is), it is readable by people. But since it is highly-structured with individual vital signs having tags, and those tags having associated values, it is also intelligible to an EMR application or other program, which can then take various actions based upon its contents.

Making exchanged data understandable to the receiving EMR application and therefore actionable, is the heart of semantic interoperability. Received data can be appended to a Master Patient Index (MPI), so that its existence is noted. Or, it might be "reading" the document and locating any (e.g.) lab values it contains, and comparing those values for specific lab tests to normal ranges, then creating alerts for any values that fall outside of the normal range. Another action might be to check whether two drug names found in the document interact with each other, and if so, create a user alert. The better structured and more unambiguous the data, the more work that can be performed on it by the EMR application without human intervention.

Emerging Practical Applications

Suppose that one of your patients is being seen at an Emergency Department (ED) and your office is notified. Assuming the patient can identify you as one of his providers, when contacted your office will need to send information on this patient to the ED – stat! If you are using paper charts, and the patient is an active patient (so the chart isn't archived) and the inquiry comes during office hours, the best you may be able to do is send a lot of faxed information to the ED. But if you have an EMR with structured data, you can create and send a CCD containing your patient's data to that ED, if they have an EMR that can accept it. Two other physicians that your patient also sees, can send similar CCD summaries – giving the ED physicians some background information to go on, including prescription interactions, allergies, disease states, doses and treatment plans. This is particularly helpful if the patient is unconscious and unable to provide such information verbally.

CCD Supports HIE

The standardized CCD document is the Health Information Exchange (HIE) pipeline from your EMR to the rest of the world, and to your patients and ultimately their Personal Health Records, (PHRs). Hopefully, you can provide a summary of your patient's encounter to them at the end of their office visit, so that your patient can take the information with them to the next care provider, or assert it to their PHR. The CCD can also be the input to your EMR, when it's received from a referring physician, or if it comes from the patient's own PHR.

The CCD gives you, in theory, a data migration pathway to the future, as long as an EMR product can import a CCD (Continuity of Care Documents) into their EMR's internal data structure and then use the data to populate the clinical database.

Therefore, it is a crucial decision whether or not to select an EMR that has fully implemented the CCD, both its export and its import, at least to the extent that is specified by CCHIT 2009 requirements. Ask yourself, how is the data in your EMR going to include specific content if you don't capture it in the first place? Any EMR developer that cannot export an encounter summary today in CCD format, and has no plans to support CCD going forward, we believe is offering a dead-end approach to EMRs (you should avoid).

When you write your purchase specifications, address the issue of what extent your EMR can both write out and read in CCD-formatted information, and use it to populate whatever internal database structure your EMR supports. Depending on the ability of an EMR to handle incoming CCD wrapped data and support for the standards used in individual sections, you have the foundation of a pathway and bridge to data independence and migration.

HL-7 Data Messaging and Integration

The data flows described above come from a series of electronic exchanges, that support data requests, provider authentication, etc. Figure 7.10 shows the answers to how well EMR products support these clinical and administrative transactions. Before finalizing on an EMR, clarify what standard transactions are included in your basic EMR/CPM price or licensing fee and what extra costs may be involved to support these standards. EMR developers that have combined, integrated EMR/CPM products, need to support a wider range of standard transactions, including all the billing transactions, than do EMRs that do not have CPM components.

Figure 7.10 EMR Support for HL7/HIPAA Standard Clinical Transactions

Standard Transaction Type	% Current Support	% Future Support
Patient ID	93%	3%
Request for Lab Results	71%	7%
Order Lab Tests	70%	10%
Patient History	63%	9%
Verify Insurance Eligibility (X12 270 & 271)	59%	10%
Get DICOM Images	46%	8%
Get ECG Test Results	40%	14%

Note: Vendors reporting support for lab results above are describing faxed results and not necessarily support for ELINCS 2 reporting. Other HIPAA transactions, which we did not inquire about, include:
- Encounter (X12 837);
- Claim status inquiry and response (X12 276 and 277);
- Referrals and prior authorizations (X12 278);
- Healthcare payment and remittance advice (X12 835);
- Health claims attachments (proposed) (X12 275).

These will be of most interest if you plan to deploy a combined EMR/CPM solution that must support both the administrative and clinical transactions.

Getting Legacy Paper Record Summaries Into EMRs

Every practice deploying an EMR faces the issue of how to get an electronic summary of current paper charts into their new EMR. One obvious answer is document scanning. On the MSP ESP™ Web site (www.ehrselector.com) is a list of paper chart scanning services that can help you migrate a summary of your paper charts into your EMR. If you don't care about populating your new EMR with your old patient records, but just want chart copies that you can recall and read, use a product like PDF Converter 6 Pro and scan everything to PDF format documents. A scanning service will provide a more structured result (at extra cost). Figure $0.09 to $0.20 cents per page if done through a scanning service, plus extra for chart pickup at your door (not all scanning contractors offer this service).

Actually, a good time to start converting your documents is before you have selected an EMR because when the HITECH/ARRA MU requirements are finalized, the logjam will burst and many practices will choose an EMR and then want paper record conversion services. This will overwhelm contractors providing such services. If you choose a PDF (OCR) format (not just pictures), you can choose any EMR that supports that format (most do now) and you will be able to expedite your EMR deployment phase because your scanning will already be done. Also, you won't overlook the cost of this conversion in your budget, which can be sizeable. Depending on your practice setting, it is not unusual to have charts with 100 to 300 pages for each doctor. In established practices most doctors have from 300 to 700 patient charts to convert. Do the math, it's a considerable cost.

Because paper record conversion is a substantial cost, some practices scan information on a just-in-time, as-needed basis, once a patient is scheduled for an office visit. The problem with this approach is that unless you have the right equipment, it will cost you more than $0.10/page just in personnel time, and may add to your office workflow. Your office staff was probably not hired to do chart scanning and may not have the experience, temperament or equipment to do this highly repetitive task. Even if they do, you still have the issue of secure disposal of your paper charts, which means your staff will be doing shredding also, a relatively noisy task.

On the other hand, if you can convert all your paper charts before "go-live," the old chart room becomes available as a potential new EMR server area or exam room. That can't be done with the just-in-time approach. Better to borrow a little more money initially than to spend years doing just-in-time paper chart conversions. If you have chosen document scanning as the primary user interface for your EMR, then the EMR itself may offer more tools for efficiently doing your paper chart conversions on an as-needed basis.

Is Document Scanning Part of Your EMR?

Even if document scanning is not your primary user interface, it may be a method supported by your EMR to bring in unstructured patient data. If you plan to scan your paper charts, account for the cost and time required to scan in your budget and implementation plan. Figure 7.11 illustrates support by EMR developers for go-live handling of paper charts.

Figure 7.11 Paper Record Conversion Services from EMR Developers

Conversion Services Available	% of EMRs Offering It
Not Integrated, but Offers as Extra Charge Service	35%
EMR Offering Integrated Scanning Services	29%
No Plans to Offer, Physician Handles Separately	27%
Doesn't Offer but Uses Third-Party who Does	6%
No, but Plan to Offer in the Future	3%

As the importance of structured data and semantic interoperability is emerging, more EMR developers are looking for ways to structure both scanned and dictated medical records, either directly or via collaboration with third parties because Optical Character Recognition (OCR) by itself is insufficient to create a structured and easily indexed patient record. EMRs with more advanced scanning features integrated can expedite capture of initial summaries for your practice's active patients. Scanning equipment and processes must be simple and intuitive, and have a short learning curve. EMRs' scan functionality is shown in Figure 7.12.

Figure 7.12 EMR Integrates the Following Scanning Features

Feature	Yes	3rd Party	Not Yet	Future
Immediate View after Scan	96%			4%
Allows Documents to be Import/Index	90%		2%	7%
Creates Audit Trail	90%			10%
Manually Rotate to Orient Page	86%	2%	5%	7%
User Customizable	80%	3%	6%	9%
Tabular View	78%		5%	11%
Switch Thumb/Full/Rotate	66%	5%	5%	24%
Tags Charts that Meet Certain Criteria	61%	3%	19%	17%
Uses Web Browser to View	60%	1%	13%	25%
Images Auto Rotate to Proper Orientation	38%	11%	24%	24%
Reassigns Misfiled Pages	24%	3%	39%	33%

OCR Approaches to Capturing Data Summaries

While basic scanning is the most common means of converting paper charts to an electronic format as unstructured images, if paper charts are typed rather than handwritten (such as from dictation and transcription), scanning plus Optical Character Recognition (OCR) can be effective.

Products that offer scan to Portable Document Format (PDF) functionality can help, as the PDF documents can be easily indexed on nearly every word. The index is stored as a catalog. The problem is meeting HIPAA privacy requirements, as the index can open the source document in context, displaying the page on which the search term occurs. We are not aware of a way to create the privacy and audit trail to make this approach fully HIPAA compliant, but Adobe or one of its competitors could certainly add that.

Images from scanned paper charts won't typically populate EMR databases in the same way that new patient encounters do. Raw scanned documents have no "hooks" to allow the information being scanned into that database to be processed them against a structured, front-end vocabulary. If scanned records are images only, you will want to see what formats your EMR handles. If they can be converted by (OCR) into characters and text, you may have more success in structuring and indexing at least some of the data.

Figure 7.13 illustrates formats which EMR/scanning services generally support for document conversion and storage. About 20 percent of all EMRs support all these formats. Many others support more than one format. Most of the EMR/scanning services support a subset of formats so check with your EMR vendor. Given products like Nuance PDF Converter Pro 6, you can scan and OCR to PDF format directly as one seamless process.

Figure 7.13 EMR/Scanning Service Uses Which Format to Save Documents?

Type of Document EMR Supports	% Supporting	Used By Program(s)
PDF	42%	Acrobat (Adobe)
RTF	25%	Word Processors
TXT	25%	Notepad & Others
DOC	24%	Microsoft Word +
XML	20%	Various
ODT	7%	Open Source Text doc
DIF	7%	Spreadsheets +
Other	13%	Various
All Listed Above	20%	All Mentioned Above

EMR With MEDCIN or SNOMED CT Support

We end this chapter with a multi-page table showing which EMRs support MEDCIN, SNOMED CT, and which EMRs were on the MSP EHR Selector (www.ehrselector.com) at the time this book was published. EMR developers change on the Selector, so check the Web site home page for a current list.

Figure 7.14 EMRs that Embed Structured Vocabularies

Product Name	EMR Developer	MEDCIN	SNOMED CT	Proprietary	EMRs on the EHR Selector
ABELMed PM – EMR	ABELSoft	N			Y
Achieve Matrix	MDI Achieve	N			
Writepad	Addison Health Systems	N			
AdvancedEMR	AdvancedMD	N			
AdvantaChart	AdvantaChart	N			
AllMeds	AllMeds	N	Y	Y	Y
Enterprise EHR	Allscripts	Y	Y	N	Y
Professional EHR	Allscripts	Y	Y	N	Y
TexTALK MD	Alma Information Systems	N			
Amazing Charts	Amazing Charts	N			
AmkaiCharts	Amkai	N			
MediPort	Assist Med	N	Y	N	
AthenaClinicals	AthenaHealth	Y			
EKiosk	AutomationMed	N			
AutoMedicWorks	AutoMedicWorks	N	N	N	
BetterHealth record	BetterHealth Global	N	N	Y	
My BetterHealth record	BetterHealth Global	N			
Wellness Connection	BlueWare	N	N	N	
Bond Clinician EHR	Bond Technologies	N	Y	N	
Medscribbler Lite	Brunmed	N	N	N	
CareData Solution	CareData Solutions	N	N	N	Y
ChartCare EMR	ChartCare				Y
ChartWare	ChartWare	N			
Essentris	CliniComp	Y	Y	Y	
CompanionEMR	Companion Technologies	N	N	Y	
CPSI System	CPSI	N	Y	Y	
CureMD EHR	CureMD	N	N	Y	Y
Medichart Express	Cyber Records	N	N	N	
Endo Express	Cyber Records	N			

Continued

Product Name	EMR Developer	MEDCIN	SNOMED CT	Proprietary	EMRs on the EHR Selector
Med-Center	Database Constructs	N	N	N	
MedInformatix	DavLong Business Solutions	N	Y	Y	Y
ScriptSure	Daw Systems	Y	Y	N	
Oacis EHR	Dinmar	N	Y	N	
Doc-U-Chart for the Tablet PC	Doc-U-Chart	N	N	N	
eDOMA for Healthcare	DOMA Technologies				
e-MDs Solution Series	e-MDs	N	N	N	Y
eClinicalWorks	eClinicalWorks	N	N	Y	
Sunrise Ambulatory Care	Eclipsys	N	Y	N	Y
CareRevolution	EHS – Electronic Healthcare Systems	Y			Y
PhastNote EMR	Elekta (formerly IMPAC)	Y			N
EMIS PCS	Emis				
EpicCare Enterprise Clinical System	Epic Systems	Y	Y	N	
Centricity EMR	GE Healthcare				Y
GEMMS One	GEMMS				Y
gGastro	gMed				Y
PrimeSuite	Greenway Medical Tech.				Y
INTERACTANT	Health Care Software	N			
Health Prove EMR/CPM	Health Probe	N	N	Y	
HMS	Healthcare Management Systems HMS	N	Y	N	
MD-Journal	HemiData	N	N	N	
MetaVision Suite	iMDsoft	N			
iMedical Patient Relationship Manager	Aprima (formerly iMedica)				Y
IMBILLS	Ingenious Med	N	N	N	
STIX	Integritas	N	N	N	
SmartDoctor	Intelligent Medical Systems	N	N	Y	
EncounterPro	JMJ Technologies	Y	Y	N	Y
KeyChart	KeyMedical Software	N	N	Y	
Kietra XPR for Clinicians	Kietra Corporation	N	N	N	

Continued

Product Name	EMR Developer	MEDCIN	SNOMED CT	Proprietary	EMRs on the EHR Selector
Mercure	Lakes Health Systems	N			
accessANYware	LanVision dba Streamline Health	N	N	N	
Life Record	Life Record	N			
Login EMR	LoginClinic	N	N	Y	
Emphasis Clinical Information Suite	M2 Information Systems	N	N	Y	Y
Horizon Ambulatory Care	McKesson	N			Y
Practice Partner	McKesson	N	Y	N	Y
InteGreat IC-Encounters	Med3000 (formerly InteGreat)	Y			Y
MedAZ	MedAZ	N			
Welford Chart Notes	MEDCOM Information Systems	N	N	Y	
mMD.net EHR	Medical Communication Systems (MCS)	N	Y	Y	
ChartMaker	Medical Information Systems	N			
Medical Office Online	Medical Office Online	N			
MedicWare EMR	MedicWare	N			
MediNotes	MediNotes	N	Y	Y	Y
Intelligent Medical Software	Meditab Software	N	N	N	
Intelligent Radiology Management Software	Meditab Software	N			
OpenVista Clinic	Medsphere	N			
MedtuityEMR	Medtuity	N	N	Y	
MyWay	Allscripts (formerly Misys)	N	N	N	Y
Momentum Healthware Care Management	Momentum Healthware	N	N	N	
Mountainside EHR	Mountainside Software	N	N	N	
NextGen EMR	Nextgen	N	Y	N	Y
Physician's Workstation	Nightingale Informatix	Y	N	N	
AHLTA	Northrop Grumman IT	Y			
CHCS II	Northrop Grumman IT	Y			
NetPractice EHR	Noteworthy Med. Systems	N			Y
NueMD	Nuesoft	N			

Continued

Product Name	EMR Developer	MEDCIN	SNOMED CT	Proprietary	EMRs on the EHR Selector
ObGynPocketPro	ObTech	N			
OmniMD	OmniMD	Y	N	Y	
Optimus EMR System	Optimus EMR	N	N	N	
Optio Healthcare QuickRecord Suite	Optio Software	N			
Optio Healthcare Medex Suite	Optio Software	N			
Concerto Medical Applications Portal	Orion Health	N			Y
Amelior ED	Patient Care Technology Systems	N			
Patient|NOW	PatientNOW	N	N	Y	
MedcomSoft Record 2006	PBFOnline (formerly Medcomsoft)	Y	Y	N	
Carevue Chart	Philips Medical Group	N			
Compurecord	Philips Medical Group	N			
OB-TV	Philips Medical Group	N			
Xtenity Enterprise	Philips Medical Systems	N			
CareSuite	Picis	N	N	N	
ED PulseCheck (Ibex)	Picis	N	N	N	
OpenChart	Point and Click Solutions	N			
Navigator Web	Poseidon Group	N	N	Y	
eIVF	PracticeHWY.com	N	N	N	
Xpert EHR	PracticeXpert	N	N	N	
ProtoCHART	Protomed Corporation	N			
Pulse Patient Relationship Management	Pulse Systems	Y	Y	N	Y
Purkinje EHR	Purkinje	N	Y	N	
QuadraMed CPR	QuadraMed	N	N	N	
RelWare's Clinical Application Solution	Reliance Software Systems	N	N	N	
RemedyMD-BariEHR	RemedyMd				Y
Intergy EHR	Sage Software	Y			Y
Sevocity EHR	Sevocity Div. Conceptual				Y
easychart	Software Performance Specialists	N	N	N	

Continued

Product Name	EMR Developer	MEDCIN	SNOMED CT	Proprietary	EMRs on the EHR Selector
SolComHealth	SolCom	N			
SpringCharts EHR	Spring Medical Systems	N			
SpringCharts Essentials	Spring Medical Systems	N			
EMRge	SSIMED	Y	Y	N	
OrthoPad EMR	Stryker (OEM)	N			Y
Systemedx EHR Navigator	Systemedx	N	Y	N	
Navigator Web	The Poseidon Group	N			Y
T-SystemEV	T-System	N			
ChartKeeper Express	VantageMed	N			
VersaForm EMR	VersaForm Systems Corporation	N	N	Y	
VersaSuite	VersaSuite	N	Y	Y	Y
SmartClinic	VIP Medicine (formerly Berdy)	N			Y
Wellogic Consult	Wellogic	Y	Y	Y	
Wellsoft	Wellsoft	N	N	N	

Wrap Up

Watch for EMR support of the latest interoperability and data standards. Many transaction standards are covered by the HL7 version 2 specs, but which ones? In 2009, the version of the HL7 specification was 2.6. In 2010, the 2.7 version will have been adopted and you will want to determine if your EMR vendor is supporting that updated version, and if not, when they will be.

Not all EMR developers list their products on the MSP EHR Selector™. If an EMR developer you are interested in is not listed, encourage them to get on, so you will have a convenient way to obtain in-depth, side-by-side feature summaries of their EMR product versus others, and to compare EMR products at more than a superficial level.

Finally, think about your paper chart conversion needs and what this will cost. The best prices and services will be available before the real demand for chart conversion services starts. If you initiate conversion services now, you have the option of sending a box of charts to two or more potential suppliers to compare the details of service. Don't authorize the destruction of your paper charts until you see the PDFs and are comfortable with the quality. At that point, you can choose the supplier with the best combination of price, service and security to complete the rest of your chart conversion.

Crucial Decision

Do you structure data at the billing code level or at the clinical level using MEDCIN, SNOMED CT® or some vendor-proprietary database structure? Should the EMR include the CCD standard? Photocopy as needed or download this Scorecard from www.ehrselector.com

Do we want our EMR to incorporate the CCD document standard? Rationale:		
We want our EMR to incorporate the following level of structure:		
	Billing Level	EMR uses ICD-9-CM, CPT, HPCPS or other billing codes
	Billing ICD-10-CM	EMR will support ICD-10 by 2013 deadline

The interaction between standards and structure comes into play here. If you select any of these standards, you can't choose a user interface that provides only unstructured data capture. There is a trade-off between structure and data-entry effort also.

Crucial Decision

Do you structure data at the billing code level or at the clinical level using MEDCIN, SNOMED CT® or some vendor-proprietary database structure? Should the EMR include the CCD standard? Photocopy as needed or download this Scorecard from www.ehrselector.com

	SNOMED CT	EMR uses SNOMED CT codes to store charted data
	MEDCIN	EMR uses MEDCIN vocabulary and code to structure data
	Vendor Proprietary	EMR uses a vendor-specific, proprietary code to store charted data
	Not Applicable	Chose to use EMR with unstructured, free-form charting
	Supports ELINCS	For lab interoperability reporting using LOINC
	Supports LOINC	Stores lab values using LOINC codes by Lab Info. Systems
	Supports DICOM	Stores imaging using DICOM codes
	Supports Drug Database	Supports standard drug database
	Vendor Proprietary	Supports vendor proprietary drug database
	Supports CCD	Can create (output) and receive and store (input) data formatted as CCD (Continuity of Care Document) standards
	Adobe 9 & 10 (CS4)	Can encode data into Adobe 9 and 10 medical wrappers

The interaction between standards and structure comes into play here. If you select any of these standards, you can't choose a user interface that provides only unstructured data capture. There is a trade-off between structure and data-entry effort also.

Crucial Decision

Do you structure data at the billing code level or at the clinical level using MEDCIN, SNOMED CT® or some vendor-proprietary database structure? Should the EMR include the CCD standard? Photocopy as needed or download this Scorecard from www.ehrselector.com

Action Item(s):

The interaction between standards and structure comes into play here. If you select any of these standards, you can't choose a user interface that provides only unstructured data capture. There is a trade-off between structure and data-entry effort also.

CHAPTER 8
Interoperability Beyond EMRs

Crucial Decision
What is your preferred level of interoperability with other EMRs, EHRs, or HIOs, PHRs, Registries and Public Health Agencies?

This chapter also addresses the following questions:

- What is the NHIN and what composes it?
- Why are PHRs, RHIOs, HIOs and Web portals important?
- Why do you need to bother with standards at all and which are important?

EMR Adventures

As Lynn walks into Dr. Alex Glass's office she remarks, "I think something strange is going on with our EMR supplier. There is a report on the Internet that the company is being acquired by Galactic EMR Healthcare systems."

"Has Galactic EMR notified us of this?" asks Dr. Glass.

"Not to my knowledge," replies Lynn (the office manager). "But I believe it because the software release from our EMR company is now nine months later than promised, and they keep hedging on when its going to be available."

"Boy, if this is true, it isn't good news," comments Dr. Glass. "It's still hard to believe. Galactic EMR already has acquired three other EMR companies, why would they want another one?" he questions.

"Perhaps they don't care about our EMR company's product, but are just after the market share," suggests Lynn. "Galactic EMR has a history of acquiring companies just to put competitors out of business and to get the support revenues and market share. They seem to grow by acquisition, rather than by product innovation," comments Lynn.

"Well, that's really bad for us. If all Galactic EMR is interested in is their market share, they aren't likely to forge ahead with the enhancements we have been waiting for. Several of the EMRs they have already acquired we dismissed when we bought our current EMR, because they weren't doing new product development on any of them, but just pushing those customers to replace the systems with the 'go forward' Costs-too-Much, Does-Everything (C2MDE) brand EMR," says Dr. Glass.

Successfully Choosing Your EMR: 15 Crucial Decisions. By © Arthur Gasch and Betty Gasch.
Published 2010 by Blackwell Publishing

"Yep, and their C2MDE product doesn't have the templates we need for our ophthalmology practice either," Lynn remarks. "We are just not a large enough specialty for Galactic to care about. Where does that leave us going forward?"

"Well, our current EMR does support all of the interoperability standards. We should be able to export encounter summaries for all of our patients in CCD format, so if we can find an alternative other than C2MDE that accepts CCD formatted records, we could migrate to that system. In fact, that may be our only alternative, because I don't think C2MDE is interoperable with our EMR. Perhaps Galactic is planning on making it so, but they aren't at present."

"I hate to think about migration – we just installed this EMR two years ago. We haven't had it long enough to get a good return on our investment. Perhaps if we end up doing that, we should look at a Web-based EMR service, rather than deploying the EMR in our office, like we did this time," says Dr. Glass. "That would at least mean we don't have to make a large up-front investment in buying an EMR application, we could just pay a monthly fee and expense it as we go along."

"That might be the best approach," agrees Lynn. "Practice revenues have increased since we deployed our system, but we haven't fully depreciated it yet, that will take two more years."

"Well, at least we did one thing right. Getting a system that supported interoperability standards helps to assure we can move patient encounter summaries to any of the other systems that support these same standards. That means we aren't locked into what Galactic EMR is pushing on us," asserts Dr. Glass.

"Right, we can wait and see what commitments Galactic EMR is willing to make once the acquisition is finalized. That will take 6-9 months anyway, maybe a year, and we will have almost depreciated our current EMR by that time. That will be the right time to make a move. By then, perhaps more EMR systems will be supporting CDA and CCR standards. Is that being pushed by CCHIT-certification and by Meaningful Use criteria under the 2009 ARRA legislation?" asks Lynn.

"I'm not sure, but I'm hoping it will help us even though we have already adopted," replies Dr. Glass.

"If so, that may be one of its best features," replies Lynn.

Communication, Communication, Communication

Hopefully, you won't find yourself in Dr. Glass's situation, but market consolidation does happen, in fact the ARRA legislation is accelerating it and big I.T. vendors with legacy hospital products are in fact always on the lookout for mid-sized EMR products. It allows them to interface one EMR product to their legacy I.T. product's lab, pharmacy and radiology systems, and promote themselves as an integrated group practice and hospital I.T. supplier. This is but one scenario that begs for better interoperability and this chapter will describe several other scenarios.

One important area for improvement is the implementation of current standards for data exchange that will allow physicians to export the essence of medical charts out of one EMR developer's system and import it into another EMR developer's system (EMR portability). In spite of all the stated support that some EMR companies publicly make about implementing standards, many of these EMR suppliers still have not achieved full support for those standards in their various EMR systems, and in some cases have not made multiple EMR systems they own, able to fully communicate with each other. This lack of interoperability makes EMR portability challenging in some cases. Physicians concerned about patient record migration will want to evaluate support for Continuity of Care Document (CCD) creation carefully, as that is the best way so far to move data out of an EMR and into another one; lean towards EMRs that support document interoperability standards.

This chapter is really all about communication – don't problems usually come down to that? (By the way, we will define and explain all of the abbreviations we have used (and more) in this chapter.)

The Nationwide Health Information Network (NHIN)

You have probably guessed that the vast realm of electronic healthcare didn't stop with the EMR at your point-of-care, which is just the first layer in a much larger venture into electronic healthcare records that the government is promoting called the Nationwide Health Information Network (NHIN). NHIN is envisioned as a means of exchanging health information via a network of state and regional systems (or networks).

These state networks are organized as Regional Health Information Organizations (RHIOs), which perform health information exchanges as the building blocks for the new NHIN. The NHIN road map describes the technologies, standards, laws, policies, programs, and practices that enable health information to be electronically shared among multiple stakeholders and decision makers to promote healthcare delivery. The work to create NHIN is on-going, most recently funded by the ARRA (HITECH) legislation and will expand the work of the 19 organizations that participated in the NHIN trial implementation projects conducted since September 2007. The Integrating the Healthcare Enterprise (IHE) organization is being proposed as a standards-based approach to verification of connectivity. In February 2009, participants from over 70 companies and 12 countries came together for a Connectathon, which is a lab-workshop where connectivity issues are identified and resolved. This was held in Chicago, a little over a month before HIMSS.

In April 2009, Nitor Group (Chester, MD) received a contract to move the project forward. Additional contracting will occur later in 2009 after this book is published. When completed, the NHIN will provide a network-of-networks foundation for an interoperable, standards-based, secure exchange of healthcare information. The Achilles heel of the program is physician adoption of EMRs; even if the NHIN existed right now, only 14-17% of the nation's group practices would be able to actually use it.[1] Many issues with this new network remain to be defined before it can succeed.

Nonetheless, we encourage physicians considering EMR adoption to look beyond their offices and consider how they can exchange information with the other "players" across this healthcare I.T. landscape. Think about your EMR as more than an office automation tool – it will eventually be a powerful way to connect to many other people and systems.

The players in the healthcare I.T. landscape include:
- Your patients (and their Personal Health Records (PHRs);
- Your colleagues in other medical offices or hospital clinics who also care for your patients;
- The hospital where your patients are admitted;
- National laboratories or other diagnostic entities;
- Your county or state public health departments;
- Any RHIOs doing Health Information Exchange (HIE) in your state;
- The Centers for Disease Control (CDC) and other federal agencies;
- The third-party payers and CMS for your Medicare/Medicaid patients;
- Any disease research or immunization registries you may be connected to;
- Drug companies and others doing healthcare research.

Stakeholders Slow to Adhere to Standards

This vast array of healthcare providers today have very little in common in the way they structure and store data, and if it weren't for standards, their (eventual) ability to exchange data would be quite limited. Currently, it's as if they all speak different languages, with a little bit of broken English thrown in.

Several registries and some other entities are enthusiastic fans of their own proprietary data formats and have resisted efforts to change them. Only recently have they become more cooperative but there is still work to be done. This may be a matter of limited finances and redevelopment expenses which ARRA funds can address.

As an example of this sporadic ability to exchange data, we spoke with one EMR user who was excited to be able to receive lab results in LOINC format (lab data standard), and spoke to both national labs about their ability to provide results using LOINC. Both claimed they could, but in the end only Quest delivered and for patients where LabCorp is mandated, full integration of lab results in a format actionable by the EMR, is not available. LabCorp is not able to report results using LOINC according to this physician. LabCorp is really a conglomeration of various different labs, so perhaps some support LOINC reporting and others do not?

We contacted LabCorp in June/July 2009 to clarify their ability to report lab results using LOINC coding. Their media contact indicated she would have to look into this issue and get back to us but never did. We contacted LabCorp a

---

[1] HIMSS Web site Definitions & Acronyms, http://www.himss.org/ASP/topics_FocusDynamic.asp?faid=143.

second time, leaving a message with the manager of media relations, mentioning the first contact and still received no response. We then sent an e-mail and followed up with a telephone call to a second media relations person, who told us that our e-mail was received and forwarded to an unnamed person at corporate, but she didn't know what LOINC codes were.

Based on this lack of response, we were unable to clarify the matter with LabCorp. If the physician account is accurate, insurance companies that mandate lab work through LabCorp are doing their patients and physicians a great disservice, since the lab is either unable or unwilling to report results using LOINC codes that could be automatically integrated into physician EMRs. Here is where intelligent pressure from third-party payors would be most helpful in promoting the adoption of standards and the elimination of the need for physicians to look in two different places in their EMRs for their patient's lab results, which creates needless extra work.

Organizations Building the NHIN

The U.S. has entitled the overall healthcare I.T. landscape the Nationwide Health Information Network (NHIN). It is an attempt by groups such as HISPC, HITSP, FHA, CCHIT, NIST, NCVHS[2] and others to create an infrastructure that can exchange data using standards derived from the HL7[3] Version-3 Reference Information Model (RIM). The standards involved for the data itself include: SNOMED CT (for clinical documentation terminology), NCPDP Scripts (for drugs), LOINC (for lab results), all wrapped into a Clinical Document Architecture (CDA) record format. When this infrastructure is completed, it will be a system of information systems that securely exchanges (using SSL encryption)[4] health information among various stakeholders. The key word is exchanges, as the NHIN is not supposedly intended to be a health data store, but an exchange mechanism. That was a lot of (probably new) acronyms, so let's make this whole idea more understandable (keep reading, it becomes clearer). Indeed, for a practical exchange of information to occur, the RHIO or message hub must support a variety of different standards including HL7, XML, SSL (mentioned above), DICOM for imaging and TLS (transport layer security), among others.

---

[2] Health Information Security and Privacy Collaboration (HISPC), Health Information Technology Standards Panel (HITSP), Federal Health Architecture (FHA), Certification Commission for Healthcare Information Technology (CCHIT), National Institute of Standards and Technology (NIST), National Committee on Vital and Health Statistics (NCVHS).

[3] HL7 is an international community of healthcare experts and information scientists collaborating to create standards for the exchange, management and integration of electronic healthcare information.

[4] SSL – Secure Socket Layer, the same encryption used for sending credit card information across the Internet now.

Overview of the Three Layers

The first layer is right above the patient at the caregiver level. This is where most source data exists, including in the patient's own Personal Health Record (PHR), if they have one. This could be called the health information source layer or data source layer. Figure 8.1 is a simplified depiction of the layers that make up the NHIN.

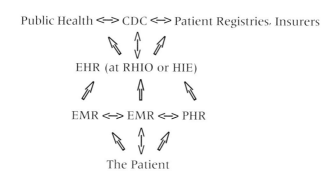

Figure 8.1 The Patient and Three Levels of Patient Data

The second layer contains the Electronic Health Records (EHRs) coordinated by regional organizations involved in Health Information Exchange (HIE), which is the abbreviation for the exchange of data. HIO (Health Information Organizations) do the exchange, and if they are regional, then they are Regional HIOs (or RHIOs). RHIOs consolidate data from one or more EMRs into EHRs. This is a subset of all patient data consolidated from more than one of the patient's caregivers. The second layer is therefore the health information exchange layer or data exchange layer.

The third layer is a conglomeration of mostly data and specialized organizations, such as: public health, immunization registries, disease registries, government, insurers, drug companies and others.

Benefits That NHIN Brings to Physicians

Why should you care about these layers and the standards they contain when choosing your EMR? One good reason is that they provide you with an exit path for your patient records if it turns out you can't live with your new EMR and need to get a divorce (or if it dies, or is kidnapped by a larger EMR developer in a merger). The ability to write episodes of care for patients in your practice allows you to take a lot (but not all) of your electronic patient record information when you want to move onto another EMR solution for whatever reason. That's only one reason, you will discover other reasons why this chapter is important to you as you read on. Let's look a bit deeper at the details of the three layers that make up NHIN.

Layer One – The Patient (Data Source) Layer

The first layer has one source of information, but is kept in potentially two different types of systems:

- EMRs, which are Electronic Medical Records with information captured by physicians from patient encounters; and
- PHRs, which are Personal Health Records that are composed of data provided by the patient directly about themselves, or patient summaries of EMR encounters provided by physicians (or any caregiver) and given to the patient at the end of their encounter, and then kept in the patient's PHR.

Both are data repositories, e.g. data exists and persists in these structures. We will discuss each of these in turn, before going to layer two.

Many EMRs and One PHR

Layer one has many EMRs, because each patient care provider creates one for the patient. If a patient has five doctors, there could be five EMRs. There could also be an EMR for each hospital or clinic where the patient is seen. Also, any home healthcare agencies or nursing homes or rehabs could create an EMR for the patient.

Patient Identification and Authentication

Each of these entities has the patient indexed under a completely different ID number, which may be some variation of the patient's current insurance ID number. However, since patients change insurance IDs, these numbers may not be based on their current ID, but some ID that existed in the past, if they are based on an ID at all. Some providers just create arbitrary ID numbers, other providers have other schemes. This makes identifying and authenticating the same patient across all of their providers, a big challenge, but only when one of these caregivers wants to exchange health information with another – which generally happens at the next layer up in the system.

Inconsistent Health Information Organization

Each care provider also has a different data structure in which the patient's health information is stored. There is not generally any commonality unless all the providers happen to be using the same EMR product and software release, which is highly unusual.

The Patient's Information About Themselves

The patient's own Personal Health Record (PHR) also exists at this level. It consists of whatever information he/she has on himself or herself, whether abstracted from an encounter from an episode of care with a professional caregiver, or just his/her own observations about their health, heart rate, state of mind or whatever, organized in no particular or consistent structure.

The key is for the EMRs that exist in the office of a caregiver to be able to read from and write to these various PHR files. There are currently over 130 PHR vendors, and quite a few of them offer Web-based solutions. Wiley-Blackwell is publishing a book on PHRs entitled *Personal Health Records – A Guide for Clinicians* by Mohammad Al-Ubaydli, we encourage you to look for that soon.

Keeping track of which EMRs connect to which PHRs is a full-time endeavor. Some of the larger PHR sites, like Microsoft or Google, list their partners; other PHR sites do not. The MSP EHR Selector has a cross-reference based on which PHRs, EMR developers claim they can read from (or write to). However, the data provided in this case is not vetted, so users of our site will need to request validation of interoperability claims. That is a challenge because of the diversity of approaches that PHR vendors have taken in storing medical information. This ranges from simple, unstructured text, to support for some document interoperability standards such as Clinical Data Architecture (CDA), Continuity of Care Record (CCR) or Continuity of Care Document (CCD). We will clarify these shortly.

There actually are specific standards for PHRs, but so many PHRs were developed before the standards existed that they are therefore not compliant with them. PHRs are a hodge-podge of various structures, that are not compatible with each other, or many EMRs. There is going to be a huge shakeout before PHRs will be very useful. Today, a physician confronted by a patient with a PHR who wants to share the data, has no idea what format it's in or how it might be structured (if at all, since it may just be freeform data that has to be read and understood by the doctor).

The PHR structures are improving now that there is a standard, but unless the EMR and PHR vendor are the same, the ability to exchange meaningful and structured PHR data is mostly unworkable at present. On the other hand, if the EMR and PHR are offered by the same developer through a patient portal (detailed shortly), then useful data can be exchanged and the flow of that data can be controlled by the patient. The portal can allow the patient to "see" any of their provider's EMR systems, so they can request an appointment, a medication refill, a summary of their previous visit, patient educational materials, or contact their physician via secured, HIPAA-compliant e-mail.

WebMD is an example of a well-known organization that did just that, but in spite of its money and reputation, less than one million Americans use the WebMD PHR functionality, mostly because there is no EMR that goes with it that any significant number of physicians have adopted. Of course 1M is not a small number, but it is less than 0.3% of Americans who could be using it. Indeed, the fact that we have to track 130 different PHR vendors means that none of them have provided a compelling case for any significant number of Americans to yet adopt and put their medical information online.

By way of contrast, use of PHR by seniors in the Kaiser Permanente Health plans is much greater. In a July 2009 press release, Danielle Paquette reported:

• Nearly half (43.7%) of Kaiser Permanente's Medicare beneficiaries are currently registered to use My Health Manager, the provider's personal health record.

- In 2008, 22.4% of lab results released online were viewed by Medicare beneficiaries, and 29.4% of all Rx refills ordered on My Health Manager were done so by Medicare patients.
- More than 87% of survey respondents are satisfied or very satisfied with My Health Manager on kp.org[5]

The contrast is pretty apparent. When coordinated by a health provider, EMR and PHR work very nicely together. Both EMR and PHR vendors are increasingly supporting HL7's CDA, CCD and ASTM's CCR document standards, and they may be able to communicate and exchange data without even realizing it. This is also why MSP maintains information on the standards that EMR developers support.

As you ponder what EMR may work in your office, you may want to expand your criteria to see what EMRs can also provide PHR and patient portal functionality. OK, just selecting and deploying EMRs may seem daunting enough for right now, but remember that information technology is rapidly expanding.

Could PDF Satisfy EMR/PHR Meaningful Use Requirements?

EMR interoperability and EMR portability, though two different subjects, are joined at the hip, both of which are going to be woven throughout the government's Meaningful Use functionality requirements. These requirements currently state, (you will) *"provide patients with electronic copies of – or electronic access to – clinical information (including lab results, problem lists, medication lists, allergies) per patient preference (e.g. through PHR)."* Now you will begin to see the practical reasons why you need to care about standards.

Fulfilling your responsibility of enabling patients to access data is another reason that standards are important to you. The ability of an EMR to write out an "encounter summary" in a usable format can be based on the Continuity of Care (CCR) standard, which allows Personal Health Records (PHRs) with CCR input capabilities to utilize your EMR information.

The Adobe PDF format, which has become a general business standard, has applications helpful to you as well. You can satisfy your patient information requirements by being able to provide an Adobe PDF document that has extensions that comply with the PDF Healthcare Standards group (that works under the auspices of the AIIM[6] organization). AIIM offers a Best Practices Guide and the Healthcare PDF Implementation Guide, which shows how PDF documents can be enhanced to contain XML-tagged (a format standard) data, based on an XSL (a style sheet standard) schema. The data to be enhanced could be DICOM (an imaging standard) or data in other formats, or be simply

---

[5] For more information about Medicare clients using Kaiser's My Health Manager PHR contact Danielle Paquette at 415 274-7927 or dpaquette@golinharris.com.

[6] AIIM is a non-profit organization focused on helping users understand challenges associated with managing documents, content, records, and business processes (www.aiim.org).

meta-tagged (tags provide structure) medical information – that can be read with Adobe's Acrobat Reader. Anyone can download Acrobat Reader free from the Adobe Web site. All of this is important to you because these standards will enable you to get data in your EMR that is not structured, into a format that allows you to access and utilize it and make it available to your patients. There are companies that now have healthcare plug-ins that empower PDF documents. One is DesAcc, Inc. (http://www.desacc.com/) which offers several products, including Health Data Explorer. This program runs transparently as an Adobe Acrobat plug-in to provide complete Document-to-DICOM interoperability, and adds DICOM and EHR connectivity and provides a simple way to integrate DICOM images into PDF files.

With an OsiriX viewer (http://www.osirix-viewer.com/), you can even view the raw file (at least on a Macintosh computer). We recommend you get an EMR that can create PDF documents that support the XFA forms/data extensions, or make sure that Acrobat Professional (or Adobe's LiveCycle Designer) is handy to create them yourself. Nothing in Meaningful Use (so far) says you can't charge the patient a little extra for providing this information but keep the charge modest, because it's not likely to be reimbursable by third parties anytime soon.

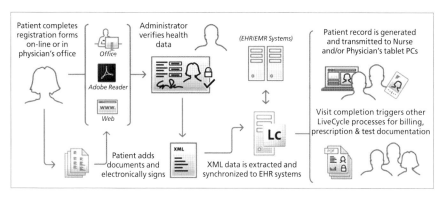

Figure 8.2 Using an Adobe PDF as a Healthcare Information Container (diagram courtesy of Adobe Software)

The point is that Adobe PDF provides a relatively quick and inexpensive way to satisfy the previously-stated patient documentation access criteria for Meaningful Use. Certainly the patient can accept the PDF record of his/her encounter and stuff it into any PHR and even have some encoded, XML-tagged data and structure to boot.

Could PDF Become the Format for the PHR Repository?

If your patient has Adobe Acrobat Professional, the PDF you provide can be cataloged (which indexes every word) and the catalog can include every other

PDF encounter summary the patient has received from all other doctors and caregivers. This makes a pretty nifty, inexpensive repository of medical data in the patient's PHR. Because each document can be password encrypted, your patient can even control who can open the document. If the same password is used for all documents, then your patient has a relatively secure data repository of medical information. This is true regardless of where it is being hosted, and any document(s) can be transmitted openly across the Internet, but not opened (too easily) by anyone else who might intercept it because they don't have the password needed to decrypt the PDF file and open it. Not bad for a one-time investment of $150 or less.

Adobe PDF documents don't have to be just CCR summaries; by the time you read this, HL7 will have released its own "Best Practices Guide" for using Adobe's PDF formatted documents to wrap data content compliant with their standard as well. Adobe is neutral about which standard organizations use their PDF format.

Personal Health Records Research

The Robert Wood Johnson Foundation, in collaboration with the University of Wisconsin, conducted research on the needs of the PHR in different care settings. The research was completed in September 2008 but how this data will be used by CCR and CDA standards organizations is unknown. It is a sure bet that PHRs will succeed only if they are integrated into already owned cell phones, PDAs, iPods, or if they are hosted on sites like Microsoft or Google that are accessible worldwide from healthcare providers who have Internet connections, but this approach leaves many security issues unanswered.

Transferring Hospital Patient Data Into Attending Physician EMRs

Hospitals don't want to support dozens of customized interfaces to different EMR products, which is why they have promoted the EMRs offered by the legacy I.T. vendors that are already located in their hospitals. However, this approach can be stifling for attending physicians who often need more flexibility in EMR functionality than the EMRs available from the legacy vendors. This is where integration companies like Medicity and Axolotl come in. Medicity provides the Novo Grid, essentially a standardized data buffer that hospitals can write into using one standard set of protocols, and which can then be accessed by a diversity of EMR solutions each supporting one customer interface. It gives hospitals the ability to write data into the Novo Grid and deliver that data to a large number of authenticated physician practices within a minute or two.

The Novo Grid (and competitive products like it) allow hospitals and physician group practices to choose integration solutions that are optimal for their respective needs – creating a win-win scenario. Hospitals continue to write data out of their laboratory and other systems, and EMR vendors can read it in one standardized format. The cost for each practice is reasonable and removes the burden of having to maintain customized interfaces to each different EMR product. Practically, it means that a physician can obtain test results for a patient he/she is seeing in the office who has had an encounter with a hospital clinic or who has had an inpatient stay. The physician accomplishes this by querying one location and then downloading and populating his/her EMR with the data from the patient's hospital stay or clinical visit.

If your hospital is offering you an EMR that comes from one of its legacy vendors, the use of a product like the Medicity Novo Grid can be the answer to the hospital achieving the one interface it needs, and at the same time allowing you to choose any of 200+ EMRs that best fit your practice needs. Determine whether your EMR is one for which an interface already exists, and if not, make it a purchase condition of any EMR you are considering.

Only four companies come close to meeting MSP EHR Selector™ requirements when 46 specialties are asserted – American Medical Software, e-MDs, Pulse Systems and the open source product from PatientOS. Note that none of these are traditional hospital legacy vendors, and most are names with which many hospital I.T. people are not familiar. There is no way of measuring whether any of these EMRs does an outstanding job with any particular specialty either, as none of them has a KLAS Research rating. NextGen and Davlong EMRs support a few less specialties, but are not hospital legacy vendors either. Hospital legacy vendors that match ratings are 67% for GE and 50% for McKesson and Cerner. The point is, don't be forced into an EMR from a legacy hospital vendor if it doesn't fit the needs of your practice specialty. Keep your EMR choices open by getting the hospital to use a central interface hub technology like Medicity, Axolotl or others.

Patient Web Portal Services

A Patient Web portal is a site on the World Wide Web that provides personalized capabilities to patients using it. It provides services that work on multiple platforms such as PCs, Personal Digital Assistants (PDAs), and cell phones, in spite of their all having potentially different user interfaces.

A 2002 Harris Interactive survey of over 2,000 online adults indicated that 90% of them would like to communicate with their physicians online, but the same survey showed that only 37% were willing to pay for it. The same study also demonstrated that 56% said that having the ability to communicate with their physician by Internet would influence their choice of doctors[7].

Portals can remain a way of communicating within layer one (patient to physician and back again), and portals can be used to communicate between layers. Figure 8.2 lists some common services that Web portals can currently provide. Some EMRs also include optional patient portals where patients

---

[7] *Patient/physician online communication: many patients want it, would pay for it, and it would influence their choice of doctors and health plans.* By Humphrey Taylor, Robert Leitman, editors. Published April 2002, Vol. 2, Issue 8, pp. 1-3 by Health Care News

can request appointments, request prescription refills, access educational materials, initiate e-mail and even host PHR functionality (this is by no means an exhaustive list). They also facilitate guided patient interviews, allowing the patient to input some data for your EMR charts before their visit. Be sure, if your EMR offers this functionality, that the author (in this case the patient) of the content is tracked separately from content you or staff members enter.

Figure 8.3 EMR/Web Portal Features

Feature	Yes	3rd Party	Xtra $	Future
Patient Able to Request Appointment	56%	9%	6%	28%
Patient Education	47%	11%	8%	28%
Patient Exchanges E-mail With MD	47%	4%	4%	18%
Patient Able to Request Rx Refill	48%	9%	9%	35%
Patient Able to Enter Data	40%	9%	6%	40%

In Figure 8.3, the service may be facilitated by the EMR vendor themselves (the YES column) or by a third party. It may be included in the basic EMR pricing or be available for an extra charge (Xtra $ column). If currently provided by a third party, the EMR vendor may be planning to directly provide these services themselves in the future (Future column).

If they do host PHR capability, the data interchange between the PHR and your EMR may be solved (at least for your practice), since the data may be kept in a single repository and a common data structure, which facilitates exchanging it.

Web Portal Middleware Providers
As Figure 8.3 shows, many EMR developers that offer patient Web portals do so by working with a Web portal middleware supplier. Portals are seen by some as the mechanism of choice for implementing RHIOs and connecting together various practices that have different types of EMRs into one integrated network that can be used by patients. Web portals can also be useful for an individual practice seeking to bring together features that a patient might wish to access, but which run on different computer systems in the office. Some of the most frequently chosen Web developers include (in order of popularity) Medfusion, Omedix, Relay Health, Axolotl, Medem, Physician Specialty and others.

To Portal or Not to Portal, or Let Hometown General Do It
Web portals raise serious security issues and dramatically increase exposure of your patient data. Brushing all such concerns aside, NCVHS appears to be poised to require that Web portals, hosted by individual practices, be deployed in the

first year of Meaningful Use, according to Paul Tang.[8] These would support a subset of such features as: reporting of lab results to patients, providing patients a convenient way to request prescription refills, making office appointments, finding and downloading patient educational material, downloading a summary of their last office encounter to their PHR, viewing some elements of the patient chart, and conducting e-mail dialog with their physician(s).

All of this is fine as long as it is secure. The exchange of e-mail and patient data has direct HIPAA implications and the use of IPSec with Virtual Private Network (VPN) tunneling is essential. Also consider that you are transferring patient data from a more secure system (your office network) to a system with unknown, and probably not very good, security. Do you want to do that?

More than half of patients in recent surveys report that they would like to access their group practice through a secure Web portal, but the key word is secure. Zero percent say that they want to communicate their confidential information over an insecure Internet connection that has already been penetrated by hackers. Check out the legal implications of offering this service and the position it will leave you in if patient records are breached.

If a breach occurs, will the patient think his/her computer was breached, or assume that the portal on your system was? While portals are all the rage nowadays, let your hospital initiate a portal first and learn lessons from how well they do. Then, get your hospital to help you if you have to institute a Web portal. As with e-Rx electronic transmissions, portals are a great capability to have as part of your EMR (and some believe will be mandated for Meaningful Use), but not necessarily one you will want to activate quickly. Enter slowly into deployment of optional or non-essential EMR components, and watch for a slip in the portal date requirement.

Layer Two – The Data Exchange Layer

PHR is one approach to having a patient and his/her various healthcare providers exchange health information encounter-by-encounter at layer one directly. In the larger world, the government is planning for most HIE (Health Information Exchanges) to occur at layer two, through the vehicle of a national Health Information Organization (HIO) that connects to various Regional Health Information Organizations (RHIOs) that build ad-hoc EHRs (Electronic Health Records) from queries to a patient's individual physician, hospital, nursing home, home healthcare or other EMR system.

The geographic footprint of a RHIO can range from a local community to a large multi-state region. The term RHIO and Health Information Exchange (HIE) are related but different entities. A HIE is information exchange (verb), while the RHIO is the organization (noun) that is managing the exchange (HIE) of health data.

---

[8] *Is the Bar Still Too High?* By David Raths. Published Sept. 2009 by Healthcare Informatics

In contrast to direct transfers at layer one, layer two provides health information consolidation, creating an ad-hoc set of electronic health information to support unplanned or emergency care by a provider who is not normally associated with the patient. This ad hoc health information supports care in emergency rooms or urgent care centers where the patient is a new encounter, and previous history, allergy, current medication, data on labs etc., is needed.

The EHR (Electronic Health Record) is an on-demand record concerning any patient, composed of data collected from one or more EMRs and from PHRs (when available). For privacy and control reasons, the EHR doesn't persist in any HIO or RHIO repository, as this simply creates one more level of potential breach, and disenfranchises the patient from having true control over their personal medical information.

Characteristic of layer two is that the patient remains identified in the EHR as long as the data is there. In contrast, when health information is moved on to layer three, patient data may be de-identified and used for population trends and other purposes.

Health Information Exchange (HIE) & Introduction to RHIOs

Regional Health Information Organizations (RHIOs) are groups of organizations and stakeholders that have come together for the purpose of electronic Health Information Exchange and are focused on improving the quality, safety, and efficiency of healthcare delivery. Regional Health Information Organizations (RHIOs) don't warehouse health information, they simply expedite its exchange as a service to their participating stakeholders. It is an important issue of governance (who controls things). Physicians and other providers are not enthusiastic about giving up patient records or control of patient records, so there is a need to adopt the approach of organizing an index to the medical records that the physician creates and controls, so that they can exchange these patient records when needed.

Master Patient Index (MPI) – Critical to Safe HIE

The challenge and key to safely exchanging health information is knowing who it belongs to. That means some sort of Master Patient Index (MPI) must exist, so that John Doe's healthcare record needed by the emergency department at Hometown General gets John Doe's health records from his various providers, and not Jonathan Doe's health records. If they get Jonathan Doe's records, from even one provider, they are as likely to hurt John Doe as they are to help him, and they will be facing a big lawsuit for negligence and malpractice. So the MPIs that track providers and patient IDs must be flawless. The whole concept of automated HIE hinges on a flawless MPI, which many argue hinges on a universal, national health information ID for every American; but there are huge privacy concerns about creating that and making it mandatory.

That being the case, there are two requirements:
- Physicians must have an EMR in the first place, as information in a paper record will never be readily indexed or retrievable by a RHIO; and
- The EMR's implemented product must be easily indexed and exchange health information in a standardized format.

Here is where the support of the Continuity of Care Record (CCR) standard is important, as it provides a well-defined structure for RHIOs to index patient records and to then retrieve data from EMRs of individual doctors when needed. ~57% of the EMR developers enable structured records to be sent to RHIOs using HL7 with 15% offering it for extra cost.

Contrasting Various HIE Methods

There are many ways to solve the same problem, and often people take different and independent approaches to doing so.

At layer one, the exchange of data is, in theory, simple. The doctor knows the patient, the patient knows the doctor and they hand each other (literally or electronically) medical information they wish to exchange, without dependence on an infallible MPI to authenticate the handoff. It's too bad that PHRs are not more standards compliant, but that's coming soon. But even when that happens, it won't solve the case of providing some basic summary of a person's healthcare status, allergies, current medications, blood type, and other information to emergency responders and hospital emergency department personnel, unless the patient carries his/her PHR with them and it's retrievable and readily printable. To make that happen, there are various schemes afoot.

- PHR is stored in patient cell phones;
- PHR is stored in patient healthcare ID cards in a chip that can be retrieved by using their fingerprint or an ID passcode;
- PHR is stored in patient USB memory stick that can be plugged into any computer and can dump a one-page summary of the information needed;
- PHR is stored on the Web and is retrievable based on a biometric ID or DL number, etc.

There are issues with all of these approaches; for example – the patient can't always remember to carry his/her wallet, or when injured may not have his/her wallet, so at the time when the patient most needs this information, any physically-carried devices may fail to meet the need.

This led to the suggestion of putting this information online and allowing some of it to be downloaded as needed, when the patient provides a passcode that can access the file. In some cases, the passcode could be biometric, so that only a patient's finger print or face print would be used to access the information. This would presumably work well in ED situations where the patient arrives unconscious or is in some other way unable to speak or is not coherent.

If any or a combination of these prove viable, then the need for the RHIO and MPI to satisfy emergency EHR needs is greatly reduced. There is still a need for quality and public health and research purposes, but these are not normally time-critical needs (except for pandemic or incidents of national significance where biological agents or weapons have been used).

Unorthodox Immunization and Disease Registries

Registries used for comparative effectiveness research are a problem unto themselves. They have patient ID information, and so fit in that sense at layer two, but they don't always work through RHIOs and they do have their own peculiar data formats. Most registries are created by independent entities focused on one disease or issue, rather than being created by some government organization, as they are in countries that have government-run healthcare. As a result of these unorthodox structures and lack of standards, many registries cannot accept data directly from some EMRs. RemedyMD is an EMR that supports several registries and is also a PQRI reporting provider.

Hopefully, as the healthcare in the U.S. shifts to a more preventative posture, various disease and immunization registries will get their standardization acts together and become partners in supporting interoperability standards, and cease being problems. In the meantime, if you want to participate in a registry, be prepared to accommodate whatever novel data structure they require, probably on a manual data entry level.

Layer Three – The Nationwide Specialized Layer

The third (nationwide) layer in the hierarchy includes various government agencies at the local, state and national levels; such as local and state public health agencies, quality organizations, the Centers for Disease Control, Homeland Security and the Department of Defense. Data at this level can be a mixture of patient-identified, and patient-de-identified information, depending on the group collecting it and the intended use.

The most important aspect of Figure 8.1 is how the data is moved from one system to another at the same or different levels in the diagram, and who controls the release and movement of that data, and is responsible for its integrity in each system it finds its way to.

The computer systems at each of these different levels and organizations in each level are all designed by different companies and organizations, so unless there are standards that all adhere to, the complexities of doing the conversion required to understand the data and move it, quickly becomes so complex and expensive, that interoperability cannot practically be achieved. That is why healthcare data standards have been defined and continue to evolve.

Patient Authorization – Clandestine Data Mining

Much patient information is already flowing among these three levels, without patients' explicit knowledge. For example, the average American is not aware that information on prescription refills (for 200 million Americans) is available automatically to insurance companies, as an aid in underwriting the risk for new policy applications. This is why underwriting that used to take a week or two, now happens in less than five minutes.

Americans implicitly give their "permission" for this transfer in the insurance policy application they fill out, often without explicitly realizing the scope of the data transfer they are authorizing or even that their prescription source data has been captured from their payment records and stored in a database in the first place.

Data going back up to five years is available on most Americans, showing their use of prescription medications, and by inference the diseases they have and are being treated for. For example, if a patient is filling antihypertensive drug prescriptions, it is presumed that they have high blood pressure by the insurance underwriter, and so on.

The point is that the collection of the data is done without informed, explicit patient awareness of what they are authorizing, and the release of the data is done with the permission they sign when they submit their insurance application form. Healthcare users must be careful about what patient-identified data is stored, the security of it, and who it can be released to.

Should such information be released to a person's employer? Should an employer be able to find out that the employee (or job candidate) is routinely taking anti-depression drugs, or drugs to slow HIV progression, or anti-seizure medications? Most people's first reaction is, no! But what if the person is applying for the position of airline pilot, or ferry boat captain, or train engineer where the safety and lives of hundreds of passengers could be at risk if they decide to commit suicide, or have a seizure while they are flying? Who decides such matters? What's the patient's role in that decision? The medication history information is already readily available to insurance companies. Think about it; when and how should a patient be notified when any of their personal information has been released by:

- The primary caregiver or hospital;
- Any secondary caregiver or specialists they have seen;
- Any company-paid-for annual physicals;
- By any RHIO that has built an ad-hoc EHR on them.

How is an audit trail created for what information has populated an EHR, where it came from, who has received this information, what specific subset of information has been received and what they have done with it? What if the audit trail is lost or destroyed? Who is the patient advocate that is the keeper of that audit trail?

Welcome to the brave new world of EMR, EHR, PHR, RHIO, HIE and flawless MPIs that exist in the NHIN. And you thought you were just automating your current paper-based office!

The Rise of Standards Committees

EMR buyers and the government are looking for a small set of well-defined and widely-adopted standards with which to harmonize communications among the diverse EMR stakeholders at all three layers in the just described Healthcare I.T. infrastructure (NHIN).

Rather than mandate a new standard and force everyone to comply with it (which as the U.K. found out, isn't so easy to accomplish), the U.S. government is encouraging all the current healthcare information players to play nice in the existing healthcare information "standards sandbox." That is exactly what has been happening at HL7 and ASTM, which have both come up with different EMR document standards, but are now harmonizing them. ASTM International is one of the largest voluntary standards development organizations in the world and are located online at www.astm.org.

How the Standards Process Operates
Standards begin with something that already works and has a following in the market. Standards typically occur when a leading vendor that has a successful way of doing something puts the word out that his way should become the "standard" way of doing it for everybody.

They then move inside the auspices of a group like HL7 or ASTM and create a "standard" that details how something is done. The general scheme is that they propose a standard based on everyone's input, then it goes for a ballot. If the ballot passes, it is tentatively accepted subject to appeasement of the negative votes on the standard. This generally results in allowing those who originally didn't support it, to get a key change or two into the tentative standard, and the process ends when they withdraw their objections. It then becomes an approved and published standard.

Standards are the glue of interoperability. Interoperability is about connecting all three layers of the U.S. healthcare system, from the patient and group practice, up to the public health, CDC, research and security uses of de-identified patient healthcare information. So standards are important.

Too Many Cooks, Too Many Non-Harmonized Standards
The problem is not that EMR developers don't support standards; rather, there are too many (sometimes conflicting) EMR data interchange standards.

The NCVHS report on Meaningful Use stated, "*Testifiers urged IHE and CAQH, as well as IHE and HITSP to reconcile their protocols.*"[9] That's bureaucrat talk for, "now get together and play nice kids." It's also great advice and will likely happen.

Until there is standards harmonization between IHE and both of these other organizations around one set of healthcare standards, no ubiquitous method to interoperability will emerge. Meaningful Use criteria could be a means of encouraging that harmonization.

As a physician who is purchasing EMR now, you need to include contract language that requires your EMR to fully support whatever harmonized standard finally emerges under Meaningful Use, within 12 months of when

[9] *Report on the Hearing on Meaningful Use of Health Information Technology.* Published May 18, 2009, p. 11 by the National Committee on Vital and Health Statistics

the MU functionality guidelines are finally issued (sometime before the end of 2009 and finalized in Q1-2010). Mark that on your issues to discuss with your lawyers.

Key Players in NHIN Standardization Efforts

If you read the earlier part of the NHIN discussion, you recall that there were a lot of organizations helping put the NHIN together. Here are some of them and what they are engaged in:

- CAQH (the Council for Affordable Quality Healthcare) www.caqh.org and their Committee on Operating Rules Exchange (CORE) supporting HIPAA X12N 270-271 transactions for patient eligibility inquiries, as well as HIPAA X12N 276-277. The organization says of itself, "*CAQH ... is a catalyst for industry collaboration on initiatives that simplify healthcare administration. CAQH solutions promote quality interactions between plans, providers and other stakeholders; reduce costs and frustrations associated with healthcare administration; facilitate administrative healthcare information exchange and encourage administrative and clinical data integration.*"
- The Healthcare Information Technology Standards Panel (HITSP) is an outgrowth of the American National Standards Institute (ANSI). Its mission is to serve as a cooperative partnership between the public and private sectors to achieve a widely accepted and useful set of standards that will support widespread interoperability among healthcare software applications and allow them to interact in a local, regional and national health information networks across the U.S.

Figure 8.4 Common HITSP Standards Summary

Standard ID	Version	Description or Purpose
IS-01	3.1	EHR Laboratory Report
IS-02	3.2	Biosurveillance
IS-03	3.1	Consumer Access to Their Healthcare Records
IS-04	2.0	Emergency Responder Electronic Health Record (ER-EHR)
IS-05	2.0	Consumer Empowerment & Access to Clinical Information Via Media
IS-06	1.1	Quality
IS-07	1.1	Medication Management
IS-08	1.0	Personalized Healthcare (Genetic Information)
IS-09	1.0	Consultation & Transfer of Care
IS-10	1.0	Immunization & Response Management

Continued

Standard ID	Version	Description or Purpose
IS-11	1.0	Public Health Case Reporting
IS-12	1.0	Patient-Provider Secure Messaging
IS-77	1.0	Remote Monitoring

CONNECT is a software solution that lets federal agencies securely link their existing systems to the NHIN. CAQH and HITSP are but two of the more than 20 federal agencies that collaborated to build CONNECT. Figure 8.4 shows some of the HITSP standards.

Web-Based EMR Interoperability

Some Web-based solutions promote interoperability between practices committed to the ASP solution, because many group practices are working out of one huge database that has a consistent structure for each. Thus, records could (in principle) be exchanged by any of the users of this Web-based EMR – offering the potential for EMR-to-EMR data transfers. If you are leaning towards a Web-based approach, be sure to broach the topic of such transfers as part of your license negotiations with the Web-based EMR developer. The mechanism used (with permission) to pass data on a Web-based EMR from one physician to another, is the same one that allows data from multiple physicians to be "consolidated" into a virtual EHR (Electronic Health Record); so Web-based EMRs potentially can be Web-based EHRs. See Doctations for an example of this approach.

There is a very important caveat however. The audit trail for the receiving EMR must maintain the fact that the data was originally captured/entered by the original physician, and not attribute it to the receiving physician. Also, it must be locked in such a way that the receiving physician cannot change it, but only append new information. While the new information would be marked with the name of the receiving physician, the copied information from the original record would not be. This is critical for medical record integrity purposes. The catch-22 is that no one Web-based EMR developer controls enough of the market to be a ubiquitous choice, so that's why emerging standards like HL7's EHR-S FM are increasingly important.

Congress and Healthcare

The U.S. healthcare system lags behind many other countries in deployment of EMRs into primary care settings. The U.S. also lags behind in deployment of Web-based portals that allow patients access to their healthcare records. Socialized healthcare systems, like those in Denmark and Finland offer both, however, achieving such integration in smaller countries is less challenging than in larger ones.

In the near future, the healthcare debate in the U.S. will intensify and this topic of patient record privacy and security may become a matter of national debate. With Democratic party control of Congress, the approaches that favor individual rights or less government control may be silenced or voted down.

There is money to be made off a patient's healthcare record and in the past, Congress has generally capitulated to special interests over empowering individuals or protecting their rights. The Meaningful Use (MU) roadmap, released in June 2009, suggests that patient access to their medical records is going to be an MU criteria for government reimbursement.

Obstacles Remain

A major focus of EMR adoption is prescription error reduction. CMS puts a 2 percent bonus in place for practices that achieve e-prescription over the next few years, but e-prescription (e-Rx) has issues particularly for controlled substances. The Drug Enforcement Administration (DEA) is trying to accommodate EMRs for controlled substance prescriptions and has recently issued new guidelines. DEA pilot programs have not removed all barriers to EMR use for controlled substances however. Moreover, since 2008, only about 6% of physician practices have adopted e-Rx systems like Surescripts/RxHub.[10]

Until the controlled substance issues are finally resolved, physicians may use e-Rx for most drugs and have to continue to hand write scripts for narcotics and other controlled substances. Look closely at the EMRs you are considering to determine whether they support Surescripts/RxHub and the latest DEA requirements that necessitate two-part authentication such as a password plus a machine-readable security token. The approach requires the equivalent of Level 4-authentication, something that many think will be burdensome to implement and inconvenient for physicians to use. If the requirements are too problematic, many practices may simply forego the use of e-Rx transmission.

Another disincentive for physicians is the breach of information of 700,000 patients by an as-yet-unidentified hacker into a major pharmacy benefits management system that was finally reported in September 2009. The breach occurred a year earlier and extortion attempts were made against the company and some of the individual patients affected. Such breaches seriously undermine public trust in having patient information available to too many organizations, some of which can't adequately protect it.

Wrap Up

While the information in this chapter goes beyond your office EMR, it is essential for you to understand the larger picture of where Washington is taking EMRs. The information in this chapter will help you firm up decisions

---

[10] *Doctors and the DEA.* By J. Moore. Published Sept. 2008, p. 17 by Government Health IT

from previous chapters and shed additional light on the question of choosing an EMR that is structured or unstructured, and that does or doesn't support standards sufficiently. The winds of change are blowing strongly now in healthcare and pressure is building towards EMRs with more structure and standards compliance. That doesn't mean that you have to comply, you can always sail against the wind, but be aware of what that decision means in light of the healthcare future envisioned by the Washington social engineers. Either way, your new EMR will empower you with the data you need to get to your destination.

Crucial Decision

What level of interoperability do you want with other EMRs, EHRs (or HIOs), PHRs and with Patient Registries and Public Health Agencies? Photocopy as needed or download this Scorecard from www.ehrselector.com

		In considering HIE beyond your practice, which of the following other entities do you want to be connected to initially, and within the next 5 years? Why?	
Connect Y/N?	**Entity**	**Approach**	**Comments/Discussion**
	Patient	My Portal	
		PHR	
	Hospital(s)	CCR/CCD/CDA	
		Shared Web-based EMR	
	Colleagues	CCR/CCD/CDA	
		Adobe PDF	
		Freeform Report	
	Disease Registry	Manual Entry	
	Immunization Registry	Manual Entry	
	Public Health	CCR/CCD/CDA	
	Rx Research Clinical Trials	Manual Entry	
	Other (specify)		
	Other (specify)		
	CDC, Homeland Security	CCR, CCD and HIPAA	

This is a Crucial Decision in which one choice eliminates others. In order to reach beyond EMR, you will need to support standards and have more structured documents. That may conflict with earlier tentative decisions and you may need to revisit them.

CHAPTER 9

Workflow Enhancement/EMR Customization

Crucial Decision
Do you want a WfME EMR or a conventional EMR?

This chapter also addresses the following questions:

- How concretely do you want workflow embedded into your EMR?
- Do you want your EMR to be mostly unchangeable or more dynamic?
- Does your previous decision on location of your EMR impact whether you can have a WfME EMR?

EMR Adventures

Smooth workflow and ease-of-use don't just happen in an EMR, nor are they attributes of every EMR. Workflow and ease of use are very much in the eye of the beholder; let's look in on Dr. Alex Glass.

Mr. Smith recently made an appointment with Dr. Glass, his ophthalmologist, because he was not seeing as clearly as he used to. Perhaps it was time for a new pair of glasses? When he arrived and had filled out all the conventional patient paperwork, he was ushered into the refraction room, where he noticed a well-known and popular EMR. He wondered if this new EMR didn't also include a patient kiosk, so that he could have entered his information directly, rather than on the paper form. Oh well, it seemed to be a new EMR, installed since his last visit a year or so ago, perhaps they were still implementing some features. When the physician assistant, Scott, was doing some initial tests, Mr. Smith asked, "That's a new EMR isn't it, how do you like it?"

"It's great," Scott replied. "I like it – I can get my work done quicker."

A bit later Dr. Glass came in to complete the eye exam. In the course of the conversation, Mr. Smith asked him the same question, "How do you like your new EMR?" Without hesitation Dr. Glass replied, "I don't like it!"

"Why not?" Smith asked, a little surprised.

"It doesn't have ophthalmology-specific templates, so it's not that easy for me to use," Dr. Glass replied, showing a bit of frustration. "Some of the information I need isn't on this screen, so I have to hunt around to other screens to find it. It slows me way down."

Mr. Smith was confused and said, "Your assistant seems to like it though."

Successfully Choosing Your EMR: 15 Crucial Decisions. By © Arthur Gasch and Betty Gasch.
Published 2010 by Blackwell Publishing

"Yes," commented Dr. Glass. "It's just fine for him, but it slows me down. It doesn't seem to have been developed for an ophthalmology specialty. I think we were one of their early ophthalmology installations. I wish I had done more research or gotten an EMR that had better thought out ophthalmology templates. I'm sure the EMR developer will offer some in time, particularly if I help them, but who has time to do that? It would have been better if the templates I needed had come with the system initially. It would have saved me a lot of time."

"How did you go about choosing your EMR?" Mr. Smith inquired.

"Well, I knew I needed to automate my charting, so I asked the service technician who takes care of my CPM system what he thought and which EMR systems he knew about. He said he also services an internal medicine practice and a pediatric practice, and both used this company and liked it fine," said Dr. Glass. "So that is the EMR developer I called. I should have done more research rather than assuming that because it worked for other specialties, it would work well for ophthalmology also. I'm sure it will get better, but it just slows me down right now."

This encounter was real, based upon an actual patient-physician encounter that occurred within the past year, and the EMR the doctor had purchased was a well-known, very popular and expensive brand name. It was also a CCHIT-certified one, so shouldn't it have been easy to use? Dr. Glass's experience was not an outright failure, but it wasn't a spectacular success either. What went wrong and how can deployments that succeed technically but don't quite live up to all user expectations be avoided?

What Went Wrong?

Dr. Glass's experience makes the point that just because an EMR is easy to use for one person (Dr. Glass's assistant), doesn't necessarily mean that it will be easy to use for another, in this case Dr. Glass himself. Ease-of-use is difficult to define and really quite personal. In essence, what Dr. Glass is saying is that his EMR isn't as easy-to-use as he would like it to be, but what is the source of the problem?

Is it that the doctor is unable to customize the workflow he is performing? The data all exists, but the EMR can't be modified to collect and present the specific information Dr. Glass needs at a particular place in his exam "workflow", he has to go hunting for it all over the EMR. EMRs don't automatically improve workflow, sometimes they make it worse; and it may take some customization to have any EMR truly enhance office workflow.

Is it that the EMR is missing key features? Perhaps he needs a field for "refraction" and one doesn't exist in the EMR's database.

So what is Dr. Glass's problem? Perhaps it is both points – he did not have some of the features he needed, and the ones that were present were difficult to locate when he needed them. What can be learned from his experience?

This chapter will point you in the direction of either a conventional EMR or an EMR with a user-accessible Workflow Management Engine (WfME). As you read this chapter realize that EMRs with WfMEs are relatively new and haven't gained that much traction yet. Over 95% of the EMRs deployed are conventional EMRs that do not have an integrated WfME. This is a technology that has not emerged as a commercial success in the U.S. EMR market as yet. We included this chapter because WfME seems to be the direction the market is moving towards and it is a potentially enabling technology. Also realize that it is difficult to assess your future electronic workflow needs when you are still working with your current, paper-based workflow. Most physician offices are not aware of their needs or all that is available in an EMR to meet those needs. Chapter 10 will help you in that area.

CCHIT Certification Doesn't Guarantee Ease-of-Use

Dr. Glass's first error was depending on CCHIT certification to provide an EMR that would meet his needs and be easy to use. While we do recommend buying EMRs with current CCHIT-certification, you may find that some non-certified EMRs are easier to operate than some of the certified ones. One reason for this is that they may intentionally provide less functionality than CCHIT specifies and therefore have simpler menu structures.

In some practice specialties, CCHIT specifications require more features than are actually needed, making CCHIT-compliant EMRs more complex with deeper menu structures to navigate. This situation is becoming worse as CCHIT continues to add more requirements for EMR certification. Meaningful Use requirements are likely to compound this problem further.

Specialty Installed Base Doesn't Guarantee Usability

The second flaw in Dr. Glass's approach is his assumption that because his EMR vendor had other installations in his specialty, it would meet all his needs. He based his decision on the belief that others in his specialty of medicine had done the preliminary work that he and his office staff should have done. Bad assumption.

Lest you think that this chapter's vignette applies to ophthalmology only, consider the following fact. The MSP ESP™ Portal (www.ehrselector.com) currently contains 43 EMR developers' product profiles. Thirty-seven of these (see Figure 9.1) have systems installed in gastroenterology practices. As you can see from the list, these are well-known and reputable EMR developers.

Yet, when we matched all 43 EMR developers' features against the 2008 list of function requirements provided by the American Gastroenterology Association (AGA), only four EMR products were CCHIT certified and a 100% match to the AGA profile of features needed! Each of the other 37 EMRs failed to provide one or more required AGA functions (recommendations that came from AGA members who had already adopted an EMR). If you chose one of the 37 other EMRs, no amount of customizing would compensate for missing (GI) features.

Would you be able to choose the four EMR products that match all GI specialty needs from the list of 37 shown in Figure 9.1? Would your hospital CIO? Would an EMR consultant that you might hire? Do you think that your CPM repair guy would know the four correct choices? Probably none of these people would without referring to an EMR feature summary check list of some sort. Even if a physician has the GI profile, evaluating its many requirements against any large cross-section of EMR developers is no small task, but it's one you can easily do yourself using the MSP EHR Selector (www.ehrselector.com).

The mismatch between EMR product solutions available and those that fit user's specialty needs and are easy-to-use, is common – not an atypical or an unusual result. This disparity highlights the differences between what features an EMR developer believes you need for your medical specialty versus what physicians actually practicing in your specialty (who have already adopted an EMR) find helpful. Since this example was extracted, we have added 23 more practice specialties (total 46) as new EMR assertions and the AGA Institute has issued their 2009 requirements list that has several key additional requirements. Things change, so make sure you are dealing with current information as you compare one EMR product to another.

Figure 9.1 EMR Developers with GI Installations

Company	Product
ABEL Medical Software	ABELMed EHR - EMR/PM V9
Allscripts	Enterprise EHR (Formerly TouchWorks)
American Medical Software	Electronic Patient Chart
CareData Solutions Corporation	The CareData Solution
Cerner Corporation	PowerChart Office
Cerner Corporation	Powerworks PM
Cerner Corporation	PowerWorks EMR
CHARTCARE	ChartCare EMR
CureMD Corporation	CureMD EMR
DavLong Business Solutions	MedInformatix
e-MDs	e-MDs Solution Series
eClinicalWorks	eClinicalWorks
Eclipsys Corporation	Sunrise Ambulatory Care
EHS	CareRevolution
Galen Corporation	Cerebella 2006
GE Healthcare	Centricity EMR
gMed	gGastro
Henry Schein Medical Systems	MicroMD EMR
iMedica Corporation	iMedica Patient Relationship Manager

Continued

iSALUS healthcare	OfficeEMR 2008
McKesson	Practice Partner Patient Records
McKesson	Horizon Ambulatory Care
MED3OOO	InteGreat EHR
Misys Healthcare Systems	Misys MyWay
Misys Healthcare Systems	Misys EMR
NextGen Healthcare Information Systems	NextGen® EHR
Noteworthy Medical Systems	NetPracticeEHR
Orion Health International	Concerto Medical Applications Portal
Pulse Systems	Pulse Patient Relationship Management
Sage Software Healthcare	Intergy EHR by Sage
Sevocity Division of Conceptual MindWorks	Sevocity EHR
VersaSuite	VersaSuite
VIP Medicine	SmartClinic

Evaluating Workflow Efficiency for Each Provider Role

Dr. Glass's third oversight is not understanding his own workflow needs; or if he did, not evaluating in sufficient detail whether his EMR optimized those workflow needs. Dr. Glass's EMR did fit his assistant's needs, but that may have been a coincidence. Dr. Glass functions in only the role of the physician in the total patient encounter workflow; other staff members fulfill different roles in the same patient encounter. Each person (role) makes up a part of the overall workflow of a physician office and it is the total workflow that an EMR ideally improves.

Dr. Glass may not appreciate the details of the tasks performed by other caregivers because that is not his role, which is why one person in an office can be perfectly happy with an EMR solution that drives another staff member absolutely nuts! This underscores the need for everyone in an office setting to evaluate how well an EMR meets their specific workflow needs, particularly if the candidate EMR has static workflow (explained shortly). Dr. Glass's experience would have been more positive if he had taken more time to research his and his staffs' workflow needs. This is important, because 20% of EMRs deployed fail to live up to their users' expectations, even today.

Workflow Transcends EMRs

Don't confuse workflow or ease-of-use with EMR or EMR-lite functionality like CPOE. Systems designed to optimize workflow are significantly different from typical EMRs. A good article about this subject appeared in a 2009 Healthcare Informatics article.[1] EMR capabilities are just a part of any overall

---

[1] *It's All About Workflow.* By Frank Poggio. Published Sept. 2009 by Healthcare Informatics

office workflow. Workflow encompasses the total encounter with a patient, from the time the appointment is made, to when the patient is scheduled and registered (not generally EMR functions), through all the documentation of the patient experience, including orders and tests, treatment and discharge plans (generally EMR functions), on until all claims have been submitted and paid (often practice management system or even third-party functions).

Workflow therefore encompasses your Computer Practice Management system (CPM), any EMR you are about to purchase and any independent systems that provide appointment confirmation reminders, insurance eligibility confirmation and even CPT coding, billing, correction, re-submission and ultimately collection. In the broadest context, workflow covers all aspects of the business process of healthcare delivery in your particular care setting, whether it be your office, the hospital, the ED, a home healthcare agency, a skilled nursing facility or wherever. However, because this book is about EMRs deployed in office settings, we will only be looking at the workflow management of the EMR component of your total office workflow.

Your Workflow Manager – Who is it Today?
Improving workflow is an important benefit that can be achieved with the right EMR (either conventional or WfME-enhanced), but it isn't automatic and it requires careful attention. In any care setting someone or some thing determines workflow. In your office today some people determine their own workflow – your office manager or billing person determines which bills are submitted when, etc. On the other hand, when you are seeing a patient and decide that an ECG needs to be run, you delegate that task to whoever is filling the role of "ECG technician." That may be the same person who is filling the role of "nurse," or it may be a diagnostic test person. In either case, you (as physician or physician assistant, nurse practitioner, etc.) are determining other's workflow. Obviously, this involves communication.

How do you handle communication like this currently? Perhaps a quick, "Could you do an ECG on the patient in room three?" as you pass in the hall, or duck your head into another exam room. How would you like to handle tasks like this using an EMR system? Would it be helpful if you could check the 12 Lead ECG box on your EMR screen, and let the system automatically add that task to the appropriate person's schedule? Is it alright with you to continue to have to seek out the person who needs to run the ECG, even while your new EMR bills for the ECG automatically?

How your EMR is designed will make a big difference in your workflow methodology – are you content with your existing manual workflow, or do you prefer a new, EMR-driven, more automated workflow? This is a place where you need to think out-of-the-box again. An EMR ideally does more than simply add a computer to your office. View an EMR as an enabling tool, one that can help you eliminate workflow bottlenecks, let you and your staff use time more efficiently and transform your entire patient encounter. It is important for you and your staff to determine whether any EMR you are seriously considering can meet your desired goals.

Workflow Learning Resources

If workflow (at least, in-depth workflow) is a new concept to you, we recommend you work through the next two chapters slowly and possibly refer to articles available from the Workflow Management Coalition that can help – go to http://www.wfmc.org/ for more information. An excellent article on workflow appeared in Advance for Health Information Executives. The Web link to this article is: http://health-care-it.advanceweb.com/Editorial/Content/Editorial.aspx?CC=171828.

The best reference however is from the "father of workflow management," Wil van der Aalst, in his book, *Workflow Management, Models, Methods and Systems*, published by MIT Press in 2002 (originally in 1997). However, it is rather technical and not healthcare specific in its discussion and illustrations. A resource that overcomes those limitations is the article, *Improving Practice Efficiency with EHR Workflow Management Systems* by Dr. Charles Webster[2]. It appeared in the V7N2 (2005) issue of Industry Alert™ newsletter and was based on the data provided from the EncounterPro EMR; it is still available on the www.medsp.com Web site. Dr. Webster has also been writing a book on this subject for the last two years; and his Web site has much useful information. He is also a frequent speaker at HIMSS. Workflow, as defined by the authors of this book, is based on a time-study approach; how much time each workflow task consumes. This is not the only approach to the topic.

Optimizing Information Workflow

Not everyone uses the time-study approach to workflow management; some look at workflow from the perspective of information flow management. In this approach, the question is, "In an ideal patient encounter, what information would you need at each step of the encounter and how would having that information expedite the actual encounter or improve its quality?" Then they make a list of the information needed, and determine:

- Is all of the information needed to diagnose and care for this patient available or not?
- If it's available, is it on the screen at present or not? If not, why not – is it a basic limitation of the EMR being considered?
- If it's not on the screen at present, where is it located and how much time and trouble does it take to find it in the EMR?

---

[2] Dr. Charles Webster, MD is Vice President of medical informatics at EncounterPro (formerly JMJ Technologies, Inc.), developers of the EncounterPro WfME EMR. He is a frequent speaker at HIMSS and TEPR on the subject of EMR workflow. Several of his presentations are viewable at http://www.encounterpro.com/online_presentations.html.

• Can the EMR be customized by someone (without programming) to bring the missing information needed to one screen, so there won't have to be time spent navigating through the EMR screens to gain access to it?

You can see where this is leading – it's another approach to determining how your current workflow could be affected after you adopt an EMR. The value of this approach is that it makes clear the issue of why EMR workflow enhancement is ultimately critical to EMR success.

If information is located and spread over various EMR screens, the EMR is going to be perceived as more difficult to operate, which is really an ease-of-use (or lack thereof) issue, which is high on the list of why EMRs fail in the market. Information needs to be in the one place where the caregiver can access and use it to provide care to the patient.

The basic idea to remember as you read on in this chapter, is that EMRs with embedded Workflow Management Engines (WfMEs) provide a means for someone in your office to modify the EMR's workflow (the provider roles and work tasks that comprise each type of patient encounter), and that most conventional EMRs do not have this ability.

Contrasting WfME and Static EMR Workflow

Let's contrast an EMR with static workflow versus an EMR with an embedded WfME that allows someone in your office to define/redefine workflow encounters, tasks, sequencing, etc. Let's call EMRs without the ability for someone in your office to change workflow, conventional EMRs. Conventional EMRs have limited abilities for change. They may allow EMR screen customization, or in some cases the ability for someone in your office to define new terms/variables, or some other minor ways to enhance usability of the EMR, but that is typically the extent of change they allow.

Sometimes conventional EMRs are designed to optimize the workflow of one particular user (often the physician who creates his/her "ideal" EMR). Sometimes conventional EMRs optimize work encounters around one practice specialty (the one that the physician who created it, works in). But total workflow design of any EMR encompasses all users, not just one physician's work items or one specialty's focus, and the limitations of this approach are obvious. In order for an EMR to be easy to use for many specialties, its workflow has to be fluid enough to accommodate the different encounters and work tasks of each specialty and each clinician associated with that specialty as well as all other clinicians and staff in the office. In order for an EMR to work well, especially in larger group practices, workflow must be designed not to inconvenience any user (nurse, receptionist, technician, physician).

So how do you distinguish between an EMR with a customer-accessible WfME and a conventional EMR? Not so much by their workflow reports, because both types of EMRs have an inherent workflow they are supporting. What ultimately distinguishes them is the ability of the user to change and redefine workflow without programming, from a high-level, user interface that the EMR with the user-accessible WfME provides. Conventional (static) EMRs do not empower this. In most other regards, they can be very much the same, as some of the features listed below reveal.

Often both static and user-accessible WfME EMRs provide similar workflow reports and some functions can also be common to both types of EMRs. Some conventional EMR sales people will point to these reports and functions as evidence that their EMR has a "workflow engine." Here are some features that either a conventional or a WfME-enabled EMR might include:

- Practice Workflow Status Summary Display – This feature will track all workflow activities and make the information available to the staff via a practice-wide, workflow summary display (sometimes called a White Board). It shows the status of each patient, what is the next activity, who is responsible for it.
- Workflow Reports – These reports (such as by encounter type) show the trend in the time consumed to complete each encounter, and the time that each component task in the encounter takes. This can help you find workflow bottlenecks that are blocking workflow productivity gains.
- Personal Task List – This feature will provide a list for each caregiver (physician, nurse, technician, etc.), showing what tasks need to be performed for which patients.

Nothing about these EMR workflow reports/functions reveals if it has a workflow engine, a tool to change the workflow the EMR provides. Nor do they show you, if the EMR does have a workflow engine, whether that workflow engine is accessible to your staff.

EMRs with User-Accessible Workflow Management Engines

You can determine if an EMR has a user-accessible WfME by looking at whether a tool exists that allows the user to get at, modify or redefine workflow. Here's what an EMR with a user-accessible WfME has to provide, as a minimum:

- Staff Role Definition Screen – A way to define what "role" everyone on staff performs. It's a table that answers the questions, "Who is/are the receptionists? Who is/are the office nurses? Who is/are the ECG or lab technicians? Who is/are the physician assistants? Who is/are the doctors?"
- Encounter Definition Screen – A way of defining what type of patient encounters your practice serves. It might be populated with items like, Annual Physical, Well-baby visit, Sick baby visit, in a pediatric practice. In an oncology practice the list would be different. In a surgical practice the list would be different again. The Encounter Definition Screen enumerates each of these types of patient encounters, and has a pointer to the work items required to complete them.
- Work Item Definition Screen – A description of each work item, and what encounters it is associated with. For example, work items might include – Greets the patient and verifies insurance coverage. Another might be – Escorts patient to exam room and takes patient's vital signs. Some work

tasks may be part of every patient encounter, like greeting the patient. Other work items may be part of only one type of encounter.

A work task can be consolidated when it is performed by one caregiver (role). For example, greets the patient and verifies insurance coverage, is combined into one task because both elements are performed by the receptionist. If in another office, the receptionist greets, but the business manager verifies insurance coverage, these would be two separate tasks, associated with two different caregiver roles (receptionist & business manager). Each office is different in how they define their workflow, based on their staff, the qualifications of the staff, how many roles each person performs, etc. An EMR with fixed workflow has a hard time combining tasks, because it has no sense of which caregivers (roles) perform which tasks.

The embedded Workflow Management Engine (WfME) uses tables that have a notion of all encounter types (and templates). The tables provide the information for all staff available to perform the encounters, all items that have to be performed in each encounter, and all information (clinical database elements) that need to be presented and completed to accomplish the task and move on to the next one.

Some user Workflow Management Engines are more sophisticated than others. The advanced WfMEs also have user-specific features, such as: when a task needs to completed, what to do if it doesn't complete on time (e.g. issue an alert), whether the task is mandatory or optional, whether the task has different pathways based on a patient variable (such as sex, age, lab values, pre-existing disease state and so on). The level of sophistication depends upon what areas the EMR with a user-accessible WfME allows the user to actually change the encounter, work items associated with an encounter, information required for each work item, the sequence of the items, their variations, what they trigger, etc.

An EMR with static workflow has no way for a physician office staff member to get into the "guts" of the EMR and tinker with workflow. Workflow is generally hard coded in by the programmer who designed the EMR, and exists in a lot of code and complicated decision structures.

Detailing WfME EMRs

So your crucial decision comes down to this. Do you want (need) this level of access to your EMR's work logic, or not? Do you want to be able to control your own workflow destiny, or not? Consider the implications of the functionality alluded to above before you decide. Consider the following:

• Automatic Screen Selection & Sequencing – Wading through dozens of templates or tabs on an EMR is time consuming, non-productive and slows down an encounter. Since a WfME EMR knows what the next task is for each caregiver (role), it also knows the next screen required to capture or document that activity. It also knows all of the clinical database items needed for that information. What if it can get all that information and present it to the caregiver responsible for doing the task, wherever he/she is working? Would that boost efficiency compared to the person figuring out what tabs the information is on, navigating to those tabs, finding the right fields to input the data to – manually?

You can think of these screens and definitions as "Information Organization Customizations," in that they are done during your EMR deployment and left alone for a time. As improvements in your workflow are discovered by the EMR users (your office staff), these functions can be redefined or modified from the initial definitions by someone in your office.

These changes can be either global to the whole practice, or particular to a specific role or even one user of the system. In fact, different users could have their own workflow tasks for the same patient encounters (if they wanted to). All this workflow definition/customization could be made by someone in your office, rather than depending on the EMR developer to accomplish. Let's look at an example.

- Alternative Actions for Work Items – These alternative actions can be user-defined in EMRs with user-accessible WfMEs. Suppose you have an Annual Physical (AP) patient encounter with all of its work items defined. Suppose you want to use this with three different patients – a 3-year-old patient, a 48-year-old female patient, and a 68-year-old male patient. Will their annual physical workflows be identical?

Not really. The 3-year-old patient would not need an ECG or prostate exam or PAP smear, but would need checks against weight and growth charts, immunizations and so on. The 48-year-old female would not need an ECG or prostate exam, but might expect a PAP smear and breast exam – different activities for the same EMR encounter. The 68-year-old male would need an ECG, a prostate check, and maybe a chest X-ray, some different lab tests and evaluation of any chronic conditions.

Three factors differentiate these patients; their gender, their age, and their chronic conditions/past medical history. It is likely that most EMRs, right out-of-the-box, don't have a separate workflow programmed in for each of these variations of the single AP encounter. In that case, you become your own workflow engine and navigate around the screens to find the items you need to include for each of these unique cases. The question is, why not let the EMR do that for you?

Think about the user-accessible definition screens, and the notion of mandatory or optional items. Think about using that information to select an "alternate action" in the work items. Some WfME EMRs give you all the tools to do this (once), so that every AP encounter thereafter can make these decisions, find and present the right information automatically.

Is defining workflow for any encounter a pain in the butt the first time? Definitely! But 5 years and hundreds, maybe thousands of encounters later, all of which are very efficient – would it be worth it?

EMRs with user-accessible WfMEs are a "new thing" in the EMR space. They represent an innovative direction that can empower your office, giving your staff the ability to modify the EMR to your actual workflow. This means both your current workflow and the smarter/better workflow you are going to evolve to, once you figure out that an EMR is not just about automating your paper-based workflow; but rather, creating a new and more efficient electronic workflow. Is this the direction you want to go?

Workflow Enhancement After Initial Deployment

Once you have automated your clinical charting with a conventional EMR, the WfME EMR or the Software-as-a-Service (SaaS) approach, you would think office workflow would go faster than charting on paper, right? Maybe or maybe not. You would also think your office would work more efficiently and therefore create time and staff resources to care for more patients. Maybe or maybe not. Obtaining these desired advantages depends upon how efficiently your office works as a "paper office" and how well you all learn to work as an "electronic, paperless practice." Reaching electronic office efficiency will take some time and practice but the possibilities with automation are many and real. If you improve your practice workflow on your initial deployment, congratulate yourself and your staff, because that isn't everyone's experience. Many practices have to return to looking at workflow issues after they have initially deployed their EMR.

There is a tendency to carry forward the systems that worked from your paper-based office, but that approach will not empower you to get the most out of your new, electronic charting system. You may deploy the paper-based way initially, but after a time you may be ready to make changes in your patient encounter workflow. How much change (and how soon) will depend on the EMR you choose, how well it is interfaced (or integrated) to your practice management system, and what level of workflow customization it supports. Workflow enhancement doesn't just happen because you convert to an EMR. For that to happen you will need to:

- Understand your current paper-based workflow. (The next chapter will help you do that); and
- Envision your new (and different) electronic-based workflow and make any adjustments needed.

None of the automation possibilities are available with your paper-based workflow, which is why so many physicians don't think about these items (initially) in their electronic workflow concept. Many EMR users don't take advantage of the more advanced functionality that their EMR may already have, because they aren't thinking "electronically." Begin to think about the right questions mentally. How can you reinvent and imagine your office workflow based on the power of this new technological tool? Answer that question correctly and you will see the largest workflow and productivity gains.

Daily Interactions with a WfME EMR

From a daily perspective, interaction with the WfME consists of identifying the specific staff on-duty that day so the EMR can "look them up" and determine what roles they fulfill. This is done as part of a staff schedule and sign-in/authentication process. Likewise, the WfME needs to know what patient encounters are scheduled, which in theory can be retrieved from your practice management system's patient schedule for that day – assuming your EMR is on "speaking terms" with your CPM. The WfME EMR then just works in the background, keeping track of where each staff member is working and what patient encounter they are working on, and what tasks are currently being done.

In a nutshell, the WfME-empowered EMR "cooperates" with every caregiver, optimizing their ability to perform the current task they are working on, for whatever patient encounter they are involved in, and keeps them informed of the next most critical task for them to start.

It all may sound too good to be true, and some physicians think it is. It takes some work, after all, to tinker with your workflow encounters. Who does that? And when, after hours? As with any EMR approach, WfME EMRs have their detractors.

WfME EMR Detractors

Not everyone is jumping on the WfME-bandwagon. WfME EMRs today only support about one-fourth of medical specialties, so this approach may not be available to you at all depending on your practice specialty. Only one hospital inpatient system – Siemens Soarian – is WfME enhanced, so there is not a large choice in the hospital arena.

A related criticism is that while WfME EMRs excel in optimizing workflow, their basic EMR functionality is sometimes lacking or in conflict with WfME features. For example, if you want highly granular structured data, and also want your EMR to use the MEDCIN front-end vocabulary, but your WfME-enhanced EMR has a proprietary front-end vocabulary, alas you will not be able to use MEDCIN (this is the case for the EncounterPro EMR, as one example). Which is more important to you – workflow enhancement or the benefits of standardized, front-end medical vocabulary, concepts, decision support?

These are real trade-offs to be considered and these trade-offs will surface conflicts in your goals. You may want the best possible workflow as a daily goal, but you may want decision support, a standard vocabulary, the ability to do longitudinal summaries of patients across the practice and other features that require a structured, front-end vocabulary too. A good, real-time, Web-based, EMR selector tool will allow you to determine which vendors can provide the functionality for each of your goals, and highlight any vendors that can satisfy all/most of them. It also allows you to run functionality scenarios where you consider the trade-offs.

WfME EMRs are mostly available from smaller and emerging companies, whose financial staying power is not well established in the market, and therefore are not as safe to deal with (the exception is Siemens' Soarian WfME EMR as they are a large company). Once an EMR application is written (in an older programming language to run on an older computing platform) it's quite a problem to "add on" a workflow engine. In fact, it takes an entire rewrite of the EMR application, which is a costly and time-consuming endeavor.

Another big issue is that WfME EMRs are deployed as in-office software and not as over-the-web, browser-based, SaaS (ASP) services. You would eliminate the ASP approach if you want a WfME EMR. There are two alternatives if you choose an EMR with static workflow; either an in-office deployment or a Web-based, Software-as-a-Service (ASP) Web server. These approaches are detailed in Chapter 6, so let's return to workflow.

A Fork-in-the-Road Decision

Physicians tend to like the WfME approach, but, as just stated, aren't typically Web-based and the Siemens Soarian WfME EMR is expensive and hospital-oriented. So what to do? Clearly there are trade-offs. What's right for your office? Only you can decide after weighing all your priorities. If you choose a conventional EMR (without a WfME) you are sentencing yourself to remain as your practice's "workflow manager." If you go with a WfME EMR, you will be giving up the ASP model, possibly a structured, front-end vocabulary, and it may not support more than 6-8 practice specialties well. Hey, no one promised that Crucial Decisions would be easy decisions! If you had begun to narrow in on the remote Web server, ASP model, you may have to revisit that decision if you want to look into a WfME EMR as your choice.

No matter what you finally decide, make sure that any candidate EMR "fits" your initial workflow well – whether or not it has an embedded WfME. Demonstrations are the way to assess that, and a workflow analysis of YOUR office is the way to document your paper-based, current workflow. Then you have something against which you can measure any candidate EMR solution you are considering. We'll help you with a process for assessing your current workflow in Chapter 10, but assume it's already done for now and let's focus on how to make EMR demonstrations meaningful to you.

Demonstrations to Assess Workflow

Relevant EMR demonstrations are key to getting a feel for a product's inherent organization of tasks and workflow. How many clicks does it take, how many screens have to be accessed to do each step in your real workflow? What if the EMR uses a template for each condition, and the patient has a primary complaint and also a chronic condition? How does each candidate EMR integrate the data that needs to be collected into one screen and eliminate the overlapping fields? If this isn't done, how many screens do you have to navigate through to actually complete the chart for both patient conditions? How much time does the navigation consume? Are the quality measures of the EMR smart enough to pull and display the primary and chronic Physician Quality Reporting Initiative (PQRI) measures, or do you have to do that manually? And so on.

Take the Controls – Fly!

No EMR salesmen are likely to cover these questions for you in their demo of their system. Have the sales people stand up while you sit down in front of the computer. Let them assist you through the EMR using several patient encounters that you see every day. Then determine, "How do you feel about using this system? Can you learn to do this everyday so that it becomes second nature to you? Will it become second nature to you in time? Are you practicing better medicine with this EMR? Are the alerts helpful or just annoying? Can they be minimized without being disabled?"

Does the EMR have a user-accessible WfME? If it does, you should be able to view a screen of the individual tasks that make up any encounter's workflow and determine whether the workflow task sequence matches the way you actually function in your practice currently.

Try changing or deleting a task or try merging two separate tasks into one using the Workflow Editor's Task Manager. Then save your new task definition(s). Next, begin charting that encounter and see if the task you deleted, changed or merged, is actually gone, altered or combined. If it is, you are probably working with an EMR that does have a WfME and will allow you to change/redefine workflow.

On the other hand, if there is no Workflow Editor that displays a list of all tasks in an encounter, you probably are seeing a demo of an EMR that has static workflow that can only be changed by the EMR developer (at extra cost) and not by you or your team.

If the EMR you are considering is one with static workflow, be sure its inherent out-of-the-box EMR workflow shown during your product demonstration is a great fit, because it will involve real dollars and time delays to get the EMR vendor to change it. All this isn't to say that an EMR with static workflow isn't a good choice. Indeed, it is the choice that the vast majority of physicians make either because they don't realize there are WfME-enhanced EMRs, or they find that such systems have other limitations that disqualify them for the specialty they practice in. These limitations can be items such as no templates for their common patient encounters, or lack of a good front-end vocabulary or any of a myriad of other details. On the other hand, if you select a WfME-enhanced EMR you can let the EMR become your workflow manager as it allows you to change some items when the EMR doesn't do what you want it to.

Wrap Up

There is no perfect EMR yet, maybe there never will be. You can't have everything you want, but you can get what you need to make your practice more efficient, safer, more profitable, more marketable. You are definitely faced with some trade-offs in selecting an EMR.

Choices highlighted in this chapter may affect decisions you thought you had settled in previous chapters. In any case, as the integration of WfMEs in EMRs becomes more common, fewer trade-offs will be required. This chapter has shown you how to determine if a candidate EMR has an embedded WfME. The next chapter will guide you through your encounter-by-encounter inventory of all your patient encounters, and to note each of the tasks associated with the workflow you are currently performing in your paper-based system.

Armed with your Physician Office Workflow (POW) information (next chapter), you will be ready to evaluate demonstrations of any candidate EMRs to determine how well they accommodate the workflow you are currently using, or would like to use in the future.

Crucial Decision

Do you want an EMR that you can easily customize and can adapt to your office workflow or can you accept a conventional EMR with out-of-the-box workflow that cannot be extensively customized by users? Photocopy as needed or download this Scorecard from www.ehrselector.com

We would like to explore office staff ability to manage the following features (without programming) on an EMR:
Ability to define/assign all staff roles.
When each person signs in and is authenticated, EMR associates person with all role(s) they may perform.
Assign personal task list to each staff member.
Supports and displays a shared task list. A task is automatically deleted on completion.
Provides a summary of workflow tasks (personal work task list) to each staff member, & updates it in real time as new tasks are triggered/added.
Support of users using different work process definitions.
For each staff person, on their terminal/PC, WfME presents all data entry fields and reference information required to finish current work task onto ONE screen.
Ability to define a patient encounter, and all the work tasks required to accomplish it.
Work tasks to be defined to work differently based on patient characteristics.
Allows any work item to have completion deadline, after which it executes optional behavior(s).

This is a Crucial Decision in which one choice eliminates the other. If you choose a WfME EMR, you eliminate all ASP SaaS vendors. You may want to read the next Chapter (10) and go through the Physician Office Workflow (POW) analysis found there before making this decision.

These are examples of what a WfME EMR can empower. If you checked any of the options, at least try out a WfME EMR. If you are not certain you need these options, go to Chapter 10 and the POW workflow analysis as this will help you decide. If you are sure you want a conventional EMR (either an ASP SaaS EMR or one with static workflow), stay with that choice (but make certain that the workflow fits your office needs like a glove!).

Any other items we need to think about now:

This is a Crucial Decision in which one choice eliminates the other. If you choose a WfME EMR, you eliminate all ASP SaaS vendors. You may want to read the next Chapter (10) and go through the Physician Office Workflow (POW) analysis found there before making this decision.

CHAPTER 10

Documenting Your Office Workflow

Crucial Decision
How can you document your current paper-based workflow so you'll better know what you need in an electronic one?

EMR Adventures

Before you decide whether to spend the time doing a paper-based workflow assessment (the subject of this chapter), read the scenario that follows and glance through the Physician Office Workflow (POW) process described.

Now let's look in on Dr. Karen Bell's practice.

Dr. Karen Bell is still in the process of determining (along with her business manager, Mary, and her receptionist, Linda), what EMR is best for the practice. In the vignette described in Chapter 3, Mary and Linda approach Dr. Bell with a sense of being overwhelmed by the thought of a new EMR, but even more so by replacing their older Computer Practice Management (CPM) system at the same time. At that point in time, Dr. Bell agreed to look at replacing their CPM system along with obtaining a new EMR, but now she is wondering whether she can really afford this. The three people are meeting to discuss their progress in making their EMR product selection decision.

Dr. Bell starts the discussion by saying, "I know I told you that we could possibly look at replacing our CPM at the same time we obtain the new EMR, but honestly, I am not sure we can afford to do both. I would really like to, especially with the concerns that you have both brought to me about how this impacts you. I am just not certain how to determine whether we can afford to right now."

Mary replies, "I may have a solution – at least a possible way to figure this out. My friend, Ann, over in Dr. Rodriguez's office, said that they took time to figure out how each person in the office worked during all their different patient encounters. That allowed their business manager to determine what they earned or lost on each of type of patient encounter. Ann said that they were advised by others that this was an important early step in their EMR decision process. She also said that they learned a lot about their office workflow that they previously did not know."

Successfully Choosing Your EMR: 15 Crucial Decisions. By © Arthur Gasch and Betty Gasch.
Published 2010 by Blackwell Publishing

"That's great, but HOW did they do this and how long did it take?" Dr. Bell wanted to know.

"Not long, a few hours spread over a couple of weeks. They made a list of all the different encounter types in their practice and gave it to everyone. Each staff person then noted the start and end time for each patient encounter type, and then they turned the information into their office manager. They only documented each type of patient encounter one time. It didn't take long to document times for the patient encounters that they saw frequently – for the patient encounters that they did not see as often, it took a couple of more weeks to get data. Once the staff got the completed forms to the office manager, she simply entered the data into a spreadsheet she found on the Internet, which totaled up the figures for her," said Mary.

"That sounds doable," commented Karen.

"There was another advantage Ann told me about. They had each person note the bottlenecks they found on each patient encounter; the places where they were getting hung up and delays were occurring. That surfaced some surprising issues such as how much time their nurses spent on the phone authorizing pharmacy refills and doing other things like that, which everyone knew was a problem but nobody realized exactly how much time these work items were taking."

"I wonder how much time we spend doing that in our practice too?" Karen thought out loud. "I also wonder how much time you spend changing billing codes and resubmitting them until we finally get paid!"

"A lot more than I would like," commented Mary. "I guess if we decide to do this workflow inventory, we will find out."

"Well, get a copy of the forms, and let's give it a try," said Dr. Bell.

Determining Practice Workflow Bottlenecks

The advice Mary brought to Dr. Bell is wise and assessing office workflow can be an eye-opening experience for many physician offices. This chapter helps you find practical ways to document both your workflow and your cash flow for each encounter. The workflow bottleneck you note may unmask some long ignored issues that you want to change before you adopt your EMR.

This chapter continues the discussion of the previous crucial decision, deciding whether you want an EMR based on a user-accessible, workflow management engine (WfME), or a conventional EMR that lacks user workflow customization. It also focuses on a process you can utilize to document your current, paper-based workflow that can be used as a guide for candidate EMR demonstrations and as a baseline for measuring post-deployment impact on workflow as a result of implementing an EMR.

It doesn't matter whether you ultimately decide to select a WfME-based EMR or a more conventional EMR, you will still be confronted with addressing workflow bottlenecks. Completing the assessment of your paper-based current workflow will take some effort and involve everyone in your practice; but it is a good way to hone in on a consensus for what your office really needs/wants from an EMR. We call the process the POW (Physician Office Workflow) Study and the details follow shortly. We recommend that you commit to do this workflow assessment for the following reasons:

- It provides a wonderful road map of how your practice works and which specific patient encounters are candidates for workflow optimization;
- It provides an excellent means of evaluating EMR product demonstrations; you can check out your actual office workflow (what you do for each of your patient encounters) against any EMR to determine how well that EMR is able to implement your workflow right out-of-the-box;
- It provides an effective way of determining what EMR customization will be required to better accommodate your office operations;
- It provides a baseline measurement for comparing your workflow AFTER your EMR is adopted, allowing you to determine and document any workflow gains achieved;
- It provides the basic information for discussing staff workflow trade-offs, so that one staff member can see how a change in their work could empower the overall efficiency of the entire office by making the work items of other staff easier or more productive.

Establishing a Workflow Efficiency Baseline

Prior to selecting an EMR is a good time to look anew at your current office workflow and document any problem areas. Ask yourself some questions. Will simply adopting an EMR alone overcome these problems? Would more problems be overcome by deploying an integrated EMR/CPM system? What will it take to reduce claim rejections, improve receivable days-outstanding, increase patient capacity, or bill for all justified services provided to your patients? Completing the Physician Office Workflow (POW) Study described in this chapter will help answer these questions.

Visualize EMR Improvements

Encourage everyone involved to begin to visualize how the adoption of an EMR could change (improve) your current office as the office goes through the POW process. What tasks are done sequentially now, that could be done simultaneously with an EMR? Any identified and resolved (by EMR adoption) will result in workflow gains. Look closely at the workflow bottlenecks your POW study identifies.

Take into account your decisions from previous chapters. If you are planning to implement a patient kiosk, how is your receptionist feeling about helping patients find and complete the "Patient Guided Interview" form on the kiosk, and showing them how to enter required data? Are you planning on adopting e-Prescribing in your new EMR, for example? What will that do to your current "approve refill requests" workflow and which of the office staff will it affect? How much time will it save? Adopting an EMR touches many staff members.

Remain sensitive to each staff person's feelings about workflow changes, because the POW will surface insecurities about the EMR adoption process. How you handle these will determine staff enthusiasm about EMR adoption. It will also help you determine what new staff training will be needed (e.g. the receptionist needs to assist patients in working with the kiosks)? Are there any staff role changes that will have to be made? Answering such questions with sensitivity and concern can quench staff fears about job security or role changes in adopting EMR. In fact, fear of needed changes may be a reason that some staff are (overtly or covertly) lukewarm about EMR deployment. Dealing with hidden fears sensitively but candidly is an important part of moving your EMR deployment forward during this critical examination of non-automated office workflow.

The POW Study reveals areas where current workflow is less than optimal and arms you to speak to EMR developers concerning their basic EMR workflow. Is it static? Does it fit your now-documented workflow? Answers will guide you in deciding whether you should adopt a conventional EMR or would be better served by a user WfME-based EMR.

Preparing for the Physician Office Workflow (POW) Study

Since this book's subject matter is EMR, the POW Study is focused primarily on the medical charting aspects of your overall office workflow, and ignores work items that are more related to your Computer Practice Management system (CPM). We did not include billing work items nor some more medically-oriented tasks such as loading of a patient's formulary prior to their arrival. However, if you are toying with the idea of replacing your current CPM, or if your CPM only provides scheduling and simple billing system functionality (it does not assist you with work items such as automatic notification of scheduled office visits, for example), by all means consider an integrated EMR/CPM rather than just an EMR solution.

The point of performing a POW Study is so that you better understand how your paper-based office currently functions, where the bottlenecks are, and how EMR adoption might improve efficiency. Therefore, both clinical and non-clinical personnel participate because all people involved in your practice will be impacted by whatever EMR is chosen (particular if it's an integrated EMR/CPM product).

Forms mentioned in conjunction with the POW Study are found at the Web site, www.ehrselector.com. Whether you are doing your POW Study totally on paper or you are going to use the POW Study Spreadsheet (the calculations needed are built in to the Spreadsheet, which improves your workflow), print out the forms so that they are in front of you as you read through the instructions that follow.

The approach is straightforward and begins with setting up the forms you will need by completing the POW Encounter Checklist. A sample portion of the POW Checklist is shown in Figure 10.1, with examples of the Encounter

Name/Description filled in. The following setup tasks can be performed by your office billing manager (or whomever), preferably by downloading the spreadsheet you can find at www.ehrselector.com (or on paper once these forms are printed).

Item No.	Encounter Task Label	Encounter Name/Description (2+ Words)	Encounters Per Month	Done
1	AP	Annual Physical	100	☐
2	WBV	Well Baby Visit	55	☐
3	SBV	Sick Baby Visit	75	☐
4	PE	Pre-School Exam	25	☐
5	SP	School Physical	25	☐
6	NA	Newborn Assessment	15	☐
7	ASO	and so on		☐

Figure 10.1 POW Checklist of All Encounter Types

Keep this spreadsheet as your master and work by using "file save as" to make copies of it. Follow these steps.

1 Enter the 10-15 (maximum 20) most frequently-performed patient encounters your office sees on the POW Checklist, (first tab in the spreadsheet) as shown in Figure 10.1. Also enter your practice name in the box provided and enter the number of Encounters of each type that occur in a month in your practice. This is your master copy.

2 Save a copy of this spreadsheet for each person participating in the study. If there are five participants, you will need to save five copies.

3 Next, open each worksheet just saved and enter the Role of one person involved. In this example – the receptionist. Each will have the name of the practice and the number of procedures, and only differ in the role of the person who will be filling out the survey. Now, your POW Checklist is ready; save each file after you have entered the Role (or person's name). One set for the receptionist, the physician(s), the nurse(s), the billing manager, the clinical specialist, the physician's assistant and whoever else will assist in gathering your office information.

4 Print out a copy of each POW Checklist and put it into a one-half inch binder to be given to the appropriate people. The only difference among POW Checklists is each person's Role (the Encounter/Name Description and Encounters per Month are the same for each person).

There are 20 tabs along the bottom of each spreadsheet, labeled 1 through 20. Each one is an Encounter Work Item List (Figure 10.2) for one of the Encounters you defined in Step 1. They have been filled in for you with all the header information – including Encounter ID, the Role Name, the Name of the Patient Encounter, and the Encounters per Month, each generated from the Encounter Name/Description area from the POW Checklist, if you use the online spreadsheet. These are all linked to the one POW Checklist (the first tab in the spreadsheet. You will have as many Encounter Name/Descriptions as you chose to fill in on the POW Checklist (up to 20) automatically generated. This will be ROLE specific, e.g. a physician will have a different list than a receptionist.

Enounter ID	Role Name		©Medical Strategic Planning - Physician Encounter Workflow Model	Page 1
AP	Receptionist	Practice Name	Your Practice Name Goes Here	
Name of Patient Encounter:		Encounters per Month	Documented Month ___ of Year ___	
Annual Physical		100		

Task ID	Item No.	DIRECT Work Item Description (entered by person doing Work Item)	Minutes Used	Document Bottlenecks Encountered Below	Gating Dep
	1	Greet Patient	0.5		
	2	Take Insurance Information	1.0		
	3	Give Patient Forms to fill out	0.5		
	4				
	5				
	6	Make Next Appointment	3.0		
	7	Receive Copayment (or entire payment)	2.0		17
	8				
	9				
	10				
	11				
	12				
	13				
	14				
	15				
		DIRECT Total	7.0	Minutes	

Task ID	Item No.	INDIRECT or SUPPORTIVE Work Item Description (entered by person doing Work Item)	Minutes Used	Document Bottlenecks Encountered Below	Gating Dep
	16	Pull Patient's Chart	2		
	17	Call Insurance Co - Verify Eligibility	7		
	18	Re-File Patient Chart	1		
	19				
	20				
		INDIRECT Total	10	Minutes	

Figure 10.2 POW Encounter Work List Form (Tab 1) for Receptionist

5   Print out each sheet (spreadsheet tab) and add it to the appropriate binder, behind the POW Checklist. The finished binder for each person will have a POW Checklist and an Encounter Work Item List page for EACH Encounter you will be studying. You will have a populated binder for the receptionist, the physician(s), the nurse(s), the billing manager, the clinical specialist, the physician's assistant and whoever else will assist in gathering your office information.

6   Hand out each binder to the appropriate person (Role) in your office and show them the forms. Instruct each person to pencil in the Work Items that they routinely perform for each type of Patient Encounter in their binder. The TOP part of the Encounter Work Item List form (Work Items 1-15) is for work done directly with the patient. Any indirect work (such as setup work done before the patient arrives or after they leave, or during their visit but when they are not actually present) is listed on the BOTTOM of the form (as Work Items 16-20). Have them complete this prior to a Kick-off Meeting to be held on whatever date you choose.

7   Include in each binder a printed announcement of your Kick-off Meeting date and instructions for all typical Work Items to be filled in by then for each person's Encounter Work Item List sheets.

The Study Kick-off Meeting

Prior to actually beginning your POW Study, once each person has filled in their Work Items for each of the 10-15 Encounter Worksheets in their binder, have a brief (luncheon) meeting and share/review the listed Work Items on each person's Encounter Work Item List (this can be a sample from each person participating rather than going into great detail). The goal of this meeting is to surface any Work Items performed routinely for any Encounter that may have been overlooked. It's also a chance to harmonize the level of detail captured in the Work Item list. The goal is not too little detail, but not too much either. Let's listen in again to Dr. Bell, Mary (the business manager), Linda (the receptionist), Amy (the billing clerk) and Julie (the nurse), as this very topic comes up at their luncheon meeting. They have just started to share, and Linda speaks first. They have put her Encounter Work Item form up on the computer-projector on the screen (whiteboard or wall) so everyone can see it (or you can pass around paper copies of the form).

As Linda quickly points out her direct and indirect Work Items, she is all set to sit down and take a deep breath – after all it's never easy to go first. A question comes quickly from Julie. "Linda, since you perform all of these tasks in rapid succession when the patient comes in, why not list them as one Work Item? After all, there aren't too many lines on these forms."

"I can do that, I'll change the form," replies Linda.

"Wait a minute," interjects Amy. "These are separate work items, not ONE work item, aren't they? There are plenty of lines, why should they be combined?" she asks.

"Seems confusing, what should Linda do, how do we handle this, I can see both points-of-view," says Mary. "We don't want to make this harder than it needs to be by putting down every little item, but we don't want to miss or overlook anything important either," she continues.

"Interesting," comments Dr. Bell. "What does The Book say about this? You know, the Successfully Choosing Your EMR Book, we have all been reading?" she asks.

"Let me look," says Mary, who turns quickly to Chapter 10 – Documenting Your Office Workflow and begins reading at the 'When Not to Combine Work Items' paragraph.

"That was helpful," comments Dr. Bell. "Now we all know what to do?"

"It clears it up for me," says Linda. "Us too," comment the others.

So what did they decide? (You do believe in the "Never Ending Story" don't you?) Read on.

When Not to Combine Work Items

Many Work Items can be combined but you may want to keep some Work Items listed separately as this will allow you better comparison of the *before and after* deployment of your EMR office workflow. You might be tempted to combine the three Work Items performed by the receptionist when the patient arrives into one Work Item. In some cases this would be fine, however in others, it could cause you to lose a valuable piece of information. For example, what if your practice is planning on rolling out patient kiosks for Guided Patient Interviews as part of your new EMR? If all three Work Items are combined, you lose information about the "handing the patient the clipboard with the information to be completed" Work Item (even though it probably only takes 30 seconds). Then, after you deploy the patient kiosk with your EMR, you may want to come back and see how much additional time it takes (if any) to: (1) orient the patient to the computer kiosk, (2) get the form on the screen and (3) help the patient get started filling in the form.

The kiosk orientation is likely to take more time than just handing the patient a clipboard, but how much more? Without the individual data, you are left to guess. In this case an educated guess might be fine (30 seconds), but in others (where the time is less certain for an existing Work Item), it is better to have it broken out in the Work Item List than integrated into several others.

To figure out which approach is best for your office, determine whether you think you will want to know specifics for any change you anticipate making to your workflow as a result of your EMR deployment. Dr. Bell's office opted to split the Work Items because they had decided to explore placing kiosks for patient-entered data, along with their new EMR. At your kick-off review meeting, discuss such issues and combine as many Work Items performed at one time as possible, as long as doing so won't eliminate data that might be useful in retrospect, after your new EMR is deployed.

Before your POW Study is completed, you will probably remember or discover some Work Items that you did not think to list when you made up each initial Encounter Work Item List. That's no problem, simply use the blank lines remaining on the form to write in the remembered task (in either the Direct or the Indirect/Supportive Work Item columns), and then note the time these newly entered Work Items require.

Populate the Encounter Form with Work List Items

Next, each person, working from their own binder, will enter the times for Work Items they actually perform for each of the types of encounters done in your office on their Encounter Work Item List form. The purpose of the binder is so that the timing of each Work Item can be filled in as the patient encounter is occurring. Each person can also briefly note any problems or bottlenecks that happen during the patient encounter. Do this using a pen or pencil but write legibly as someone will be transcribing what is written into the spreadsheet previously mentioned.

The sample case in Figure 10.2 shows that the receptionist has entered some Work Items in the Direct (patient care) Work Item Description area (at the top of the form) and some in the Indirect/Supportive Work Item Description section (at the lower part of the form). For the receptionist, the Direct Work Items fall into two groups – those performed when the patient arrives and those performed when the patient has completed his/her visit. That is the way the receptionist has listed her Work Items, leaving a couple of lines between each of her entries in order to write in any Work Items that she may have overlooked during her setup phase but which she discovers when the POW Study is actually performed.

In this specific case there were three such tasks: (1) pulling the patient's paper chart, (2) filing the patient's paper chart, and (3) calling the insurance company to verify the patient is still covered by the plan listed on their insurance card. They have all been entered (see Figure 10.2).

Dependencies and Gating Factors

In some cases, a Work Item may depend on some other Work Item being completed and is, therefore, a gating factor. In the case of the receptionist's Work Items, the "Call Insurance Company – Verify Eligibility" is a gating factor (shown on the form in red in Figure 10.2), as it determines when direct Work Item 7 – "Receive co-payment (or entire payment)" can actually be done. Unless Work Item 17 is completed before the patient arrives at the check out/payment area, the receptionist won't know what payment amount to collect. Enter the number of any gating factors in the "Gating/Dep" column of the Encounter Work Item list, just as the receptionist did by Work Item 7.

Any Work Item, either indirect or direct, that is a gating factor for other Work Items, has a strong potential to become (or may already have become) a bottleneck in your office's workflow process. It is a Work Item ripe for attention and some sort of automation.

Enhanced Workflow Opportunities

In many offices the insurance verification task is done automatically the day before a patient visit by an integrated EMR/CPM system. In this alternate, electronic workflow, the payment status is already known when the patient arrives. Likewise, a well-integrated EMR/CPM can download the patient's drug formulary at the same time, so it's available to the physician/clinician during the patient encounter in the exam room. This enhances office productivity – in this example, for the receptionist (and for others as well).

In our receptionist's case, Work Item Seven (Verifying Insurance) could be eliminated for every patient (across all encounters). This would not only eliminate the dependency (Work Item 17), but also Work Item Two (Take Insurance Information) – saving a total of eight minutes (in case of the sample shown in Figure 10.2). That's eight minutes times the number of encounters per year. If a physician sees an average of 30 patients per day and works 220 days per year, that's a savings of four hours per day – or 0.5 FTEs! Not bad.

The point is, whatever receptionist time is freed up can be reinvested in some other worthwhile Work Items; for example, helping patients become oriented to the patient kiosk for the Guided Patient Interview. The patient-entered data on the kiosk, in turn, saves time for the physician and office nurse while they are with the patient in the exam room, freeing up the minutes they would have spent re-entering the data from the paper form into the medical record. They simply review the patient-entered information with the patient as part of the exam, and make any edits or corrections. This illustrates the positive ripple-effects of changing a couple of Work Items in the receptionist's workflow. A similar gain can happen with conversion from manual to EMR-based prescription refill authorizations, for example.

The bottlenecks section of the POW Encounter Work Item List provides an area where any slowdowns (or wild variations in task times) are noted and should include anything that is worthy of discussion when the study is completed. Once you have documented your workflow completely, look for areas where these type of savings could be realized.

What to Do When You Finish Documenting

As previously noted, during the actual collection of patient encounter data, as you go about your normal work, simply enter the times required for completion of each Work Item and note any bottlenecks or dependencies you come across. That's it, except for special cases.

When your Encounter Work Item List is complete for one Encounter type, go to the POW Checklist in the front of your binder and check off that Encounter type. When every Encounter Work Item List for every Encounter type in your binder has been checked off, your part of the Study is over and you can return your binder to the person who will be consolidating the data. It's not that hard actually, the proper setup makes the execution phase simple. The spreadsheet provided helps make the cost process straightforward also.

(You can help make the spreadsheet better. If you find some spreadsheet enhancements you need (for example, you don't think there are enough lines in the Direct & Indirect sections for your practice), let us know. The spreadsheet is on the Web and can be changed rather quickly! Drop an e-mail to betty@medsp.com with any suggested changes you have.)

Handling Variations of a Single Encounter Type

Real world workflow is all about "exceptions," those little variations from what the form lists. These are, by the way, VERY important to your EMR data gathering because in your new EMR, you are going to have to handle exceptions to how the EMR typically flows, and these places can drive you nuts. This is one area in which the WfME EMRs have an advantage as they empower someone in your office to change the workflow of your EMR – a conventional EMR will not allow you to make dramatic changes.

One reason for doing this workflow study is to help you evaluate how easily your workflow can be supported by your candidate EMR systems. You should demo these workflows-with-variations on each EMR, to see how easily they accommodate them. How does the EMR work with a patient who has a co-morbidity (or chronic condition)? How many extra screens do you have to navigate to get the encounter documented? Want to find out in advance how easy-to-use your EMR will be? Try it out on encounters that have significant workflow variations.

To illustrate capturing these variations, look at the bottom of the Encounter Work List form (shown (cropped) in Figure 10.3). There is a section for up to three variations of standard workflow done for the majority of your patients. This example is taken from the Physician's Encounter Work Item List (and is hypothetical – since the MD would order, not do the 12-lead ECG).

The physician filling in the Encounter Work List form has determined that there are variations to the Annual Physical encounter. These variations are different Work Items for male and female patients, and different Work Items for elderly and very young patients. The physician writes in the variation names – Child, Woman, Elderly Man (in the brown-highlighted areas for data entry on the form). The physician then writes in just the additional tasks to be performed beyond those already entered in the Work Item sequence for all Annual Physicals (listed at the top of this form). If there are more than a few additional Work Items discovered, a separate Encounter Work List should be made up, rather than variations to an existing one.

Patient Encounter: (Work List Variation 1 Below) — Encounters per month: 15

Task ID	Child	— Annual Physical			

Item No.	Enter Encounter Unique Variation Work Items Below	Minutes Used	Document Bottlenecks Encountered Below	Gating Dep	Encounters per Month	Add'l Hours
25	Developmental Assessment	5			15	1.25
26	Immunization Assessment	3			15	0.75
27	**Subtotal Variation 1**	8	Minutes		Hours =	2.00

Patient Encounter: (Work List Variation 2 Below) — Encounters per month: 10

Task ID	Women	— Annual Physical			

Item No.	Enter Encounter Unique Variation Work Items Below	Minutes Used	Document Bottlenecks Encountered Below	Gating Dep	Encounters per Month	Total Hours
28	Pap Smear	3			10	0.50
29	Breast Exam	5			10	0.83
30	Bone Density (if post-menopausal)	2			10	0.33
	Subtotal Variation 2	10	Minutes		Hours =	1.67

Patient Encounter: (Work List Variation 3 Below) — Encounters per month: 6

Task ID	Elderly	— Annual Physical			

Item No.	Enter Encounter Unique Variation Work Items Below	Minutes Used	Document Bottlenecks Encountered Below	Gating Dep	Encounters per Month	Total Hours
31	12-Lead ECG	8			6	0.80
32	Prostate Exam	3			6	0.30
33	**Subtotal Variation 3**	11	Minutes		Hours =	1.10

Encounter Variation Summaries

Variation No.		Total Minutes	Encounters per Month	Add'l Hours
1	Child	8	15	2.00
2	Women	10	10	1.67
3	Elderly	11	6	1.10
			Hours =	4.77

Figure 10.3 Encounter Work List with Data Entered and Automatic Totals

Once the variations are written in, note the time it takes to complete each new Work Item. That's it. The billing manager will need to enter the frequency with which each variation occurs per month in the box provided for each type of variation. At the very bottom of the form, there is an Encounter Variation Summary which is calculated automatically once the times have been entered into the spreadsheet. The variations also automatically carried over into the Task Cost Section of each Encounter Work Item List, as shown in Figure 10.4.

Handling More Than Three Variations

If there are more than three variations or if the Work Item variations are significant, you will then need to make up an individual encounter form for each special case – perhaps, "Annual Physical-Elderly Male," and "Annual Physical-Post-menopausal Female," and "Annual Physical-Pre-Menopausal Female," and so on.

Notice in Figure 10.3 that the extra time associated with each variation is totaled for you and automatically goes into the variation summary table at the bottom of the spreadsheet. The spreadsheet also calculates the total (in this case monthly) time, by multiplying the number of encounters times the time/encounter – which calculates the total times for each encounter for each provider (role) involved. These calculations will appear only on the spreadsheet, of course, you won't see them on your paper forms.

Costing Your Office Workflow

Because the spreadsheet already includes the formulas, the costing of each type of Encounter Work Item is straightforward. Costing is automatically calculated on the spreadsheet once the business manager or whoever has access to employee pay scales, enters that number into the Role Cost/Hour column on the right of each Encounter Work List form, as shown in Figure 10.4.

Note that the hourly rate for whatever ROLE the person fills (in this case $20/hour) has been entered at the top right of the Encounter Work List form. This allows all costs to be calculated for the Direct, Indirect/Supportive and all Variations of the Encounter Work List. Also provided is a TOTAL cost for each Encounter, shown at the top (in this case $662 for the receptionist).

Summing Up the Encounter Work Lists

What remains is to sum up ALL Encounter Work List forms for each person in each role. That is the function of the LAST tab on the POW Study form in the Excel spreadsheet. It takes the totals from the 20 Encounter Work List forms for each person and consolidates them onto a Summary Worksheet. Again, the data is picked up automatically by the spreadsheet (the Summary Worksheet is not shown).

The Grand Total Affair

Summing it up by ROLE doesn't show the total cost for each patient encounter type seen by your office; that requires adding each participating person's data together. Since each office's staffing and roles will be different, we could not anticipate and link these for you in advance. However, the shell of a Worksheet to do that is provided (also at www.ehrselector.com). You will need to simply LINK the appropriate cells in the Encounter Total Worksheet (Figure 10.4), to the totals from each person's (Role's) individual worksheets (last tab on the POW Study), to arrive at a Grand Total for each encounter type seen in your office. 90% of the work has been done for you and someone with Excel skills can complete the final linkages in 30-60 minutes (probably your business manager, as this has sensitive employee salary information on it).

©Medical Strategic Planning - Physician Encounter Workflow Model — Page 1

Enounter ID	Role Name	Practice Name		Role Cost/Hour
AP	Receptionist		Your Practice Name Goes Here	$ 662

Name of Patient Encounter:	Encounters per Month	Documented Month ___ of Year ______	Enter=>	$ 20.00
Annual Physical	100			

Task ID	Item No.	DIRECT Work Item Description (entered by person doing Work Item)	Minutes Used	Document Bottlenecks Encountered Below	Gating Dep	Encounters per Month	Total Hours	Task Cost
	1	Greet Patient	0.5			100	0.83	$ 16.67
	2	Take Insurance Information	1.0			100	1.67	$ 33.33
	3	Give Patient Forms to fill out	0.5			100	0.83	$ 16.67
	4							
	5							
	6	Make Next Appointment	3.0			100	5.00	$ 100.00
	7	Receive Copayment (or entire payment)	2.0		17	100	3.33	$ 66.67
	8							
	9							
	10							
	11							
	12							
	13							
	14							
	15							
		DIRECT Total	7.0	Minutes		Hours =	9.17	$ 233.33

Task ID	Item No.	INDIRECT or SUPPORTIVE Work Item Description (entered by person doing Work Item)	Minutes Used	Document Bottlenecks Encountered Below	Gating Dep	Encounters per Month	Total Hours	Task Cost
	16	Pull Patient's Chart	2			100	3.33	$ 66.67
	17	Call Insurance Co - Verify Eligibility	7			100	11.67	$ 233.33
	18	Re-File Patient Chart	1			100	1.67	$ 33.33
	19							
	20							
		INDIRECT Total	10	Minutes		Hours =	16.67	$ 333.33
								$ 566.67

Patient Encounter: (Work List Variation 1 Below)		Encounters per month
Child	- Annual Physical	15

Task ID	Item No.	Enter Encounter Unique Variation Work Items Below	Minutes Used	Document Bottlenecks Encountered Below	Gating Dep	Encounters per Month	Add'l Hours	Task Cost
	25	Developmental Assessment	5			15	1.25	$ 25.00
	26	Immunization Assessment	3			15	0.75	$ 15.00
	27							
		Subtotal Variation 1	8	Minutes		Hours =	2.00	$ 40.00

Figure 10.4 Encounter Total Worksheet

When the Grand Totals are all done, compare the total cost to your practice for each patient encounter type to what you are reimbursed (based on E&M codes) for that encounter type, and you will see whether or not you are profitable for that particular type of patient encounter. That can be an eye-opener for some encounter types. It's an important eye-opener however, because it underscores the fact that your clinical documentation (your new EMR) needs to capture ALL of the clinical work you are actually doing, along with those all-important variations you documented, so that you are billing at appropriate levels. The E&M calculator within your new EMR will tell you what level of billing is justified by the work you have performed for each encounter (including the variations). If it's integrated with your CPM, that billing will be captured. If it isn't linked to your CPM, be sure someone manually adjusts the E&M codes submitted for these "special cases" so that you get paid all you are entitled to.

EMRs & Medicare Fraud – Friend or Foe?

An EMR, used improperly, is an invitation for a Recovery Audit Contractor (RAC) and all of the hassles that entails. There is a difference between billing for all the work that medically needs to be done, and doing extra work for which there is no medical need, so that you can bill at a higher E&M level. Be sure you understand that difference. Billing for extra work won't happen if you use your EMR properly, but it can just as easily be used as a tool to rip off CMS. The point is that, either way, your EMR will document what you are doing. If it's all above board, the EMR will be a powerful ally in defending you during any audit and will justify all you have done.

One More Thing

One other question that is asked of us frequently (for which this chapter provides the answer) is whether it is wise to accept the EMR that your hospital is offering under the Stark Safe Harbor deal, or should you go your own way? The answer is – Any EMR that doesn't enhance your workflow and provide ease-of-use in your office setting with your staff, even if it's FREE, isn't a good deal. Not only don't take it – run from it. There is no one, perfect EMR. Even an expensive EMR (Epic, GE, McKesson, Allscripts) may not be right for your practice – or it may be just right. Use this book and tools like the MSP EHR Selector to make the correct decision for you and your practice.

Understand the motivations of anyone who offers you an EMR under the Stark Safe Harbor deal or as a "free" open-source, public-domain EMR. Look at the vested interest of whoever is making the offer and make certain that it also supports YOUR vested interest. Be cautious about anyone talking about "universal EMR solutions" – even if they are CCHIT-certified. Almost every EMR today was CCHIT-certified sometime between 2006 and now. So what? One CCHIT-certified EMR may be a good fit for you, and the next one, a disaster.

Far too often, the EMRs offered by hospitals are only the ones that the hospital's existing legacy I.T. vendors either have created or partner with because these EMRs interface with the hospital's lab, pharmacy, radiology and other legacy systems. This approach means that the I.T. people don't have to create a new interface to link the EMRs offered (which of course, is a very nice situation for the hospital's overworked I.T. department). But should the fact that choosing a particular EMR doesn't inconvenience the hospital's I.T. department be the determining factor in what EMR your practice adopts? Definitely not! What's important to you is always gated by two things: Is it easy for everyone in your office to use? Does it fit your current and future workflow well?

Here are some other EMR facts. NO EMR developer (of the 104 we have data on) supports all 45 practice specialties and two-thirds of all EMR developers support six or fewer practice specialties. While that number is growing, it isn't growing rapidly, and efforts like CCHIT (which determines what a specialty functionality must be in order for EMR developers to be certified) is slowing down the entire process. If you are a physician who practices in a specialty supported by one of the few EMRs most hospitals offer under these Stark programs, take a good look and perhaps adopt what the hospital offers you. But if you aren't, then the Stark offer is really not designed for you, and your hospital should know that and work with you instead of ignoring your needs in deference to their own.

Wrap Up

These last two chapters (9 and 10) have given you several ways of looking at how customization and workflow enhancement will impact your satisfaction with the EMR you ultimately select and deploy. Hopefully, we have conveyed the benefits that can be yours from doing an office Workflow Study.

Use the information in Chapter 9, along with your POW Study data, as criteria to test any final candidate EMRs against, during your demonstration of them. Each EMR has a particular type of workflow it is organized around. Some do SOAP-oriented charting; others are more encounter-oriented. Some have the ability to merge templates for two different patient encounter types, others don't. Some can handle the encounter variations that occur in your office (found during your Workflow Study), others can't. Ease-of-use is intimately integrated with workflow and workflow enhancement is the bottom line for EMR.

Know your workflow and learn the workflow of any candidate EMRs, then look for a match. Use this book, the MSP EHR Selector or any other tool that protects your anonymity to narrow your search to 4-5 qualified EMR products. Only then should you seek in-depth demos – you doing your workflow on their system in your office. Use your POW Study Encounter Work Item Summaries to guide these demos to determine where each EMR bottleneck is, where dependencies are, what links need to exist to your CPM system to make the workflow smooth, etc. Does that EMR developer support those links to your CPM or will you have to abandon your CPM and buy an integrated solution? You'll be armed with much more information to determine the answers to these (and other) questions based on what you learned in Chapters 9 and 10.

Crucial Decision

Do you want to use a process for assessing your current paper-based workflow so that you will better understand how your office currently functions and have a basis for determining what features you need in an EMR? Photocopy as needed or download this Scorecard from www.ehrselector.com

	We did the POW Study and are so happy to be finished!!
	We did not do the POW Study, we're just going to put down Work Items and places in our Patient Encounters where we already know we have a problem.

Here is our list of problem areas/bottlenecks that we discovered or already know exist:

Here are some EMR functions that we want to ask each candidate EMR vendor about and TRY OUT on our problem areas:

Your Crucial Decision is whether you will simply fill in this form based on the quick observations of your office personnel or you have actually performed the POW Study of your office workflow. Either way, use this Scorecard to document your bottleneck areas and think about how an EMR might improve these places.

CHAPTER 11

Essential Medical Record Content

Crucial Decision
What core medical record content do you need and what specialty-specific features do you require?
This chapter also addresses the following questions:
- Do you need decision support features available during your patient encounter?
- Do you need quality controls that reject bad data?
- Do you need real-time clinical alerts?
- Do you want medication/pharmacy features beyond MU requirements?
- Do you want to actually block unsafe orders?
- What patient-entered data content do EMR developers support?

EMR Adventures

Dr. Rodriguez is out of town on a fishing vacation in a remote area of Montana. One of his patients, Ruth Dean, had recent surgery for a torn cartilage in her left knee and is currently in physical therapy as part of her rehab. On the second week of physical therapy, her primary therapist is off for the day and Ruth is seen by a therapist who does not know her well. The substitute therapist takes Ruth through a new set of exercises and instructs her to do the same exercises daily at home. Wanting to get better quickly, Ruth does the exercises religiously, even through pain, until on the third day of the new routine, her left thigh/hip area become so inflamed that she cannot sit, move or sleep without great discomfort.

Ruth calls Dr. Rodriguez's office on Saturday, hoping that he is in and can see her, or that she can at least speak to him. She could call her orthopedic surgeon but she trusts Dr. Rodriguez – especially in light of her chronic ulcerative colitis. Ruth knows that she does not tolerate anti-inflammatory drugs and has had rectal bleeding with past use of them. At this point though, Ruth is so uncomfortable that she is willing to put up with some rectal bleeding but she would prefer that Dr. Rodriguez choose a drug with the least side effects for her. She is disappointed to learn that not only is Dr. Rodriguez out of the office but the office is closed until Monday. She makes the decision to go to her local walk-in clinic, where she is seen by Dr. Sunny Day.

Successfully Choosing Your EMR: 15 Crucial Decisions. By © Arthur Gasch and Betty Gasch. Published 2010 by Blackwell Publishing

"I just can't take this pain anymore," says Ruth. "I need something to help me but I also have ulcerative colitis and will probably bleed with any of the NSAID medications."

Dr. Day examines Ruth and is able to pull up her chart electronically because Dr. Rodriguez's office and the walk-in clinic are part of same integrated delivery network and RHIO. While Dr. Day is looking at the history of Ruth's ulcerative colitis and her need for relief from her probably inflamed sciatic nerve, a screen pops up advising Dr. Day that a 2007 Mayo Clinic study of ulcerative colitis patients found it safe for Celebrex to be used for short-term indications.

"I have great news for you," comments Dr. Day. "You can use Celebrex for a short time to relieve your inflamed nerve and you will most likely not suffer bleeding side effects. I will prescribe the dose for you to try over the weekend. You can call Dr. Rodriguez or your surgeon on Monday, or you can call me back if you experience any bleeding or an increase in pain over the weekend. I also want you to continue your icing of the area and you should not do any further exercises until you see your surgeon."

"Thanks so much," says a relieved Ruth. "I didn't think it would be this easy. I am so glad Dr. Rodriguez has an EMR and is part of this network!"

Medical Record Content: The Heart of the EMR

Because EMRs are a new tool and paradigm change, they raise other issues to be considered when selecting and deploying them.

- Can the EMR directly (or in conjunction with the CPM) access practice schedules to make patient appointments?
- Does the EMR assure that ICD and CPT codes used are correct and reimbursable?
- Does the EMR produce CMS-required documentation for all patient encounters?
- Can the EMR directly obtain authorization for specific procedures?
- Does the EMR provide access to different parts of the EMR at the same time for more than one authorized and authenticated user?
- Does the EMR require two types of identification to initially authenticate a user and provide access to both the EMR and CPM systems (if they are separate systems)?
- Can the EMR provide a secure mechanism for users to change data in existing, signed records, or append information to them, such as e-mail messages sent by patients or other providers to your office?
- Does the EMR provide an "outlined" or brief record that can be expanded to present any selected data in the outline?
- Does the EMR's patient history section include occupational exposures, habits and compulsive behaviors (e.g. alcohol or cigarette use), past injuries, operations, inpatient admissions, immunizations and genetic information?
- Does the EMR provide a means to electronically communicate with other staff members during the encounter via secure, instant messaging?

- Does the EMR preserve the audit trail showing author, date and so on, for all third-party medical records that are merged into the EMR?
- Does the EMR track which methods of communication the patient has authorized you to use, such as secure e-mail, secure fax or other means?

These are just a few of the issues that EMRs introduce, which don't exist for paper-based charts, that staff must now handle in an EMR-enabled practice.

Verifying Medical Content With EMR Demos

Whatever medical content you ultimately decide upon, demos are essential for evaluating medical record content that is important to you. We encourage you to do thorough demos, but timing is key. Don't conduct demos too early in the decision process. A recommended sequence would be:

- Determine practice-wide and personal EMR goals;
- Establish a budget for the entire project;
- Conduct your workflow analysis of each type of patient encounter;
- Build your EMR medical content feature/requirements list;
- Compare EMRs to identify a few, qualified candidate EMRs;
- Make a literature request;
- Choose three to four EMRs and schedule demos;
- Narrow the field further and conduct site visits;
- Generate final requirements (with legal advice) and issue an RFP;
- Evaluate RFP responses and enter final contracting;
- Award the order or licensing agreement.

Many physicians use the EHR Selector™ criteria to build a list of features they ask each EMR developer to demonstrate. Some of these features would definitely go unaddressed if your EMR demonstration is left to EMR salesmen, who will not go out of their way to demo features their systems don't have.

One good demo approach is to use your own paper charts from a recent patient visit and put in all the data for the encounter you actually performed. Choose an encounter that you perform very frequently, because if the EMR isn't fast at doing this, your office workflow will be compromised. If the EMR isn't fast at performing patient encounters that occur infrequently, perhaps you can live with that.

Don't take demo shortcuts, if some data has to be scanned into the EMR, scan it in. How long did that take? See how well the scanning process is integrated. Does it add barcodes to each page that identify the section of the chart? Is scanning a single-page or a batch-document process? Who will do the scanning and where will it be done? Can it be done after the patient encounter? How many scanners will be required? What type of scanners? Can a keyboard scanner combination work? This may be an eye-opener, and will surface some additional issues that would have remained hidden if the demo had simply been conducted with pre-attached images that would have otherwise been used. Make sure your demo is specialty specific. Make a list of the requirements to be included in your purchasing or licensing agreement.

Different Care Settings Need Different EMR Solutions

There are no one-type-fits-all EMR solutions, in spite of what your hospital CIO or any EMR consulting firm tells you. When deciding what is "essential" medical record content, take your practice specialty into account. Not all EMRs are a good match for all care settings or practice specialties. Figure 11.1 shows what care setting EMRs were first designed to serve.

Figure 11.1 Care Settings EMR Applications Initially Were Designed to Serve

EMR Serving	% of EMRs Available
MD Office	47%
MD Office & Hospital Clinics	9%
Hospital In-patient Areas	11%
Hospital Out-patient Areas	3%
Skilled Nursing Facilities	3%
All of the Above Settings	27%

There is some crossover between physician office EMRs and EMRs used in hospital clinics or hospital inpatient areas, but each care setting has its own unique issues. Developers of hospital I.T. products, like Cerner, McKesson, Siemens, GE and others, are increasingly moving into the physician office EMR space.

When an EMR developer does move into a new care setting, the specialties they initially support are the larger ones. Figure 11.2 shows the specialties in which over 100 EMR developers first introduced their products.

Figure 11.2 Practice Specialties EMR Developers First Served

EMR Product Clinical-Specialty Focus When EMR was Introduced	% of EMR Products
General & Family Practice	45%
Internal Medicine	9%
Emergency Medicine	8%
Orthopedic Surgery	3.5%
Ophthalmology	3.5%
OB/GYN	3.5%
Cardiology	3.5%
Ear, Nose and Throat	3%
Pediatrics	3%
Other	14%

There are still many EMRs that are intended mostly for hospital settings. They are available from companies including: Philips, Meditech, Picis, CliniComp, iMDSoft, T-Systems, Wellsoft, MedHost and others. Some of these serve the entire hospital, while others serve one or more clinical settings like: OR, Labor & Delivery, ED or some ICU areas. The MSP EHR Selector has a growing number of EMR developers that focus on these non-physician-office EMR segments, but is looking for more. Some developers that offered EMRs initially for physician group practices, are now migrating into the hospital EMR space.

When you are considering an EMR developer, get a sense of their future product development focus. If you are considering an EMR developer that currently supports two or more EMR solutions, rest assured that some of these may not be supported in the future. Find the primary "go-forward" product and give it a good look. If you choose a product that is not going to be developed aggressively in the future, you may find yourself having to prematurely migrate to a new EMR all too soon!

Prioritizing Your Medical Record Content Requirements

Until you work with an EMR, it's challenging to envision how an EMR could assist you with your clinical decisions or other new elements it will introduce into your patient exam, and therefore you may overlook some features that you later discover you may have wanted. Other new capabilities may be compelling and you decide that you must have them now. We suggest you organize EMR features into one of three preference lists:
- Must-Have features (MH);
- Like-to-Have features (LH), if budget permits;
- Maybe-Later features (ML), in a future deployment phase.

Use this chapter's Scorecard to document items by these preferences. There is a column to check for items that need to be in your purchasing/licensing agreement. Check this column for any MH items, and for any LH items you are not sure exist in the EMR. Make them individual items on any RFI or RFP so that any extra costs associated with these items are identified.

Medical Content Requirements
To support medical content, an EMR must accomplish four tasks:
1 It must *collect and gather* all available patient data (requires excellent standards support);
2 It must *organize and present* all gathered data to you effectively, on the screen and on the printer;
3 It must *correlate and enhance* all data, providing notices, alerts and enforcing blocks to unsafe actions;
4 It must *share appropriate medical content* with other authenticated providers within the boundaries of the permissions that have been granted for that data by the patient.

The balance of this chapter is broadly organized around discussing these tasks.

Task 1 – Data Collection & Reporting

In a JAMA article by Peter Smith (et al.) clinicians indicated that one of seven paper-based charts are incomplete, missing everything from lab results, radiology and other imaging results, history and physical exam data, and medications[1]. One purpose of adopting an EMR is to eliminate (or minimize) missing information.

Medical record content must include complete patient demographics, problem lists, medical history, clinical encounter notes, documented patient consents and medical directives and powers of attorney, approved formularies, refill histories, all results from tests ordered from labs, imaging studies, ECG, pulmonary function and other procedures and studies that are ordered; and any information you wish to transfer from your patients' PHRs into your EMR.

Each part of the record can be directly interfaced (ideally) or can be scanned in and kept as an image (not desirable). Therefore, the first task is to determine whether all diagnostic devices can send data that your EMR can assimilate directly without scanning. You will need to ask around and consult your EMR developer. For example, do all lab providers send test results in ELINCS format with LOINC encoding? It's likely that some do (particularly national labs) and others don't (usually hospital lab vendors).

If (some or all of) the labs indicate that they can send results in ELINCS format, then your next question for the EMR developer is whether his or her particular EMR can accept and process lab results in that format. Again, you are looking for a "yes" answer. Any mixed solutions are less than ideal and will affect ease-of-use and workflow. Harder-to-use systems are more likely to have incomplete data.

Specific EMR content requirements for medication and diagnostic tests are discussed later on.

Previous Encounter Data Loading & Serial Comparison

Data collection issues can impact data organization and presentation capabilities. For example, it's often helpful in patient encounters to rapidly check all current observations against those observed and retrieved from previous visits. EMRs differ in how they implement such functionality. Some EMRs force you to go to a different tab in the EMR (and sometimes several new screens) to display previous patient results, making it hard to compare current and previous data. Others let you see current and previous data side-by-side.

Likewise, if some lab results are faxed in or have to be scanned into your EMR, they usually end up in the Scanned Information section, perhaps under a Lab Results tab. But the directly-interfaced lab results (from labs supporting

---

[1] *Missing Information During Primary Care Visits.* By Peter C. Smith. Published 2005, Vol. 293, pp. 565-571, by JAMA

ELINCS and LOINC) will end up on the summary sheet, along with the other structured results.

In such cases, you will have to refer to two different sections of the chart to see all lab results. How well does the EMR user interface facilitate that? In this case organization and presentation are somewhat undermined by data collection issues.

Automatic Data Collection – Direct Device Interfaces

Whatever your specialty, there may be a few devices you use (like an ECG machine, pulmonary function device, treadmill, endoscope, ultrasound, or whatever) that generate data or test results for your patient chart. If at all possible, you want to find an EMR that supports direct interfaces to all devices used in your practice, so that the data they generate comes into the EMR directly, rather than having to be scanned in.

Scanned-in images (like scanned-in lab reports) are not structured and therefore their data is not actionable by the EMR software directly and may also have to be stored as unstructured data blobs. However, if diagnostic devices like ECG machines are directly interfaced and the data is structured, it can be processed directly by the EMR to provide alerts, initiate action blocks and provide decision support. Therefore, investigate whether or not an EMR can interface well to devices used in your specialty. If not, it may add new workflow items (like scanning) to your workflow process, slowing down overall workflow.

When you evaluate interfaces, check the brand and model of equipment you have to assure that any interfaces the EMR developer has available will work with your specific models. An EMR may have an interface to a GE and Philips ECG machine, but not to a Burdick or Siemens ECG machine, for instance. In any demonstrations, hook-up your device and let the EMR developer demonstrate that it works. Also, carefully clarify any additional costs associated with interfacing your devices. Don't settle for a simple, "Yes, we have/can interface it," type answer.

Tracking Patient–Entered (PHR) Data

Here's an unsettling but real scenario. Your patient comes in for his/her routine appointment and says, "Hey doc, I've compiled all my medical information in my new Personal Health Record (PHR), and I want to load it into your new EMR system, how do I do that?" Guess what? That has already started to happen. Besides throwing up your hands and mumbling, "I'm not sure," what's your answer? One approach is to take control in the first place and offer a patient portal/PHR combination for your patient to use, but if you are just deploying your first EMR, that may be more than you can initially manage.

We have covered patient-entered data in a number of earlier chapters, so we won't belabor the point, we address it again only as a reminder that patients can enhance your essential medical record content. In addition to patient history, EMRs should support various assessments, such as the Nottingham

Health Profile[2], SF-36[3] or other standardized health profiles. Determine what health profiles any candidate EMR is able to capture and provide.

Consider also whether a patient portal is something that you would like to have and determine if your candidate EMR developer can support portals.

Harvard Medical School estimated as early as 1997, that one-of-two people in the U.S. between the ages of 35 and 49 used at least one alternative therapy. Also in 1997, Americans made 386 million visits to see a physician, but 627 million Americans sought alternative therapies (at a cost of $27 billion of their own dollars). The same study found that those seeking alternative therapy were primarily the educated and prosperous.[4] Add to these findings, lists on the Internet that not only inform potential patients of your physician contact information, but that use current (or former) patients to rate you as a provider. Like it or not, you are in competition with your colleagues, not only across the hall, but also in some cases – across the nation.

There may be an abundance of patients (and reimbursement) to go around currently, but the U.S. government will begin penalizing practices that cannot document patient-centered, quality care at some point in the future. We believe that there will be growing emphasis on patients as data-entry partners in healthcare, as PHRs are more widely adopted.

Patient-Entered History and Reason(s) for Visit
You might start with allowing your patients to enter their emergency contact, health insurance, and some family history information. The majority of the EMR developers from the MSP/Andrew EMR Benchmark had systems that allowed this level of input by patients.

For physicians/clinicians who are more comfortable with patient data entry into the EMR, some EMRs allow details of the patient history and physical to be entered directly by patients. Many EMR developers enable patients to add details about infectious diseases they have contracted, their medical problems and family medical history, any childhood diseases or inherited conditions, and any emergency department visits they have had since their last office visit. Fewer EMR systems allow patients to enter details on their diets, any other physicians they are seeing, their vital signs (e.g. patient-tracked blood pressure), or any exercise programs they participate in. Even fewer EMRs allow patients to enter information on such details as their wound care or any goals they have for improving their health.

---

[2] The Nottingham Health Profile is intended to provide a brief indication of a patient's perceived emotional, social and physical health problems.

[3] The SF-36 is a multi-purpose, short-form health survey with only 36 questions.

[4] *Trends in Alternative Medicine use in the United States 1990-1997*. By David M. Eisenberg, et al. Published Nov. 11, 1998, Vol. 280, pp. 1569-75, by JAMA

Hey, Who Entered That Data?

Any time an EMR incorporates data from more than one care provider (or a patient), medical-legal issues can surface. Mixing patient-entered data with data entered by various caregivers clouds the issue of who entered which data. Some EMRs attribute all documentation entered to the physician who signs the chart, no matter who did the charting. How does the EMR maintain an absolute audit trail or prevent one person from being credited for another's work and observations? If the audit trail can be disabled in any way, the legality of the EMR as a medical-business record is called into question. If any inconsistent data can be included in the EMR, it calls the credibility of the entire record into question. How is inconsistent or impossible data corrected and who has the authority to do so?

EMRs with such flaws are an open invitation to presumed fraud and huge penalties, if it is discovered during Recovery Audit Contractor (RAC) audits. Unless you modify most standard vendor agreements, you – not the EMR developer – will be held accountable for the fraud. See Chapter 13 for discussion of this important topic.

Patient–Entered Medical and Test Results

Practices that include a number of diabetic patients will appreciate the need for an EMR that allows patients to enter their lab data. Diabetic patients manage their care on a daily basis with physician/clinician guidance. If you have an endocrinology practice, patient-entered lab results could be important. For those EMRs that did allow lab data to be entered by patients, it is good news that blood glucose was the test most often enabled. However, not all EMR developers included patient-entered lab data, so if this is important to your practice, check this feature carefully. Other lab data that some EMR developers enabled patients to enter (in order of how many EMR developers included the feature), were cholesterol, PAP smear results, mammography results and Prostate-Specific Antigen (PSA) results.

Patient–Entered Medication Information

In spite of the governmental and other emphasis on medication errors and their impact on patient care, the ability for patients to enter information on medication allergies and general medication information is not a common feature offered in EMRs. About half of the EMR developers that participated in the MSP/Andrew EMR Benchmark offered patients the ability to enter medication and allergy information on their EMRs. Less than half offered patients the option of listing any vitamins or supplements that they were on or any medication side effects patients suffered while on a particular medication. Even fewer EMRs offered patients the ability to enter the reason that they were on a particular medication or dietary supplement.

Clinical Documentation Inconsistencies and Tampering

Another aspect of clinical decision support is alerting clinicians to inappropriate or erroneous data entered. Many EMRs that use speech recognition without NLP (Natural Language Processing) or EMRs that allow typed or other freeform text entry, will not be able to discern charting inconsistencies because they aren't actually indexing information entered. In a typical speech recognition (SR) system, during the initial exam, you chart that the patient being seen is "not febrile." Later, in your summary statement – when you have assessed your patient further – you state that the patient, "has a temperature of 102 degrees." Obviously, one of these statements is not true, but since some SR EMRs don't index the vital signs, the EMR accepts both statements without flagging this glaring inconsistency. Good luck if you find yourself in court with that record! Only EMRs using structured data entry can catch such errors and allow you to correct them, rather than let you contradict yourself in your charting. Careful attention to documentation inconsistency checking is highly desirable, but not that many EMRs offer it. As a result, it's a vetted feature assertion on the www.ehrselector.com (MSP ESP) Web portal.

Inaccurate Vital Signs Accepted Without User Warning

Some EMRs also allow the entry of blood pressure readings with reversed systolic and diastolic value (e.g. 70/120) to be accepted. This problem has existed for more than a decade. Some EMR systems (including some CCHIT-certified ones) accept manually-entered, but physiologically-impossible clinical data, without generating any sort of clinical alert or warning. Other EMRs with both proprietary and embedded third-party drug middleware systems allow users to chart ointments administered by IV or IV-only agents administered by intramuscular injection.

Data Inconsistency Invites Litigation

Figure 11.3 underscores the magnitude of the clinical inconsistency problem. Such errors are finally attracting the attention of AHCPR[5], JCAHO, quality organizations and yes – trial lawyers during litigation. Such inconsistencies are time-bombs waiting to be ignited. When will EMR developers wake up?

Physicians adopting EMRs must check such problems as part of product demonstrations. If you find them, get a firm commitment in writing that they will be addressed by a particular date, or scratch the EMR developer from your EMR short list. Any electronic medical records created by such EMRs are subject to being challenged in court for lack of document integrity.

---

[5] The Agency for Health Care Policy and Research.

Figure 11.3 Quality Controls for Entered Data

Common Data Integrity Issues	Yes	No	Uncertain
Alerts About Impossible Drug Admin. Routes	52%	41%	7%
Accept BMI Entry w/o Check Age of Patient	52%	38%	9%
Accept Reverse BP Data Entries	51%	42%	7%
Accept Dropped BP Digits	45%	51%	4%
Hi/Lo Check for Manual Entered Data	41%	56%	3%

Tools to Enhance Data Structure

Since not all EMRs support ELINCS (LOINC) lab reporting, technology exists to help you transform character-based, relatively-unstructured lab data into more-structured information that can be indexed. One such tool is a keyboard scanner like the Keyscan product we discussed in Chapter 5. It delivers Optical Character Recognition (OCR) recognized words in a PDF format as its output, all without user intervention. Portable Document Format (PDF) documents may be cataloged if you have Acrobat Professional (~$150 list), which provides an index to every word, including lab-test labels, although the labels and values are not associated by such indexing approaches.

If you have a high volume of lab or other paper reports to scan, a faster, duplex-capable scanner may serve you better. Having a separate scanning area is helpful if there is a large volume of scanning, since scanners are sometimes noisy contraptions. There are several good, relatively-inexpensive scanners.

Also, don't simply assume that Adobe software is best for creating and processing PDF documents. We had a two-page Word document that, when sent to the Acrobat printer, crashed Microsoft Word after less than 10 seconds of processing. When the same Word document was opened in Open Office 3.1 (which has PDF creation as a free, integrated function), in less than 6 seconds it created the PDF file without incident. You can't beat the price of Open Office and the current 3.1 version has many fixes and is very Microsoft Office format compatible. It also provides an excellent Microsoft Office bridge for users operating on Unix, Linux, or MacIntosh systems.

Another notable product is Abbyy's FineReader, now at Version 9. We've not yet evaluated Version 9, but Version 8 had some medical form processing features that allowed it to screen-scrape any report with a fixed format. It is possible to create "macros" that would tag such data, making structured information possible.

Talk to your EMR vendor and see what support they provide for PDF documents in their EMRs. Many EMRs that don't use document scanning as their primary input type; nonetheless, they have reasonable scanning capabilities.

Task 2 – Chart Content Organization & Presentation

How intuitive are any dashboard and all EMR screen layouts? Do screens appear cluttered? Is the organization of the data collected immediately apparent and arranged to be easy to interact with? Is there appropriate textual labeling or is everything just icons? How is color used? Is there too much use of color? Does the EMR support the Pantone color chart? Is the font size too small to be easily read at the screen size and resolution you prefer? Do you have any control over the amount of information presented on one screen? What type of content is presented on each screen and how many different screens are required to enter all needed information for each type of patient encounter? What help screens are available and is the help provided concise and easily understood? Are help screens role-specific or is there one help screen for every user?

Now consider whether the EMR supports all the content of your common medical records and how it's organized. Does it include specialty-specific content, such as genomic profiles, disease registry reports or other non-standard content required in your practice setting?

Next determine what approach to charting will best meet your needs, depending upon your specialty and practice setting.

SOAP-Oriented Charting

Structured charting supports problem lists, but some EMRs are more SOAP-organized than others. That's because some are intended more for inpatient, single-problem type encounters, where care is focused on one (or a few) diagnosed medical condition(s); while others are more focused for the outpatient setting, where you may prefer an EMR that is less SOAP-like since the patients encountered may have multiple problems and conditions. What works in an oncology unit doesn't fit an urgent care or hospital emergency department setting. Both SOAP and non-SOAP EMRs exist, but they organize charting differently.

Charting by Exception

Closely related to loading and editing previous data is charting by exception. Some EMRs bring past encounter patient data forward to your current screen and then enable you to chart by exception, which is the approach that many chronic disease clinicians prefer. It is often much faster than reentering information that hasn't changed. Going tab-by-tab and charting by exception are approaches to clinical decision support, but not having charting by exception forces more user interaction and many more mouse clicks to chart patient data.

Query & Data Retrieval/Reporting

While putting accurate information into an EMR is important, getting it back out is even more so. What good is information that can't be retrieved? Within the Health Insurance Portability and Accountability Act (HIPAA) privacy and security constraints, data retrieval for a patient record, or from all patients, should be equally simple. Most quality reports require a longitudinal view of multiple patients across your entire practice or disease population. If you have multiple doctors, you will need summaries by physician as well. In terms of record content, retrieval for multiple episodes for one patient is what's needed. So your EMR data retrieval capabilities must empower queries that are both broad and deep – yet simple and quick. Robust EMR reporting is crucial to recognizing problems and making office workflow improvements. There are two report destinations to be considered.

- Retrieval to the EMR screen (viewing data on screen); and
- Printing documentation.

These two abilities are linked, as a screen display is simply a report that is sent to the screen, not the printer. Often screen reports are summary reports, while printed reports are detail reports. Who wants to look through a 200-page report on the computer screen?

Variations in the Ability to View the EMR Data

The ability to view the patient data by patient visit is the most common approach offered in EMRs. Next is the ability to view data in chronological or reverse-chronological order. Fewer EMRs enable viewing progress notes by provider and even fewer have the ability to view medical records based on billing codes (perhaps because unless your EMR is also your CPM, or your CPM has a bidirectional interface to your EMR, there is no way to get the necessary billing codes back to the EMR). Very few EMRs listed the ability to view progress notes by office or progress notes by specialist, which may be of great interest if you have several doctors and at least two offices.

Figure 11.4 How Medical Record Content Can Be Viewed

How Data Can Be Viewed	Current EMR
By Patient Visit	87%
By Chronological Order	80%
By Reverse Chronological Order	73%
By Provider Progress Note	69%
By Billing Code	62%
By Office Progress Note	53%
By Specialist Progress Note	41%

Medical record content must be reportable to be truly useful. The more limited an EMR's query and reporting capabilities, the less useful it is to you.

Special Medical Content Needs – Medical Research

If your practice (or hospital) is part of a medical research group, you need the ability to query more than patient name, chart ID number, encounter date and patient date-of-birth. Research queries may also require: medication (and dose), provider, diagnosis and research protocol, as well as procedure followed by combinations of data, summary pages, and lab tests.

Even if you are not involved in research, the patient demographic data set needs to capture full name, gender, race, and date-of-birth, among other items and associate it with no more than one unique, personal identifier across your entire office. Data sets should also include any membership in a family group, e.g. children, step children and biological and step parents for all patients who are minors. Any healthcare power of attorney should be linked and on file in your office. Figure 11.5 shows the capabilities of more than 100 EMRs.

Figure 11.5 Patient Information Retrieval Parameters

Data	EMRs Supporting
Full Name	100%
Partial Name	100%
Patient Record #	97%
Social Security Number	95%
Age	84%
Sex	81%
Primary Diagnosis	81%
MD Name	78%
Insurance	76%
Admit Date	74%
Responsible Party	73%
Lab Test Name	69%
Radiology Test Name	69%
Billing Date	68%
Radiology Test #	65%
Lab Test #	64%
MD Specialty	57%
Pay Schedule	57%
Office Folder Heading	54%

Few EMRs support query by diagnosis acronym, patient pharmacy preference, appended data and patient lab preference.

Molecular Biology & Genetic Testing

Molecular biology is an exploding area. Genetic testing raises special EMR issues, from both content and legal perspectives. From a content perspective, there are over 3,000 tests available now and counting. Structuring data from these tests is a challenge for every EMR because there is not yet a general agreement and consensus on terms, making data integration a problem.

Complicating matters further, we are not aware of any EMR comparison dataset that includes these particular features, so physicians (who need access to such information) are essentially on their own when it comes to evaluating this area. It is likely to be several years before there is any consensus approach about capturing such data.

Additionally, most of this information is highly sensitive and should not be available to all providers. Releasing it raises authorization, tracking and legal issues. Definitely seek specialized legal advice if your practice requires storing such information. If you want to mitigate litigation risks, be sure your system is hardened (safe from being hacked), provides a full access audit trail and is accessible only by authorized researchers (users).

Task 3 – Clinical Decision Support

Associated with the EMR are some new things to reflect upon, as they weren't possible with paper-based charting. Real-time reminders, alerts, blocks, decision-support information and best practice guidelines are such capabilities.

A Decision Support Vignette

Suppose your patient of 10 years comes to you one day because she "just isn't feeling quite right," the clinical decision support your EMR offers could be a great resource. Perhaps you determine that your patient's heart rate is 100 at rest (her blood pressure is 124/80, only slightly higher than her usual 108/70). This first piece of information is simply vital signs data.

Now you use your EMR to recall her previous visit record, a subtle form of decision support. Some EMRs can simply display all vitals from a previous visit alongside of the current ones. Data from previous encounters shows that her heart rates have ranged from 66 to 72. Now you have information but not much else. You ask your patient about specific symptoms and they are all negative – no bleeding, dark stools, but she mentions slight abdominal cramping. She also remarks that she gained a little weight over the holidays and that a friend at the gym suggested that she take green tea to help her lose some of it. Your patient took that advice to heart and began consuming multiple cups/bottles of green tea a day.

That's interesting. You think back to your "green tea course" in med school. What – your med school didn't offer that course? So, now what? You Google or Bing (green tea + side effects) and what pops up? Tea has about half the quantity of caffeine as coffee, but people often drink more of it than coffee, particularly iced tea in the summer months. So maybe caffeine overdose is the issue.

More in-depth problems are (according to this Web site) that, a 2001 study reports that "green tea extract reduces the absorption of non-heme iron by 25 percent." Another (2005) study found that long-term tea drinkers develop protective mechanisms by having heavier parotid glands.[6] This same Web site identifies Lipton Instant Iced Tea as containing fluoride, and cites a 2005 study in which a middle-aged woman was diagnosed with skeletal fluorosis after drinking up to two gallons of iced tea daily. Why? Because her green tea contained too much fluoride. How much is too much fluoride? The USDA database, which contains the fluoride content of more than 400 foods and beverages, may be just what you need.[7]

Turning your EMR screen so your patient can see it, you let the Internet help you with your patient education to the side effects of green tea in large quantities. This last step transforms your encounter from data collection to actual clinical decision support and adds credibility when you suggest the patient back off on the quantity of green tea being consumed.

As the green tea example makes clear, not all real-time clinical-decision support has to be integrated into your EMR in a formal way. If you are using an ASP model EMR, or even if you are not but have an Internet connection on a tablet PC, you have live access to WebMD, Bing, Google, PubMed and other more specialized search engines. A few doctors we know actually Google while they are seeing a patient or go to a pre-determined medical content site that can offer current information on diagnosis, medications and treatments. Most don't.

Sixty-five percent of EMR developers said that they support a vendor-maintained knowledgebase that guides physicians/clinicians during the patient exam. By the way, you may not have needed a computer to alert you to caffeine in tea, but how current are you on the effects of pomegranate, noni berry juice, fenugreek seed, cinnamon bark powder, or the other over-the-counter products that your patients are consuming in addition to any prescribed meds for chronic conditions, they may be taking?

Decision Support Approaches

Clinical Decision Support (CDS) systems ideally offer diagnostic and other clinical assistance at the point-of-care when and how the clinician wants it – but is this realistic or is it still science fiction? CDS covers a wide landscape of capabilities from the exotic and esoteric to everyday applications. The CDS spectrum ranges from help with differential diagnoses, notifications and alerts, suggested tests to rule out some diagnoses or conditions, or evidence-based treatment alternatives with expected outcomes – it's all part of CDS.

---

[6] http://www.amazing-green-tea.com/green-tea-side-effects.html.

[7] Ibid

Some EMRs support real-time, evidence-based decision support and make it available for every encounter. If the EMR you are considering does not, you may still be able to use some Web-based CDS resources. As with e-prescription, just asking, "Does your EMR have Clinical Decision Support (CDS)?", is too broad a question to be useful. Again, break it down into the specific capabilities that you want, including Alerts and Blocks. We discuss some of the available CDS features in the sections that follow.

Decision support has been approached in three primary ways and is still very much an evolving area.

- The most common approach is through use of Bayesian logic which calculates a probability of a set of conditions for a specific diagnosis;
- The second approach uses combinatorial logic, which lists all diagnostic or management options based on facts contained in a knowledgebase rather than options filtered and ranked according to probability. For more information on these two approaches, a good orientation article has been written by Julie McGoaan[8];
- The third approach, described below, is the most cutting-edge and where we believe CDS is heading.

EMRs that automatically link available clinical support capabilities to current diagnosis and symptoms are most useful to physicians during the patient encounter, as demonstrated in our vignette. However, the current level of integration that exists between an EMR and evidence-based clinical knowledgebases are still limited in most cases.

Commonly-Available Decision Support Functionality

The bullet list below shows features available in most EMRs now.

- Links to decision support information such as a medical dictionary or other physician reference resources;
- Disease management or other guidelines – specifics of what to include in each visit for a newly diagnosed congestive heart failure patient, for example. PQRI quality standards are also important and related;
- Suggests appropriate or alternate tests or procedures;
- Provides reference information based on payor information. If you wanted to send your Medicare patient for a special procedure, these EMRs would let both of you know if the procedure was covered by CMS, for example;
- Supports a context-sensitive search by condition – with transmission to PubMed or other resource.

This last feature, context-sensitive searches by condition, is much less widely available in EMRs than the others.

---

[8] *Problem Knowledge Couplers: re-engineering evidence-based medicine through interdisciplinary development, decision support, and research.* By Julie J. McGoaan, Ph.D. Published October 1999, pp. 462-470, by AHIP

Decision Support Update Frequency

How current is any reference information used for decision support? The Web does a poor job revealing the currency of data presented, so be careful about that. If your query returns three "hits," you sometimes have no idea if you are looking at data from 2001, 2009 or even pre-2000 information?

By the way, Google now offers a filter to return only data posted in the last year, but that doesn't guarantee the information is new, or that it was posted in that time frame.

Clinical Reminders/Alerts/Blocks/Notifications

Closely aligned to the clinical decision support are:
- Clinical reminders;
- Clinical Alerts (CAs), included in EMRs for a variety of medical situations because they also help you make or modify decisions; and
- Clinical Blocks – which actually stop certain actions.

Clinical Reminders

The use of reminders is the lowest level of clinical alert; reminders are more a means of encouraging you (or your patient) to do something you might otherwise have overlooked. Reminders can be based on clinical guidelines or protocols embedded in an EMR's documentation system, which guide care and documentation, safeguard medical necessity, or help you capture complete medical data. On some EMRs, you can set your own reminders, which is a desirable feature.

Clinical Alerts

An alert is based on a problem or possible adverse outcome recognized by the EMR application and sent to a physician/clinician intended to alter their action (unless it is overridden). The only way an alert can be generated is if an out-of-range value can be detected. The only way an out-of-range value can be detected is if it's encoded in the first place. That happens if someone enters it manually or it comes over electronically from a lab or directly from a device (ECG, e.g.) that is interfaced to your EMR. As you might expect, speech recognition EMRs and EMRs that use freeform typing or document scanning, offer fewer alerts than those based on care templates, pick lists and structured data.

How well is your EMR able to alert you concerning features that are safety factors in your practice's patient care? Consider a lab value that is out of normal range; how is an out-of-range value displayed on any EMR being considered? On the paper lab report it may only appear as an "*" next to the specific value, but how do you want it to appear on your EMR?

On some EMRs you won't have a choice and it will appear however it was on the printed lab results that were scanned in. On other EMRs, you will have a configuration option that allows you to indicate its urgency (which also means its level of annoyance). That might include appearance in a different color, flashing the value on your screen, or a message in a box – it's up to the EMR designer to provide you the capability to adjust such factors. The same is true for drug alerts. How do you want these alerts to appear – in some fixed and modest (non-intrusive) manner or more aggressively, in a way that is sure to catch your attention? Put your preference on your demo list to explore for any EMR(s) you are considering.

Clinical Blocks

Clinical blocks are like clinical alerts on steroids – rather than just getting your attention about a matter, they proactively block or otherwise interfere with something you are doing when a "rule" determines that your actions indicate a dangerous situation; and require you to take a conscious action and note the reason in the chart, in order to overrule them. For example, if a child who has allergic asthma is prescribed certain drugs, the orders would be blocked, not just alerted, until intentionally over-ridden by the physician. Not all EMRs support clinical blocks or allow the user to determine whether an intervention is an alert or significant enough to be a clinical block to some EMR action (like prescribing).

Explanation of Reminders, Alerts & Blocks

The following list provides examples of EMR clinical decision support, but is not an exhaustive list. If you see a criterion that interests you but is not exactly what you want, ask any EMR developers being considered about your specific need. Many EMR developers offer most items on this list:

- Alerts triggered by health maintenance guidelines, such as reminding your patient to schedule an annual mammogram or Pap smear (Reminder);
- Alerts based on diagnosis or specific patient problem. This could include a chronic condition that is recorded for your patient that you haven't specifically addressed within a set time period. An alert will pop up at your patient's next visit reminding you to follow up and document the status of your patient's condition related to that diagnosis (Reminder);
- Alerts triggered by the CPOE can decrease insurance denials. Some EMRs issue alerts when your orders are incomplete or do not meet the reimbursement billing standards of third-party payers (Reminder);
- Alerts based on a pending report or referral that is not in the EMR or available for review that, based on predetermined time periods, should have been completed already (Reminder);
- Alerts for either missed or pending patient appointments. Missed appointments can be billed for, if that is your policy, and are not likely to be overlooked by your busy office staff if there is an alert issued (Reminder);
- Alerts for lab reports that show abnormal lab results, usually in a different color from normal lab results (Alert);
- Alerts for non-compliance with care guidelines is important because government agencies are becoming increasingly interested in these. The later versions of CCHIT, and the Agency for Health Care Policy and Research

(AHCPR) standards, are increasingly requiring EMRs to alert clinicians about out-of-range lab, prescription and manually entered information in EMRs (Alert);

- Alerts for pending lab work not received within a specified time (Alert);
- Alerts with filters for patient age, gender or specific diagnosis. When you enter the symptoms of fever and rash on a 6-year-old patient, you could receive an alert from a public health agency (or the CDC) about a local measles outbreak, if you are connected to the NHIN (Alert);
- Alerts based on a combination of data; lab work and diagnosis (i.e. Alert);
- Alerts and blocks ordering a standard dose of a medication for your patient newly diagnosed with renal impairment (Block).

Figure 11.6 lists some reminders and alerts in descending order by availability.

Figure 11.6 Real-Time Alerts Offered by EMRs

Alert	% Offering
For Pending Lab Work Not Done	98%
Filtered on Age, Gender, Diagnosis	95%
Triggered by Health Maintenance Guidelines	95%
Triggered by Diagnosis or Problem	93%
Triggered by Lab Report	92%
Triggered by Orders	85%
For Pending Referral/Other Report	83%
For Pending or Missed Appointments	74%
Criticality can be Assigned by User	72%
Triggered by Combination of Diagnosis, Labs	63%

The alerts that are of importance to you are those that should be discussed with any EMR developer being considered. This is not an exhaustive list, so think about other alerts that would be helpful to you.

Alert Fatigue and User Alert Suppression

Finally, there is nothing as annoying as an alert that continues to pop up when you do not want it to, or one that issues an alert that you really do not require. Some EMRs offer the ability for you to determine which non-life-threatening reminders and alerts are displayed and which are suppressed. The ability to suppress various alerts is a very desirable feature.

e-Prescription (Part of CPOE) Decision Support

Meaningful Use is likely to require some e-prescription (e-Rx) functions to be part of the overall Computerized Provider Order Entry (CPOE) functionality.

If you ask an EMR developer, "Does your EMR support e-prescribing functionality?", and are not more specific, EMR developers will generally reply, "Sure, our EMR does that." But what does that really tell you about their CPOE or e-prescribing (e-Rx) capabilities?

E-prescribing can provide more than 16 separate functions (see Figure 11.5). Proposed Meaningful Use (MU) standards (6-16-09) state, "*Uses CPOE for all order types including medications.*" Is your e-Rx functionality part of a general CPOE module? In the bullet list that follows, only the four italicized MU e-prescription functions were required (by the 6-16-09 draft). Is that all you want from your EMR or do you want more?

EMRs that support Surescripts/RxHub offer other important capabilities. Which of these features are Must-Have, Like-to-Haves, or Maybe-Later e-Rx capabilities for your practice?

Don't accept vague assertions that any EMR offers e-prescribing at face value. Instead, check an e-Rx functionality list item-by-item. Here are some specific capabilities to look for:

- Gets the patient's formulary (from payer or CPM) before the visit and loads it into the EMR record;
- Loads the prescription filling history from the patient's pharmacies;
- Loads a past history of active and discontinued medications;
- *Checks each prescription to see if it's on the patient's formulary;*
- *Checks each prescription for allergic reactions – from the patient allergy list;*
- *Checks each prescription for interactions with other patient medications;*
- **Checks prescription against a patient's chronic disease states;**
- **Checks prescription against the patient's age and BMI;**
- **Checks prescription against current lab values** and alerting when hepatic or renal function is impaired and a "normal" dose would become an overdose for that patient (note: simply having an EMR that loads lab results does not mean that medications are checked against them);
- Maintains a list of the patient's preferred pharmacies online;
- *Sends each prescription as an electronic transaction to the designated pharmacy;*
- Creates an e-fax and sends it to the pharmacy;
- Creates a typed prescription to hand to the patient who carries it to their pharmacy (a very basic capability, but claimed by some EMRs as an e-prescribing capability – very misleading);
- Obtains electronic confirmation that the Rx transaction has been received by the pharmacy and is in the queue to be filled.

Three other e-prescribing functions (indicated in **bold** above) are common causes of adverse drug events and in some cases patient deaths, yet MU (to date) is silent about them. The items listed above aren't all of the e-prescription functions to be considered, but may be the most significant ones.

Always Evaluate Individual Functionality, Not Combined Functionality

The e-prescribing methodology example illustrates the basic approach to use in determining what content you want for other sections in your medical record.

Consider each content area separately – e.g. clinical alerts, administrative and file management, security, audit trail and privacy, clinical encounter content, reports and correspondence, signatures and authentication, discharge plan and follow-up, qualifying criteria, interfaces and auto-population of data from medical diagnostic devices and equipment, staff messaging, and patient profile content. Then make an informed decision on the specifics and note any items that require verification during product demonstrations.

This avoids confusion about overall functionality. For example, "Does your EMR support Physician Quality Reporting Initiative (PQRI) measures?", is not a good question, because few systems support all of them. The same is true for Healthcare Effectiveness Data and Information Set (HEDIS) criteria evaluations. Always list the specific PQRI or HEDIS measures your practice uses separately.

Integration of Medication & Pharmacy Decision Support

Many physicians are investigating EMRs because of the incentives for physician offices to have e-prescribing capabilities (as part of the federal government's CPOE adoption and push to make healthcare paperless). Physicians using e-prescribing adopted Rx identification using their National Provider Identifier (NPI). This is a step towards the government's goal of achieving universal e-prescribing under Medicare by 2011.

CPOE is also a hospital EMR issue. Most hospitals have adopted some Computer Pharmacy System (CPS). If it isn't part of the overall infrastructure supplied by McKesson, Cerner or Siemens, it may have been deployed by smaller pharmacy information system vendors. Check interoperability between your EMR and whatever system the hospital where you admit patients has adopted.

In a study conducted by the FDA that evaluated reports of fatal medication errors from 1993 to 1998, the most common error involving medications was related to administration of an improper dose of medicine, accounting for 41 percent of fatal medication errors[9]. All EMRs have the ability to keep track of the date, the dosage and the instructions for each medication you prescribe; however, only 67 percent of EMRs have the ability to alert you to a dosage that is not within the expected dosing range.

Ninety-eight percent of EMRs alert for drug-allergy incompatibility and drug-drug interactions but only 55 percent alert for drug-disease (say asthma) interactions. This would include alerts such as our example in Chapter 4 that involved Long Acting Beta-2 Agonist (LABA) inhalers. If you are a general practitioner or family physician, these type of alerts can be especially important to you because it is difficult to keep up with everything that is changing for all of the varied patient conditions you see in your practice.

Ninety-eight percent of EMRs offer frequent medication updates from the developer; however, you need to check this area carefully. What is frequent?

---

[9] *Strategies to Reduce Medication Errors*. By M. Meadows. Published May-June 2003, Vol. 37, pp. 20-27, by FDA Consumer magazine

Shorter is better. Medication updates should be posted to your EMR within a few days of being issued. Don't assume that all EMRs update with the same frequency; get the update frequency in writing.

Be cautious about EMR developers that do not use one of the common, third-party drug interaction middleware databases, as maintaining a drug interaction database in a timely manner is a formidable task.

Over 83 percent of EMR developers incorporate medication middleware into their EMR systems. The First Data Bank product is chosen most often, followed by the National Drug Classification (NDC) database, RxHub/Sure-scripts, Multum (Cerner), Medispan, vendor-proprietary systems, Infoscan, NewCropRx, Thomson-Micromedex and Gold. Think seriously about giving preference to EMRs that use any of these embedded drug databases over those EMRs that rely on their own, proprietary built-in databases that an EMR developer must maintain themselves.

Because of the government e-prescribing push, most EMR developers have included medication-related features in their EMRs, but it's still important to check on this. Figure 11.7 shows our survey results for medication integration by EMRs.

Figure 11.7 EMR Integrates the Following Medication Features

Alerts	% Offering
Keeps Date/Dose/Instructions for Each Medication	100%
Alerts for Drug-Allergy Incompatibility	98%
Alerts for Drug-Drug Interactions	98%
Frequent Medication Updates from Developer	98%
Prescriptions Print from Med List	98%
Maintains Active/Inactive Med List	95%
Tracks History of Discontinued Meds	95%
Can Enter Allergies in Free Text	95%
Keeps Patient's Preferred Pharmacies	93%
Medication Renewal Pulls Prior Data/Allows Edit	93%
Med List Shows Which Provider Prescribed	93%
Can Track Patient Prescription Refills	90%
Alerts for Unexpected Dosage	90%

Widely-Supported e-Prescription Features

Ninety-eight percent of EMRs offer the ability to print prescriptions from the patient's medication list; while 95 percent maintain both active and inactive med lists, allowing you to see (ideally on one page) what meds your patient is currently taking, as well as what meds have been prescribed in the past. Ninety-five percent keep a history of discontinued medications – a feature that can avoid problems if previous meds were stopped due to drug intolerance.

Ninety-five percent of EMRs allow entry of allergens as free text; while 93 percent track patients' preferred pharmacies, including telephone and fax numbers. Ninety-three percent retrieve prior Rx data, so you can just edit it. Ninety-three percent show who prescribed each medication; while 98 percent track Rx refills, alerting your staff before your patient calls, so you can proactively schedule any needed office visit. Eighty-one percent allow the entry of meds as free text, but only 67 percent alert for a medication dosage in excess of standard maximums. Sixty-four percent offer an alert for nonstandard dosing intervals; while 60 percent offer automatic dosage calculations.

Some EMRs don't provide a field for a second user's (nurse's) initials for drug calculations on high-risk drug therapies, in spite of JCAHO mandates to do so. Such limitations can contribute to preventable ADEs in oncology practice and hospital emergency department settings. Only 26 percent of EMRs alert you to the possible need for medication dosage adjustments based on Dx or renal/hepatic functional status.

Formularies and Medication Education Materials

Look for e-prescription, formulary-specific medication education materials available to patients. Your e-prescription system should load the patient's formulary from their third-party payor. Figure 11.8 shows the percentage of EMR products that support formulary and other features.

Figure 11.8 Percent of EMR Products Offering Supporting Features

Feature	% EMRs Offering
Prints Rx Education Tracts for Patients	83%
Sorts by Rx Name, Disease, Date, Rx Date	81%
Medication Flowsheets Are Created	76%
Formularies Are Available	63%
Deviation from Rx/Formulary Comments	58%
Indicates Off-Formulary Effective Drugs	55%
Patient Specific Formulary	45%

With 83 percent of EMRs having the ability to print prescription education material for patients, there is no reason for patients not to receive drug utilization information, yet the patient education area is one that often gets cut short in a busy office. That can come back to haunt both you and your patients. If your

EMR developer does not offer education as an option, there are a number of quality patient education software packages available for separate purchase.

Eighty-one percent of EMRs can be sorted by prescription name, disease, or the date of the prescription. This would have been an ideal feature for practices that had patients for whom they had prescribed Vioxx, once the drug was recalled. Seventy-six percent of EMRs have included the ability to create medication flowsheets which can be valuable tools for keeping track of what medication a patient is on or has been on. Flowsheets indicate a patient's complete drug history and can be used to reconcile his/her medication usage across multiple patient visits. Flowsheets can be of particular assistance in clinics when a variety of clinicians see a patient on different office visits.

Patient-Specific Formulary Details

A formulary is a list of prescription drugs that has been approved by a state, health plan, or hospital that can be dispensed without prior authorization, which is a real time saver. Some formularies are more restrictive than others. Open formularies provide coverage for both listed and non-listed drugs while closed formularies generally provide coverage only for drugs that are included on their list. Other formulary approaches fall somewhere in between. Under a tiered cost-sharing approach, for example, generic and preferred drugs require lower co-payments than brand name and non-preferred drugs.[10]

Formularies often employ the notion of tiers of drugs. Many national and near-national plans use at least a three-tier system; the first tier is populated with generic drugs, the second tier with brand-name drugs and the third tier with high cost drugs. Some plans have a special, fourth tier for specific expensive drugs. Many of the Medicare drug plans use a specialty tier, which includes biotechnology or injectable drugs. Other plans use a two-tiered approach – one for generic drugs and one for brand-name drugs; based upon these tiers of medication, a patient's co-pay amount changes. These factors assist physicians/clinicians with prescription choices and enable decisions based on generic versus brand-name drugs, cost of co-pay for each prescription and so on.

Seventy-six percent of EMRs offer multiple formularies, an important feature if you have patients from a variety of health insurance plans. Sixty-five percent of EMRs include formularies of some sort, but it is important to know what formulary the EMRs you are looking at include. Fifty-eight percent of EMRs alert you to the fact that a drug you are prescribing is a deviation from what is prescribed on the patient's formulary. And 55 percent of EMRs indicate off-formulary effective drugs; while 45 percent will download a patient-specific formulary. The inclusion of formularies in an EMR could be very important if you are seeing primarily Medicare/Medicaid patients or for occupational health practices.

---

[10]Information adapted from the National Health Policy Forum Web page, www.nhpf.org/pdfs_basics/Basics_Formulary.pdf.

Lab Results Reporting

Once you have thought through the e-prescription functions required for decision support, do the same thing for your lab orders and results. Think through how to handle the fact that some labs can report data to your EMR in an ELINCS-2 format using Logical Observation Identifiers Names and Codes (LOINC), and others provide lab results as faxed data that is appended to the EMR as unstructured images. If possible, you want to avoid situations where you have to check two places in the EMR to review your patient lab results.

Radiology Reporting

The Digital Imaging and Communications in Medicine (DICOM) 3.0 standard makes full provision for encapsulating Adobe PDF files within a DICOM wrapper, allowing them to be archived to PACS (Picture Archiving and Communication Systems) and transmitted with the same network protocols used by magnetic resonance, computed tomography, ultrasound, and other medical imaging devices. DICOM is a standard for handling, storing, printing, and transmitting information in medical imaging. It includes a file format definition and a network communications protocol. Physicians who rely on images will find DICOM widely adopted by hospitals and making inroads into physician offices, clinics and other patient care areas.

Nailing Down Update Frequency

The MSP/Andrew EMR Benchmark asked how often EMR developers update standards, and over half of the participating developers didn't answer this question.

   For those that did answer, 11 percent said every three months, 10 percent said once a year, 7 percent said every 24 hours and the remainder of the answers varied from there. It would appear that this is one area in which the EMR developers are not helping physicians to keep as current as they could be, so be sure to address it in your EMR contracting documents. Physicians depend upon the information in their EMR systems to be current, so check this out carefully.

Task 4 – Sharing Data With Other Providers

This last function is discussed and elaborated in Chapter 7 – Vocabularies, Standards and Interoperability and in Chapter 8 – Interoperability Beyond the EMR. The objective is to pick an EMR that supports as many interoperability standards as possible. This means one with CCHIT certification granted in either 2008 or 2009, or within the last 18 months – whichever is more current.

Wrap Up

When putting your medical record content requirements list together you can often leverage requirements prepared by third parties. The MSP EHR Selector provides a requirement list; the COPIC Insurance Company (CO, IA, NB) provides another. The HL7-EMR-FM specification is a third source. There are several others. The longer a list has been around, the more likely it is to be somewhat obsolete, unless it has been continually used and updated.

The COPIC list of EMR functionality (285 items) is now in its third revision. The MSP EHR Selector requirements list (700+ criteria) has been continuously revised since its inception in 2003. The MSP/Andrew EHR Benchmark list (2,200 items currently) has been updated annually 13 times. Some specialty organizations also have lists. Don't overlook your specialty organization. Much of the AGA Institute's EMR functional list is also embedded in the MSP EHR Selector. Minnesota has an EMR requirement list, as does Georgia. Some of these lists are copyrighted by the organizations that created them, so check with specific organizations about use rights granted or copyright fees required.

These various lists contain many duplications (or slight variations in statements), so you need to cross-walk all lists you are using to harmonize the language. Be concise and make every word meaningful, specific and make every criteria measurable.

Once your medical content requirement list is assembled, it needs to be compared against all the EMR developers' products you are considering. This is where a tool that facilitates side-by-side feature comparisons of all criteria for EMR developers that serve over 46 practice specialties is helpful. On the MSP EHR Selector, such a comparison consumes 34 pages to print out, item-by-item – if every item is included. Normally, you would only do a printout of a subset of the items that would be on your specific list.

There are other important medical record requirements that space prevents discussing in detail, but follow the same methodology for assessing each one and move from general features to more specific criteria. Medical record content is up to you and we encourage you to show your list of important criteria to any EMR developer you are considering, and discuss it with them so you are both on the same page about what the list is trying to express/specify. It should also be discussed with your healthcare legal advisor.

When you locate an EMR developer whose system matches your current needs, ask the vendor to describe their developmental plans. Think carefully about what EMR features are essential for you now and might be in the future. You can always get an EMR with more functionality than you need today, and simply not deploy some features; but getting one with fewer features than you need and hoping that the EMR developer will have more features when you want them, is an invitation to future disappointment.

If you acquire a system that lacks state-of-the-art medical content features today, there's no guarantee that it will be enhanced by its developer to have state-of-the-art features in the future.

Watch Out for Vaporware

Many early EMR adopters have experienced vaporware burn. Vaporware features are those promised by EMR developers, often in response to an inquiry from someone about to adopt their system, that do not exist currently but the developer promises verbally that the "company should have it in the next release." Too frequently, the feature is not in the next release and not even on the new feature development schedule.

Cutting down on vaporware is one primary reason why the most important features on the MSP EHR Selector are vetted. Printing out the criteria that vendors have asserted they can provide, and then attaching that list to your RFP as functional requirements (so the are incorporated by your legal advisor into the purchasing/licensing agreement), also help eliminate vaporware.

Seeking specific details concerning what any candidate EMR developer offers is crucial to obtaining what you consider essential medical record content.

Use the Scorecard that follows to assist you in determining the components of each feature that you consider essential and share what you want with any EMR developers you are considering.

Crucial Decision

What core medical record content do you need? What specialty-specific features are required? Photocopy as needed or download this Scorecard from www.ehrselector.com

Indicate the level of importance for the EMR attribute listed below with the following codes: **MH = Must Have, LH = Like to Have, ML = Maybe Later.**

EMR Attribute	Demo Date	Extra Cost? (Amount)	Legal (Covered in Contract)
Real-Time Clinical Alerts (List Desired)			
Medication Features (List Desired)			
Rx Information Source (List Desired Source)			
Medical Alerts (List Desired)			
Drug Formulary Features (List Desired)			
Decision Support Features (List Desired)			
Patient-entered Features (List Desired)			

Medical record content is the heart of your EMR. Use this Scorecard to move from general features to more specific criteria that are important to you. Make your list, then evaluate each feature personally during demonstrations in your office.

Crucial Decision
What core medical record content do you need? What specialty-specific features are required? Photocopy as needed or download this Scorecard from www.ehrselector.com

How Often is EMR Data Updated or Up-to-Date?

Ability to Query EMR (List Desired)

Ability to View EMR (List Desired)

Medical record content is the heart of your EMR. Use this Scorecard to move from general features to more specific criteria that are important to you. Make your list, then evaluate each feature personally during demonstrations in your office.

CHAPTER 12
Evaluating Vendor Stability

Crucial Decision
What makes an EMR developer a stable business partner?

This chapter also addresses the following questions:

- How do you know a vendor will be in business in 5 years?
- How do you know an EMR solution will continue to be enhanced?
- What factors are driving EMR market consolidation?

EMR Adventures

Let's check in on our friend, Dr. Alex Glass, the ophthalmologist who purchased an EMR based on the recommendations of his service technician and some physician friends. If you remember, Dr. Glass did not like his EMR much at all, while his assistant, Scott, thought it was great. Today, Dr. Glass and Scott are grabbing a quick sandwich in between patients on a busy Monday AM.

"I wanted to catch you later today but now is as good a time as any to let you know that our EMR vendor called and the call has me a little rattled. The guy said that we shouldn't worry about anything we read concerning their not staying in the EMR business," Scott reported to Dr. Glass. "He indicated something about being bought by a larger vendor and something else about rumors of a lawsuit, but he assured me that we would have continued support for our EMR – I hope so..."

"What do you mean?" asks Dr. Glass. "When are they to go out of business? What assurance did he give that any new company would support us? Can we have access to the EMR source code? Oh, this is not good news!"

"I know, I asked him to call you back after hours and he said he would. I did an Internet search and there were a couple of articles that hinted at something about our EMR vendor being in trouble financially but there was nothing specific," answers Scott.

"Still, the call bothers me. What does our purchasing agreement say about how we can obtain the EMR source code?" asks Dr. Glass.

"I don't know," answers Scott, "but even if we get it, what are you planning to do with it? You don't have time to learn to become a programmer, you're busy enough being a doctor and where would you find a programmer, and if you did, what would that cost?" continued Scott.

Successfully Choosing Your EMR: 15 Crucial Decisions. By © Arthur Gasch and Betty Gasch.
Published 2010 by Blackwell Publishing

"I have no idea what to do with the code, but I know that unless we have it, we have nothing if this EMR company goes out of business," laments Dr. Glass. "I think you better get the receptionist to cancel our afternoon appointments so that I can look into this further. Can you help me?"

Approaching the Topic of Stability

Stability is a delicate balance. Instability and consolidation in the EMR (and any) market is the norm, as Dr. Glass found out all too clearly. Size of a vendor alone offers no assurance that they will remain in the market. Neither does selecting a mid-sized EMR vendor guarantee that the company will be around under its present corporate structure in the next 5 years. Obviously, asking a vendor if their company is stable is of little help because every EMR vendor will tell you that they are. Therefore, in order to determine EMR vendor stability, we looked at the question from a different perspective.

The first areas we researched were the traditional measures of company stability, such as revenue growth, efficiency (ratio of revenues/employees), brand identity, potential for becoming an acquisition target, type of funding and so on. Then we went further and looked at stability from the perspective of the entire EMR industry, developing measures for it as a whole and comparing individual companies against that benchmark to see how they measured up. There are never any guarantees in business, but with this approach, you can arrive at a fairly accurate picture of EMR vendor viability.

Market Consolidation Implications

How likely is it that an EMR vendor will go out of business or become part of the continuing EMR market consolidation? To begin to answer that, we will list some EMR consolidations that occurred during the last 3 years; listed here are but a few:

- GE Healthcare acquired IDX. IDX was GE's third major EMR acquisition, as GE had previously acquired SEC (Ann Arbor) which became its original Centricity product, along with the Millbrook system.
- Allscripts acquired A4 Healthcare Systems and later Misys (its third major acquisition).
- McKesson acquired Practice Partner (formerly known as PMSI).
- Cerner has made two acquisitions and now has three different EMRs.
- Nuance/Scansoft acquired Dictaphone and later Philips Speech Systems.
- Sage Software acquired Emdeon (formerly WebMD).
- Henry Schein acquired both Cliniflow and MicroMD.
- Siemens created a partnership and marketing relationship with NextGen. That in fact is more interesting, because both companies were healthy but in complementary segments – Siemens primarily in the inpatient segment and NextGen in the physician office segment.

While consolidations may bring to mind small companies being acquired by larger ones, the examples cited were some pretty big companies being acquired by their larger competitors (who intentionally overlooked smaller alternatives). Certainly, such acquisitions will continue but at a slower pace.

An EMR company that is acquired in many ways poses a risk to its installed base of hospital departments or physician group practices. Even as the acquiring company continues on, there is no assurance that its current product line will be the "go ahead" EMR that remains intact or receives future development. The purpose of some acquisitions is simply to obtain and consolidate market share, and to afford the acquiring company an opportunity to market a competing product of their own to you when your current EMR ages and you want to replace it, or the client base gets frustrated because their EMR is no longer being kept current. Other times the desire is to integrate two complementary products, such as an EMR with a CPM so that a company is in a better competitive position in the market.

The worst case is where there is no acquisition at all, only a corporate failure, such as an EMR developer going into bankruptcy. This happened a while ago to Acermed and Dr. Notes. When the physicians licensing these EMRs needed additional EMR functionality, their next move was to purchase and migrate existing patient records to a new EMR. On rare occasions an EMR developer will go into bankruptcy, but then emerge later (under the same or different name) having reorganized or newly incorporated. In those cases the development of your EMR product might continue. This happened with Berdy Medical, which reorganized and was reintroduced to the market as VIP Medical.

Integration of EMR/CPM Drives Developer Consolidation

The viability of current CPM (Computer Practice Management) systems affects EMR purchases and is thus driving some acquisition in both directions (e.g. EMR companies are acquiring CPM business and vice versa). This happened, as mentioned in an earlier chapter, with Cliniflow, when it was acquired by Henry Schein. There are real benefits in functionality in the tighter integration between the clinical observations, diagnosis and therapeutic interventions with the optimization of ICD and CPT coding and potential reimbursement. Most EMRs that have been around 6-10 years weren't originally designed to be part of an integrated CPM solution, so those EMR developers are buying ones that are a reasonable fit, and then interfacing them to get some first level benefits of an integrated product. Newer EMR+CPM products however are now being designed from scratch, so that they work together seamlessly, out of a single database and with a consistent user interface.

If you are the owner of either a purchased EMR or CPM, you can expect to see some significant changes (and perhaps some inconsistencies with your current design) in newer versions of the interfaced products. That is OK and a good thing as long as the developer is committed to a backward EMR chart compatibility or at least to a migration path into whatever the new chart (internal) structure may become. Since this is the trend for the future, some of these endeavors are attracting venture capital money, so they may be well financed, but that presents the possibility that the company developing the interfaced/integrated products may ultimately be sold to generate the ROI on the venture capital investment.

Source Code License or Open Source EMR?

To plan for the contingency that your EMR developer might go belly up, it's a good idea to include specific provisions in your purchase (or licensing) agreement to provide you with access to all source code. For some larger EMR developers this can be a difficult, to near impossible, condition to get into the sales contract or licensing agreement. Some agreements state that the EMR developer must keep their latest source code in escrow, and transfer it to their licensees, in the event of their failure and some even require that in the event of their acquisition by another company (very few larger EMR developers will agree to the latter provision).

One initial way to assure that you have access to your EMR code, is to forgo any of the proprietary EMR products and instead choose an open source EMR. Open source is an important alternative to proprietary systems because with proprietary EMRs, if the company fails, you have no option to go forward unless you have required that source code transfer to you in such circumstances. With open source EMR approaches (like VistA) you have the source code always available. This provides you some flexibility in making customizations or even developing your own EMR open source version.

Open source provides various operating system choices, mostly in the Unix family of operating systems. Current versions can run under Apache, Artistic license/GPL, Eclipse Public License (EPL), GNU General Public License (GPL), Affero GNU General Public License (AGPL), GNU Lessor General Public License (LGPL), MIT License, Mozilla Public License and the New BSD License. There are several open source licenses that exist. One such open sourced EMR is Medsphere (Carlsbad, CA).

Medsphere demonstrated upgrades to its OpenVistA, an electronic health record developed for the VA Hospitals, and later abandoned by them. Since then it has been given an enhanced medication reconciliation, pharmacy functionality with a pharmacy dashboard, a pricing engine and a patient drug information library. We have previously listed the down side to open source EMRs, so let's return to the topic of determining vendor stability.

How to Determine the Stability of an EMR Developer

Data from the MSP/Andrew EMR Benchmark affords a number of measures for determining the stability of EMR developers and we used a combination of measures from the Benchmark. The first criterion we looked at was the relationship between the date a developer entered the market and the amount of revenue they had. Our thought is, if we compare EMR developers that have been in the market for the same period of time, if a company has more revenue, then it is growing faster and is more likely to survive.

The number of years an EMR vendor has been in business is the first feature that people typically consider when thinking of stability/viability. However, this criterion is a little tricky in the EMR arena because EMRs have not been around for that long, and products from those vendors that have been around the longest are sometimes based on fairly archaic platforms and languages.

How Long in the Market and Revenue

If an EMR developer is successful, then there should be a correlation between the year they entered the market and their revenues. Companies that entered the market 10 or more years ago but still have small revenues, may not have a value equation or product that appeals to the market or may be lacking capital or some other critical element. Companies that have offered EMRs for at least a decade should not be reluctant to share their revenues, unless they have a problem in this area.

Figure 12.1 illustrates findings for revenue growth and length of time in the EMR market. Five years ago, 71 percent of EMR companies had revenues below $2M. Five years later, 24 percent of those small companies had grown in revenue (47.7 percent remained in the <$2M category). Likewise, another 11 percent had moved out of the $2-5M revenue range, while 6 percent more had moved beyond the $5-10M category.

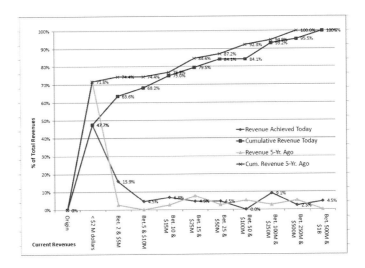

Figure 12.1 EMR Developer 5-Year Growth in Revenues (by Revenue Cluster)

Looking at the graph overall, revenues of $5-10M represent a drop in risk for an EMR company, and presumably risk is reduced as revenues increase, yet over 68 percent of EMR vendors fall below this threshold. Of the newcomers to the EMR market in the last 5 years, 83 percent have not achieved revenues in excess of $2M, and only 6 percent have achieved revenues of more than $10M. This group is presumably more viable than the other newcomers.

More than half of the current EMR developers entered the market after 1998 and almost 30 percent of the EMR developers entered the market less than 5 years ago[1]. A couple of years ago, 15 percent of the EMR developers (approximately 30 companies assuming 200 EMR developers) had been in the EMR market for 3 years or less! That's amazing when you think about it. In order to demonstrate to you that they are safe to purchase from, they need to show you their revenue trends for the last 3 years. A few of these companies are public and all of the public companies should have revenues over $2M. Some private EMR firms are not as easy to locate revenues for.

How Long has EMR Been Marketed

Entry of new EMR developers in the market is a healthy sign, because it means that more players are realizing the potential in the market and investing in the product development needed to enter it, but at the same time it would be naïve to believe that a strong EMR product with a competitive feature set (even one with CCHIT certification) is enough for long-term success.

Between 2001 and 2005, the U.S. EMR market evolved from having many very small, startup EMR developers (less than 35 employees) to more mid-sized and larger EMR developers. Smaller vendors are particularly aware that you will look for some measure of company size in order to determine if they are likely to grow and remain a viable competitor over the next few years. Of 29 companies with under 15 employees in 2001, only 19 of them existed 5 years later, and only 10 of the 29 (about 33 percent) exhibited the growth that would be needed to assure risk-sensitive physicians.

Again, 19 companies (with less than 15 employees after 5 years in the market) is about 10 percent of the total number of EMR developers in the U.S. market. Companies that remained small (not identified in this book) are unlikely to be able to continue to respond to a rapidly expanding EMR market or to obtain sufficient brand identity to even participate in the market. Length of time in the market versus number of active licenses is sometimes a good indicator of stability. Being too new (say less than 2 years), or too old with too few site licenses, seems to us to be troubling indications.

There are newer, innovative EMR products coming to the market that are perhaps worthy of your attention, but if you prefer a company that has been tested, know that just over 40 percent of the EMR products have been marketed for over 10 years with another ~20 percent having been marketed for between five and 10 years. Over one third (37 percent) of the EMR

---

[1] MSP/Andrew EMR Benchmark – Q1-9

developers have been marketing their products for less than 5 years and may be the more affordable ones, and perhaps the more innovative or specialty-specific ones. Nonetheless, the length of time a product has been marketed is one criterion which you can determine the importance of on your Stability/ Viability Scorecard (at the end of the chapter).

Number of Employees

The number of employees can also be an indicator of stability/viability and it is always interesting to look at the number of employees in an EMR company, and compare that to the company revenues. However, in the past few years, a number of larger companies have merged and become even larger. Again, there is no guarantee, but asking any EMR company you are interested in how many employees they have can be an important part of your Stability/ Viability Scorecard. As a company's revenues grow, they typically hire more employees, so tracking employees is an indication of growth, as long as the company isn't financing that hiring by incurring losses. Figure 12.2 shows the comparison between the number of employees that EMR companies gained (or lost) over a 5-year period for a sample of 81 EMR companies. It suggests that about 16-20 employees are needed to sustain a critical mass; while companies that reach over 75 employees tended to consistently grow, which suggests there is still too large a percentage of very small EMR firms entering the market (see Figure 12.3).

While this data is only a snapshot at a point in time of the market, it would be a concern if companies with less than 35 employees today, still have less than 35 in another 2 to 3 years. EMR developers that are smaller are likely to either leave the market, or if their EMR solution is sufficiently robust, to be acquired by a CPM provider or other larger entities looking for a quick entry into this expanding market.

Figure 12.2 Growth in EMR Developer Division (Company) Size Over Five Years

Number of Employees	Companies 5 Years Ago	Companies Today
≤15	29	19
16-35	9	14
36-75	12	12
76-250	8	14
251-500	4	8
501-1000	2	4
1001-5000	3	4

We can't give you a hard-and-fast rule of thumb for what's too small, but there clearly is a critical mass that an EMR developer needs to achieve to remain viable and support growth in this market. If a vendor cannot achieve business growth sufficient to support 30-40 personnel within 3-5 years of entering the market, no matter who their corporate parent or partner may be, they need to seriously reexamine their value proposition as it relates to pricing, support, basic features, size of the market niche being addressed and access to capital. Such reexamination is due for nearly 40 percent of all EMR developers currently participating in the U.S. market.

Revenue Growth and Employee Growth In Sync?

Revenue growth is more significant than employment growth (that one-third of companies achieved). Physicians often perceive two choices: Believing that they can deal with a small EMR developer that offers a system they can afford, but has a 5 in 6 chance of not being (financially) viable in the next 5 years, or dealing with a large, viable EMR developer that offers only systems that are way beyond the physician's budget limits, and getting more expensive all the time. This chapter offers focus on this belief.

Number of Employees	% of All EMR Companies
≤15	24%
16-35	18%
36-75	16%
76-150	18%
151-250	9%
251-500	9%
501-1000	5%
1001-5000	5%

Figure 12.3 Number of Employees in Selected EMR Developers

A relatively new EMR developer must show that it has revenues of more than $10M (or at least greater than $5M) in order to differentiate itself from other startup EMR developers, although this by itself may be insufficient to sustain a critical mass in the market. An EMR developer that chooses to use revenues, however, should be prepared to support revenue claims from an independent source.

A good source of this data is the Harris Infosource Selectory database, which lists revenue (est.), number of employees and year established (although not always for the EMR division of larger corporate entities). Many of the EMR developers are listed here, but companies with under $1M in annual revenues may not be listed, and small private companies generally self-report data to D&B, which collects the data for this product. All that aside, for larger private and public companies, this resource can be helpful. We have listed in Figure

12.4 the profile for NextGen. Realize that these change frequently, so this does not reflect the company's situation at the time you read this book.

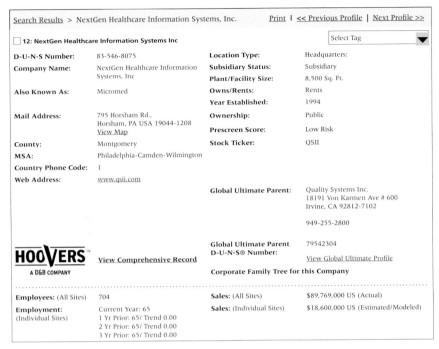

Search Results > NextGen Healthcare Information Systems, Inc.   Print I << Previous Profile | Next Profile >>

☐ 12: NextGen Healthcare Information Systems Inc

D-U-N-S Number:	83-546-8075	**Location Type:**	Headquarters:
Company Name:	NextGen Healthcare Information Systems, Inc	**Subsidiary Status:**	Subsidiary
		Plant/Facility Size:	8,500 Sq. Ft.
Also Known As:	Micromed	**Owns/Rents:**	Rents
		Year Established:	1994
Mail Address:	795 Horsham Rd., Horsham, PA USA 19044-1208 View Map	**Ownership:**	Public
		Prescreen Score:	Low Risk
County:	Montgomery	**Stock Ticker:**	QSII
MSA:	Philadelphia-Camden-Wilmington		
Country Phone Code:	1		
Web Address:	www.qsii.com		
		Global Ultimate Parent:	Quality Systems Inc. 18191 Von Karmen Ave # 600 Irvine, CA 92812-7102 949-255-2800
		Global Ultimate Parent D-U-N-S® Number:	79542304 View Global Ultimate Profile
	View Comprehensive Record	**Corporate Family Tree for this Company**	

HOOVERS™
A D&B COMPANY

Employees: (All Sites)	704	**Sales:** (All Sites)	$89,769,000 US (Actual)
Employment: (Individual Sites)	Current Year: 65 1 Yr Prior: 65/ Trend 0.00 2 Yr Prior: 65/ Trend 0.00 3 Yr Prior: 65/ Trend 0.00	**Sales:** (Individual Sites)	$18,600,000 US (Estimated/Modeled)

Figure 12.4 A Typical EMR Developer Listing from Harris Infosource Selectory

Shown is a part of the data available from Selectory on NextGen, a well-known EMR developer located in Horsham, PA. One of the features of this data is its Pre-screen Score, in this case "low risk," indicating that Harris believes NextGen is financially stable. There is much other useful information, including the D-U-N-S number, the Employee Count (704), yielding a revenue/employee of a bit over $127K. That tends to confirm other stability indicators.

These records can also show corporate relationships, if the EMR developer is part of a larger venture or has a silent parent organization. The latter reveals a NextGen/Siemens partnership and has a link to follow for more information. A bit more research on Google (using key words like "acquired," "acquired by," "partnership") can turn up additional information of interest.

Revenue/Employee Value Ratio
Another marker of stability is the revenues/employee value. A ratio of $200,000 or above is generally healthy. Ratios between $100K and $200K are good also, but ratios of $100K or less require a second look. This might be fine during the first year or two of a company's start-up phase, but is not that healthy an indicator 10 years later.

The revenues that an EMR developer has can help determine stability/ viability and is a question that the company should readily answer. Almost half (47.7 percent) of EMR developers had revenues of $2M or less although by the time of this book's publication that number should have increased. About 16 had achieved revenue levels of between $10 and $15 million. The rest of the companies made less.

If you predefine a revenue level in your stability/viability definition you will be quickly narrowing the field of EMR developers to include in your search. What EMR developer revenue level you are comfortable with is one criterion on your Stability/Viability Scorecard at the end of this chapter.

A general rule of thumb for the relationship between number of employees and company revenues is that a company will need about $125,000 to $175,000 per employee to grow and thrive in the medical electronics or technology business. A company with 15 employees would need to achieve at least yearly revenues in the range of $1.8 to $2.6 million in yearly revenues to be self-sustaining.

If you are really feeling ambitious, to determine what number of software licenses an EMR developer would need to sell each year to achieve such revenues, add the revenues from their first year sales (new systems) multiplied by the list price or 12 times their monthly maintenance fees, to 20 percent of that cost per system, times the number of system/licenses in their installed base. Twenty percent is not a hard number, as some companies charge as little as 15 percent and others as much as 25 percent per year of the initial system price for ongoing support and product enhancement.

Such calculations begin to reveal whether a developer's installed base plus new installs is likely to sustain them in a positive cash flow position, or whether they have not yet achieved critical mass and may be more risky a venture. While a developer may refuse to report revenues, it is usually possible to find out what they charge for EMR licenses, and usually to get an estimate of the number of employees on staff (from the company itself or from a qualified EMR systems analyst). Some of this information is tracked in the POMIS report, which is written by Vinson Hudson, Jewson Enterprises, and distributed through our Web site, www.medsp.com. The POMIS report includes a database on 403 POMIS vendors, including almost 200 EMR developers.

Revenues of New EMR Vendors

There is another way of looking at the issue of vendor stability/viability – through early revenue growth achieved. When companies first enter the EMR market they generally have negative cash flow but work hard to achieve a rapid increase in sales. During the first few years there should be dramatic revenue growth (whether or not there is positive net income).

The MSP/Andrew EMR Benchmark looked at the revenue size of EMR developers that had entered the EMR market in the last 2 years. Only about 6 percent of the EMR developers that entered the market in the last 5 years have achieved revenues in excess of $10 million. These were the most successful of the newcomer EMR developers.

Another 11 percent have achieved revenues in excess of $2M. These were the moderately successful newcomers. The vast majority (83 percent) have not yet achieved revenues of $2M, which raises questions about their success in this market. Given the estimate of critical size, this suggests that companies under $2M in revenue are probably struggling to stay afloat, and may be more focused on that than upon what features should be developed for the next release of their EMR software, or may be grossly undercapitalized and needing to hold down expenditures due to limited funding. This is an ominous sign for the future of these companies as only 6 percent or so are safe and another 11 percent are on the cusp of viability.

Source of EMR Developer Revenues

An EMR developer's revenue source can reveal a measure of stability/viability as well. Those companies funded mainly by venture capital money typically have a five year time frame in which to become successful and one of the definitions of successful is being sold to a larger medically-oriented company.

Fifty-two percent of the EMR developers stated that they had no long-term debt, financed their growth out of gross income, and are financially stable companies. Forty percent stated that their funding came from bank loans or venture capital or angel funding. These vendors are somewhat less stable than those that have a lower percentage of funding from these areas. This is another question that is worth asking any EMR developer whose product you are interested in, also included on the Stability/Viability Scorecard.

Focus and Leadership of EMR Developer

Another factor we use to determine vendor stability is where the EMR developer is located and where they are marketing their products. For example, a U.S. developer, selling to the U.S. market exclusively, is probably more focused than a Canadian EMR developer that is selling to both the U.S. and the Canadian EMR markets (which have somewhat different EMR feature requirements). Several of the companies in our opening acquisition list were larger U.S. EMR companies that got involved in the ill-fated U.K. EMR project and lost millions trying to get U.K. doctors to adopt technologies they hadn't asked for, (the mid-sized and smaller EMR developers involved were considered to be too small to bother with).

Another measure we use is whether the visionary responsible for the EMR is still with the EMR company and actively engaged in enhancing the product. If not, who is spearheading the on-going EMR development?

Website Information

Press releases from various Web sites can also be informative (see Figure 12.5). As noted by Scott in Dr. Glass's office, the Web will alert you to some rumors prior to anything concrete, but you cannot build a reliable response to rumors, especially early ones. The Web will offer specifics of information that has already occurred, and is a good place to look for general EMR vendor information.

NextGen Healthcare | Strategic Partnerships
NextGen Healthcare partners with leading information & technology companies to ensure our EHR, EMR & practice management software keeps our customers ...
www.nextgen.com/com_partners.asp - Cached - Similar

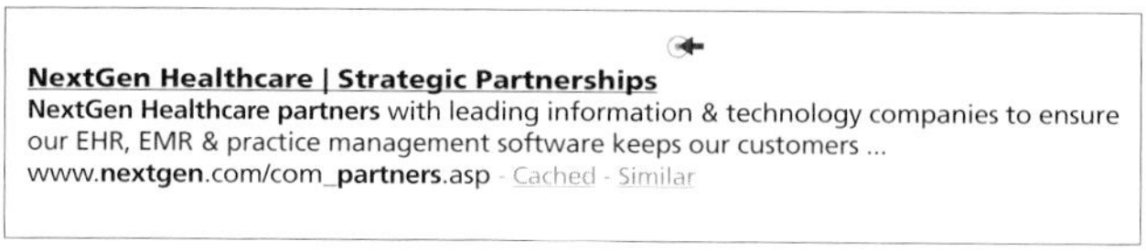

Figure 12.5 Press Releases From the Web are Also Informative

Check out EMR developer Web sites, as you will want to test your initial reaction to it, particularly if the developer is offering an ASP-based EMR solution. Websites that are difficult to navigate, lack complete contact information (like a physical address), lack helpful product descriptions or focus exclusively on marketing hyperbole etc. allow you to draw inferences about the EMR product. Would the EMR solution be any easier to use?

CCHIT Certification

Basic functionality to nationally-established standards is important. The government has established CCHIT (the Commission for Certification of Health Information Technology) to institute basic functionality standards for EMRs. Currently over 90 EMRs are CCHIT-certified. By the end of 2009 that number will have increased again so that, while CCHIT is a necessary certification for any EMR, it tells you little about the differences in EMR solutions that are actually available. A tool that drills down to details not covered by CCHIT is what is necessary to choose an EMR that is right for your practice specialty, number of offices, preferred input type, budget and other requirements.

We recommend you choose a system that is CCHIT-certified; but not just any EMR, one that also meets your budget, specialty focus, practice size and many other practice-specific issues that are important to your practice, patients, delivery style and workflow preferences.

The CCHIT mission is to accelerate the adoption of health information technology by creating an efficient, credible and sustainable product certification program. The CCHIT commission approached this goal by establishing standards to be used for reviewing electronic health record products for their ability to carry out fundamental tasks they felt were common to EMRs in all care settings. A growing number of organizations are requiring CCHIT certification in order for an EMR to be recommended for their members, qualify for malpractice insurance reductions or obtain state assistance for EMR funding, so the basic functionality of this standard is gaining traction in the market.

We believe that one criterion of a stable/viable EMR developer is CCHIT certification but that there is a danger that many physicians will assume that buying a CCHIT-certified EMR product is an assurance that there are no issues with the solution.

Conclusions and Recommendations

So what is the critical mass (in terms of revenues) that an EMR vendor must reach to be viable? MSP believes that developers with sales of $15M or more have reached critical mass in the EMR market, although that in itself does not guarantee brand identity or access resources to complete in a large number of negotiations should the number of sales in the market suddenly accelerate.

Figure 12.6 Emerging EMR Developers That Have Achieved $10M-20M in Revenues

EMR Product Name	EMR Developer Name
e-MDs	e-MDs
MediNotes	MediNotes
Pulse Patient Relationship Management	Pulse Systems
CPSI System	CPSI
EMIS PCS	Emis
NextGen EMR	NextGen
INTERACTANT	Health Care Software
accessANYware	LanVision dba Streamline Health

The companies in Figure 12.6 are some newer ones that have achieved between $10M and $15M in sales and therefore represent a good base for continued growth among the emerging EMR developers. Of course many of the larger, more established companies have substantially greater revenues and are not listed in Figure 12.6, companies like McKesson, GE, and others. Data in the above table was self-reported by the EMR developers, and many developers declined to report even revenue estimates. Unless they are large, public companies require any prospective EMR developer to provide audited revenue information before considering acquiring a system from them.

Wrap Up

If an EMR developer is perceived as risky, that developer has probably already lost your sale, even if they attempt to pursue the sale to its conclusion. Few EMR developers provide good financial or other data from which you can infer vendor stability or their market risk. You will need to look at multiple indirect indicators and draw your own conclusions. Use the Stability Scorecard to compile some information. Be diligent and you will gain sufficient information to determine which EMR vendors are stable. As data interchange standards are increasingly supported, there is better potential to migrate from one EMR to another, if you find that your current EMR developer is not "keeping up with the industry" to your satisfaction.

Crucial Decision

Indicate which EMR Stability/Viability attribute you chose and briefly note the rationale for the choice. Photocopy as needed or download this Scorecard from www.ehrselector.com

EMR Attribute	Importance (1=min/10=max.)	Verbal	Docu./Demo
Years Vendor in Business			
# of Vendor Employees			
Year Vendor Entered Market			
Vendor Size Compared to 5 Years Ago			
Vendor Revenues			
Source of Revenues			
Revenue Growth			
At Critical Revenue Mass?			
Length of Time EMR Has Been Marketed			
Primary Care Setting Focus			
Internal Code Development			
# of Middleware Partners			
CCHIT Certification			
Other			

CHAPTER 13

Lawyer-Proofing Your EMR

Crucial Decision

Do you need legal advice to mitigate risks of EMR purchasing or licensing agreements?

This chapter also addresses the following questions:

- Can you rely on an EMR that is CCHIT certified to be legal in all aspects?
- What expertise do you need to assure that your EMR records will stand up to legal challenges?
- Is the lawyer who covers your general practice issues adequate for EMR legal issues?

Acknowledgment

This chapter was contributed by Dr. Reed Gelzer, MD, a principal of Advocates for Documentation Integrity and Compliance. Reed is a contributor to *How to Evaluate Electronic Health Record (EHR) Systems*, by Patricia A. Trites, MPA, and Reed D. Gelzer, MD, MPH (more information at the end of this chapter). I have known Reed for several years, and he consistently and widely advocates EHR compliance with well-established records management requirements and tighter standards for making charts generated by EMRs trustworthy medical records that are also not fraudulent, thereby keeping the physicians who use them out of trouble.

Reed has worked tirelessly, through his participation on CCHIT-committees and work with standards groups like HL7, to both develop standards and requirements as well as to raise awareness of risks associated with poorly-designed EMR systems. He has promoted the adoption of due-diligence testing by purchasers and users, against basic records management and medical records performance criteria that would mitigate downstream risks of EMR adoption – only to be thwarted by some of the largest EMR developers and largest physician member organizations. It would be prudent to review and utilize *How to Evaluate EHR Systems* prior to purchasing any EMR.

EMR Adventures

Dr. Jonas was proud of his office's minimally disruptive, painless changeover to their office EMR system. By taking advantage of resources available through his

Successfully Choosing Your EMR: 15 Crucial Decisions. By © Arthur Gasch and Betty Gasch.
Published 2010 by Blackwell Publishing

physician association, his entire office staff had been involved in the planning and preparation – and now they were reaping all the promised benefits of this new tool. Charting was faster, easier, and timely, he'd also seen his practice income go up while he and his wife were going home earlier, and so were his three partners. Everything was going great – or so it seemed.

Today, though, he's scratching his head a bit. A worried patient called asking whether one of his office employees, who happens to be an in-law, may have sneaked a peek at her past medical history which revealed some long-ago marital discord and indiscretions. The patient is so concerned that she is requesting a HIPAA Security Audit Report.

Dr. Jonas logs into his EMR and checks the reports available, but none of the names seem to be what he's looking for. He phones his EMR developer's support line and learns how to search for the information he needs. Launching the required reports, he's surprised to find them very scanty – there just isn't much information here. Checking for a patient whose record he knows he himself viewed earlier in the day, he's unnerved by the absence of any indication that he had looked at that record. Perhaps the system isn't working correctly – some setting has been messed up?

He calls the support line back and is further disturbed when he finds that the system was installed and configured with key audit functions disabled by default. When he asks the support person how this would happen, he's told, "Users often turn the audit functions off because they slow down the system so much."

Now he's really feeling uncomfortable. What's he going to do? He didn't recall that the developer or the EMR install team had said anything about audit trails being disabled. Now he realizes that he doesn't know who has looked at which patient records and perhaps who may have altered them! With some anxiety, he calls his attorney and explains the situation. His attorney doesn't have a medical records practice and says he'll have to get back to him. An hour later his attorney calls back and suggests that a local Compliance Specialist be engaged to help identify the extent of legal issues he might be confronting.

"Why didn't the EMR developer turn on that audit trail setting? They didn't ask me about it when it went live. This is going to be really expensive and it's going to take a lot of time!" Dr. Jonas frets.

On the first visit by the Compliance Specialist, Dr. Jonas executes appropriate business agreements so that the specialist has access to the EMR system without creating a HIPAA violation. Then the two sit down for what the Compliance Specialist calls a "simple EMR stress test." Dr. Jonas is becoming increasingly apprehensive as he wonders what an EMR "stress test" is and why is he hearing about it for the first time now? The Compliance Specialist asks, "Didn't you do this as part of your acceptance testing?"

"What acceptance testing?" replies Dr. Jonas, "The EMR developer just installed the system and we started using it. We spent more money than I wanted to in order to purchase from a well-known, larger vendor – one that had more installations and had been developing EMRs for many years. I figured that they installed a safe and reliant system." The Compliance Specialist nods but doesn't say a word.

As they test the system together, the initial discovery is that the EMR does not produce a standard encounter record. The Compliance Specialist explains that a standard encounter includes basic CMS documentation requirements such as identifying authorship of each section of the patient record, but apparently that isn't what his EMR system does. Instead, his EMR attributes all the available sections, records and reports only to Dr. Jonas, showing him as the sole author of the whole record. None of the documentation entered by his nurse, or by the patient at the new kiosk, are attributed to them. The problem in the EMR design was beginning to sink in.

"Do your medical assistants do the chief complaint and History of Present Illness (HPI) for any of your Medicare patients?" asks his Compliance Specialist. "Of course," replies Dr. Jonas. "They do that for some patients, particularly on busy days. We've worked that way for years."

"But do your records document any of that?" asks his Compliance Specialist.

Dr. Jonas pulls up a recent patient record where he recalls that his medical assistant had filled in some of the Medicare data. It indicates that he alone provided all the services, including the chief complaint and HPI, which were actually done by his assistant. "Oh, this isn't good... ," says a little voice in his head, "this is trouble!"

Looking through other, more sophisticated reports available from the underlying database software that actually stores the EMR's data, more detail becomes available. Although the record does not show who did what, the system does show time-stamps for each section that was entered, including the HPI. Looking at the log-in and log-out times for Dr. Jonas' assistant, it is clear that one of the assistant's log-out times is the same as when the HPI was completed, appearing to show that a curious auditor with some basic database knowledge could reconstruct who did what. The EMR simple stress test was not seeming so simple now.

Dr. Jonas' thoughts are interrupted by his Compliance Specialist's next statement. "Look, these default templates you're using generate extensive documentation for even simple visits like a healthy patient's viral respiratory infection, which the EMR's coding engine bullet-counts to a 99215 code. You seem to be billing for services as if you provided them yourself and in these cases, coding high without consideration of medical necessity," he remarks.

Dr. Jonas is now really feeling concerned, along with a mixture of frustration and fear. He had noticed that the practice income had increased, which he thought was good because that's one of the reasons he wanted to purchase an EMR in the first place. "The EMR developer said we were probably missing some reimbursable charges by under-coding for the services we provide," he thinks out loud.

The Compliance Specialist replies, "Yes, under-coding for complex procedures where there is medical necessity is quite common in many practices, but that isn't the same thing as up-coding for simple encounters by adding unneeded services – that's fraud and it's covered by the False Claims Act. The False Claims Act provides for fines of $5,500 to $11,000 per incident. Let me see your purchasing contract."

Dr. Jonas calls his wife who retrieves the EMR contract from the office safe. As she hands it to him, his fear is turning into anger towards his EMR developer. He hands the contract to the Compliance Specialist, who scans it briefly and points out a particular area to Dr. Jonas, who is mentally bracing himself for what he is about to hear.

"Hmm, like most EMR contracts I see, this one has a 'Hold Harmless' paragraph. Did your lawyer who helped you negotiate this agreement, not point this out to you?" he asks. Dr. Jonas lets the question pass.

"Do you realize that if a Recovery Audit Contractor (RAC) finds these routine up-coding events and misinterpretations of who actually provided the services, you're on your own, since you've agreed in the contract not to blame the EMR developer for any problems the EMR system has?" he asks. "Who did this purchasing contract for you anyway?"

"Well, we didn't want to agree to the purchasing terms offered by the EMR developer because we thought they would be too favorable to them – after all, this company is a giant enterprise and they must have a ton of lawyers. The EMR was stretching our budget and we were trying to save some money, so we took some terms from their agreement and some terms from the boilerplate legal agreement in our medical organization's 'White Paper' and sort of merged them together. In retrospect, it was probably a bad approach," reflects Dr. Jonas.

"Do you know what it would have cost you for some front-end legal advice on the purchasing agreement when you were buying this?" inquires the Compliance Specialist.

"We got two quotes, one came in at about $5,500 and the other was more like $12,000, as I recall. They both seemed like a lot of extra money at the time. I can't believe the EMR developer didn't bring up the legal aspects and how their system actually merges together all who contribute to collecting the patient information, and attributes it to me," complains Dr. Jonas.

"Why would they?" remarks the Compliance Specialist. "I've found in my practice that some EMR developers tend not to bring up certain topics, rather than shine a light on them, because they are afraid that doing so will mess up the deal and cause you to choose another vendor's system."

"Yeah, but I trusted these guys – and apart from this issue, the EMR has performed very well," says Dr. Jonas. "What can I do?"

"My advice is to come up with a mitigation plan immediately. Let me help you with that, we can quantify the potential damages and discuss them with your attorney for the best course out of this mess."

"How bad can it be?" asks Dr. Jonas.

"It can be quite expensive – a hospital in Florida paid an $11 million settlement due, in part, to defects in their anesthesiology EMR system,[1] and there was a recent article about how outpatient practices had paid fines up to $175,000 per physician due to problems with their EMR-sourced documentation,"[2] noted the Compliance Specialist.

"Unbelievable! How can this be?" Dr. Jonas replies – despondently, "I have no idea what I am going to do. I don't have that kind of money, even with the increased revenues we have received, it's not like we have kept the additional funds in a savings account; we have invested most of them back into the practice. How will I tell my partners about this? I am just so angry at my EMR developer for not pointing this out. And so angry at myself for saving a few thousand bucks on the front end by not retaining a legal firm that specializes in negotiating EMR purchase agreements."

"Well, if it's any consolation, you aren't alone. Many EMRs come with their audit tracking functions turned off by default, and some, like yours, don't properly attribute entries into the patient record to anyone but the physician who signs it," adds the Compliance Specialist. "Even getting legal advice isn't going to help unless that law firm has knowledge about EMR contracting issues and is a medical law practice."

"I realize that now," says Dr. Jonas. "I called the attorney that handles our general operations and he didn't know what I was talking about."

As the Compliance Specialist prepares to leave, he thinks, "There are other items here we need to discuss, e-Discovery and metadata-associated risks for starters, but today's not the time to bring them up. Dr. Jonas already looks overwhelmed and I don't want to distract him from his patient care. For today, I can help by passing him the name of a law firm that specializes in medical liability and fraud issues."

Dr. Jonas felt sick himself and didn't want to see patients today, but what could he do, his waiting room was full because his new EMR had allowed the practice to take new patients again. Dr. Jonas was really upset and anxious, but he couldn't let his patients see that. "What am I going to do now?" he thought. "What?"

"One thing I need to do is make sure the audit trail reports are turned on, now that I realize they were off. I'm so glad my Compliance Specialist suggested a law firm to call, and gave me their business card on the way out. He also offered to return to help me to perform more vigorous compliance testing, he seems sympathetic and like he wants to help," thought Dr. Jonas.

These are some of the thoughts and emotions swirling around in his head as Dr. Jonas makes his way into the exam room to see his first patient of

---

[1] *Failure to Recognize Loss of Incoming Data in an Anesthesia Record-Keeping System May Have Increased Medical Liability.* By Michael M. Vigoda, MD, MBA and David A. Lubarsky, MD, MBA. Published 2006, Vol. 102, by Anesthesia & Analgesia

[2] *The problem with EHRs and coding.* By Deborah Grider, CPC, et al. Published April 3, 2009, by Medical Economics

the day, who turns out to be the woman who complained that her personal information had been leaked. She looks like she wants to talk about it too. "How could this day get any worse?" thinks poor Dr. Jonas as he tries to greet her with a smile.

The Current Legal Context for EMRs

This vignette well-illustrates the case for obtaining proper, specialized legal assistance when delving into EMR purchases and deployments. Knowing how strictly your EMR follows well-established records creation, management, and output tasks is critical to making sure that all of your hard work isn't automatically converted into less-than-legal records that can be readily challenged or impeached. In all cases, electronic documentation systems must also provide means to prove that the record system is doing its job, by virtue of its access and documentation audit trails.

Even specific and basic EMR system requirements well known in law, such as a HIPAA Security Audit report, cannot be presumed to exist in all EMRs. EMRs with well-designed reports and audit trails do exist, but even the best-designed system can be improperly configured or wrongly used, and naturally these are things that many EMR developers don't bring up or dwell upon. Getting the contract right on the front end is crucial and far more effective than trying to fix details on the back end, as Dr. Jonas discovered.

Important Legal Functionality

Issues like "e-Discovery" and "metadata-associated risks" are also important, and only now drawing the attention of the legal community, and there are many details left to be clarified. There is the potential to oversimplify the issues surrounding EMR deployment; however, much of the apparent confusion can be addressed by starting with what doctors already know about paper-based, medical record documentation.

For example, the record must accurately show who did what and when. With a handwritten paper chart, the handwriting and the color of the ink can often identify who wrote it, or at least that several people contributed to the charting. That isn't always so easy in an electronic chart. Also, any changes to a completed record must be accurately captured and such an altered record must be clearly identified as changed, indicating by whom and when.

Are Electronic Records Credible?

The remainder of this chapter was written by Arthur and Betty Gasch. Credibility is essential to the successful adoption of EMRs as a foundational technology for the serious healthcare reform that is now being discussed in the U.S. Congress. Technology can enable the changes that the president and congress are calling for – but it must do so in a manner that instills trust among all stakeholders, especially patients and insurance companies.

Having seen many reports of hackers breaking into banking and other computers, the average American isn't convinced that electronic medical records are really safe, or accurate either. And then there is the issue of being able to change data once it is stored electronically. Americans have become suspicious, for example, of technology such as electronic balloting, with many believing that voting results can be altered. Balancing the negative side of automation are the many advantages to practicing medicine using an EMR.

Because of the government's EMR stimulus, positive or negative (or a blend of the two), the EMR will soon be a widespread reality. The need for EMR credibility is fundamental to developing a responsible electronic process, one in which the physician/patient relationship continues based on trust. The area of EMR credibility is still presently in flux, as explained in the following example.

The Legal Status of an EMR Medical Record

When a clinician enters a patient's blood pressure on a paper form, the form is signed and becomes part of the patient's chart; it's a legal record and an original document. If you look at an original paper record, you can see what is written on it, determine if anything has been crossed out, any new information appended, and even if more than one person wrote in the document.

But when a clinician enters information onto a screen form that stores information entered in a computer database – what is that? It isn't a document. Is it a legal record of the care provided? There has been some confusion surrounding EMR legality, and audit trails in particular. Some EMRs (including some well-known, larger ones) allow clinicians to change information after the fact. This is very dangerous and a practice that is fraught with potential problems, as pointed out in the opening vignette.

(Dr. Reed Gelzer has been telling the EMR industry for sometime that the thin ice of allowing audit trails to be disabled is not only a problem, but may actually be illegal). There is an established set of federal rules of evidence that apply not only to EMRs, but also to paper charts. These rules are part of the Business Records Exception 803(6)[3]. Here are Reed's derived guidelines for assessing whether an EMR will support these established federal rules:

- The information in the EMR has to be recorded by someone who was at the patient encounter, such as the physician, rather than another physician who was not present;
- The information must be recorded in a timely way because it will be less valuable if written down six months after the patient was seen;
- The information must be stored in a secure and protected area, but the EMR must also be easily accessible;

[3] *Foundation of Digital Evidence.* By George Paul. Published 2008 by American Bar Association

• The information recorded must be part of the normal course of business.[4] We'll next look at the audit trail aspect of these rules in more detail. We chose the audit trail feature because EMRs vary greatly in how they address this. (Like Dr. Gelzer, we think it is important for you to purchase an EMR that legally-admissible patient charts. The other points, and a more in-depth accounting of audit trails, are covered in Patricia Trites' and Dr. Gelzer's book mentioned in the beginning of this chapter).

Data Integrity

To track the sequence of data stored in an EMR database, its entries must be time-stamped, at the individual item level (creating an incremental "snapshot" of the database). The database must contain fields indicating the logged-in user who updated it and the template or form-ID that was displayed during data entry. This information, in addition to the patient data itself, should be stored in some encrypted format by the EMR program, so that it is not directly readable or alterable by humans, but only by the EMR program. This minimizes the potential for tampering or adulterating the database records, at least for users who do not have the source code of the EMR program. Users with EMR source code can adulterate anything.

Without such audit trail data, you can't say with any certainty, when any data in any instance of the EMR database was actually added, changed or deleted, and therefore the integrity of the EMR to document the sequence of care remains questionable. Quite a few currently available EMRs do not satisfy audit trail requirements that would prevent data tampering. Many don't record enough information in the audit log and some EMRs are missing the pointer to the previous state of the database. Some EMRs are missing an entry for the user who asserted data, others are missing what form was displayed while the data was captured and some simply allow the user to disable the audit log and then enter or modify data. In any of these situations, reports generated by the EMR fail to meet the criteria for being a medical-legal document that substantiates care provided.

How Audit Trail Function Impacts You

Even if you are an honest physician, one who would not go back and change your charting after the fact, if you purchase an EMR that does not satisfy audit trail requirements, this could affect you. Consider the following scenario.

A patient comes to your office complaining of not being able to sleep, and you perform an exam and conclude that the patient would benefit from some anti-anxiety medication, so you prescribe it. The patient isn't sure if anxiety is the problem, but he knows he cannot sleep so he takes more than the prescribed dose of this anti-anxiety medication and ends up in the emergency department because his wife cannot wake him.

---

[4] *The Legal EMR – Avoiding the Appearance of Fraud and Abuse.* By Dr. Reed Gelzer, MD, MPH, CHCC. Published June 2007, Vol. 2, No. 6, by HIMSS in The Digital Office

With an EMR that disables the audit trail, a physician could go back into the EMR and indicate that the patient educational materials and warnings on that drug were provided to this patient during the office visit, when in fact – none were. You might be tempted to do this because the patient is now suing you, claiming that you didn't tell him about the potential problems of an overdose, or the side effects or whatever.

But, suppose you actually did discuss this very topic with your patient and gave him all of the medication information, as well as a handout on depression, all of which is documented in your EMR. A clever attorney could indicate that you might be lying about your valid entry by showing that your EMR allows you to adulterate audit trail data, and then suggesting that the actual entries were adulterated entries and not those made by the EMR software during that patient encounter.

That is the situation that an EMR with the ability to disable the audit trail leaves you in. An EMR that allows the audit trail to be adulterated or one that doesn't snapshot the EMR to document each caregiver's entries, or doesn't log the form displayed, just might make you the next Dr. Jonas – check the audit trail details out carefully and make certain that you specify data integrity characteristics in your final EMR sales or licensing contract.

Who is Addressing This Issue?

To its credit, CCHIT (a government-created entity) at least took up this issue, but after two years of committee deliberations about it, dissolved the committee that was considering it. CCHIT then said that the issue was transferred to their Quality Committee to be addressed in 2009. CCHIT has the mandate to assure a minimally functioning EMR, so we look forward to seeing the Quality Committee address this issue and for CCHIT to make this part of (2010) CCHIT certification.

Several years ago, HL7 also took up this issue in its committee working on a Record Management Evidence Support Standard that would apply to EMR-created medical records. This resulted in a new standard initiative that was balloted and passed in January 2009. However, a large physician organization initially refused to close its negative ballot, and so did one of the largest EMR developers. Therefore, the HL7 initiative (at the time of this writing) was not a fully adopted standard as yet. Without this standard, data from many EMRs won't qualify as admissible medical-legal evidence in legal proceedings.

The FDA claims an EMR is not a medical device, even though it makes medical calculations, decides what decision support is available and searches for it, and flags real-time alerts to users. Yet the FDA ignores EMRs. The only federal agency that has not yet weighed in on this issue of audit trails is the NCVHS sub-committee that sets the Meaningful Use standards. What will they do? Will NCVHS choose to address this issue by requiring that only EMRs that demonstrate that they don't allow adulteration of the medical record, be qualified for reimbursement under ARRA legislation; or will they duck the issue as the FDA continues to do?

It's a Good News – Bad News Scenario
The good news is that well-designed EMR products without such flaws do exist. In many EMRs, creating unalterable audit trails is quite easy, but in the older EMRs with archaic data structures, there can be system gaps or design flaws that make enforcing audit trails difficult or impossible to achieve without time-consuming or awkward work-arounds or product redesigns.

The bad news is that antifraud investigators, RAC auditors, judges, and medical malpractice carriers are becoming increasingly aware of the risks posed by faulty EMR designs, inattentiveness to even the most basic rules for medical record integrity and circumvention of fundamental principles of records management.

At the end of the day, healthcare transformation is built on the foundation of EMR. Healthcare looks to EMRs to improve efficiency, provide real-time alerts, search for, find, organize and present decision support information during the encounter, and increase practice capacity to accommodate the 31 million Americans that the government will create health insurance for. If the credibility of the EMR data is in question, it will in time create huge problems and make EMR a weak foundation and underpinning of healthcare reform and a huge waste of taxpayer money.

EMRs with flawed audit trails pose a risk for conscientious physicians who do everything right, but just happened to choose an EMR designed to make it impossible to differentiate improper from proper documentation. Don't become one of the physicians in this last category.

One way to mitigate your risk is to have your legal advisors include clauses in purchasing or licensing agreements, that put liability for such flaws back on the shoulders of EMR developers. Don't blindly accept agreements offered by any EMR developer, which favor the seller and have clauses that excuse their company and EMR products from any liability issues. The larger EMR developers are less likely to be willing to negotiate such points, in which case going with a more flexible EMR company may be a better choice.

Learn More, Get Help – Excellent Resources

In automating your practice, you are establishing a long-term association with your EMR developer. It needs to get off on the right foot and with everyone on the same expectations page, so that the relationship doesn't end in an early divorce, which will be both expensive and painful.

We recommend that you obtain a copy of *How to Evaluate Electronic Health Record (EHR) Systems*, by Patricia A. Trites, MPA, and Reed D. Gelzer, MD, MPH, which is available from AHIMA for $129. Read it and discuss it with your attorney. If your attorney doesn't have the time or expertise, contact an attorney listed on www.ehrselector.com who does.

The MSP EHR Selector has begun including Legal Alerts™ paragraphs in its user HELP screens for appropriate criteria that have important legal considerations. It is one of many unique features of this resource. When you read the HELP screen, there is a link to a third party legal resource that provides further clarification.

Protect Your Patients From Medical Identity Theft

Medical identity theft is on the rise. The Federal Trade Commission (FTC) indicated that 8.3 million people had their identities stolen in 2005 and about 250,000 of these included their medical identities. When a person's medical identity is stolen and used by someone else, the accuracy of electronic and paper records can become compromised and dangerous to the actual patient.

Consider the case reported in the September 2008 Government Health IT magazine of a Colorado man who received a bill for $44,000 for colon surgery that he did not have. Apart from the bill itself, the person who did receive the operation obviously had colon cancer. How do the imposter's medical records get deleted when he/she has the same name, social security number, address, etc. as the real person? What prevents these false records from being sent in an emergency by an EMR in response to an HIE request from a RHIO?

With 250,000 occurrences of this a year, there are already conflicting paper-based records. As a practitioner, you need to be very careful that you know the patients you are treating routinely and that you are sure of the authentication of patients you treat on an emergency basis or who are newly admitted to your practice. Here again is where biometric ID (such as fingerprints) can be very helpful in sorting out imposters using someone else's identity from a real patient whose medical identity has been stolen. One simple and inexpensive biometric identifier is to have a picture of the patient in their chart. Almost any EMR can accommodate such functionality. New technologies from Fujitsu Computer Products of America are available that read infrared images of vein patterns in a person's palms to identify them.

Consultants are also available to help you in this area of medical identity theft. One such company is ID Theft Security, located on the Web at www. IDTheftSecurity.com. Confer with your EMR vendor as to how an identity once created, can be de-identified if it turns out the identity is false. This may be difficult to accomplish in some EMR products, particularly those without biometric markers.

Cloud Computing/Web-based ASP EMRs Complicate Matters

If your patient data is in your office, then you are subject to the laws of your state. However, if your browser is in your office and your ASP provider is in another state, which state privacy laws apply to your patient data? Some experts suggest that the data might be subject to the laws of every state that your data passes through between the time it leaves your browser and arrives at your Web-based EMR provider. If these two states are distant, the path between them may vary from transmission to transmission – it's just the way routers work, which would tend to undermine this perspective.

This complicates the notion of an audit trail and being able to prove where your data is and how it's being secured. There are solutions such as multi-level authentication and use of IPsec protocol that create a Virtual Private Network (VPN) between two systems connected across the Internet. These are especially important for Web-based, ASP solutions. Specify such points in your licensing agreement and make sure that the liability falls on the individual where the breach occurs, and is not shifted totally onto your shoulders. Achieving full HIPAA compliance may prove more challenging under the Web-based ASP model compared to the in-office model, particularly if you are required to prove it. See Dr. Gelzer's book for more information.

Wrap Up

Obtaining outside legal advice and guidance is prudent and a Crucial Decision you face in selecting your EMR. The take-away from this chapter is simple. Bottom line – identify and avoid the legal problems discussed before you acquire and license your EMR. Don't sign standard legal boilerplates provided by your EMR developer. Include money in your EMR budget for legal services. Legal services will cost between $6K and $12K depending on the type of EMR you select and the scope of the issues involved.

In recent years, the legal importance of electronic record functions have become more widely appreciated and discussed. This has spurred the legal community to take a closer look at all types of electronic record and messaging systems, including EMRs. MSP has included legal comments provided to us by law firm(s) that have healthcare specialty practices. These HELP screens alert subscribers to links that provide additional discussion or clarification of the legal issues. Discuss all of these issues with the law firm you select to do your contracting.

The final contract should include the functional criteria you listed in your RFP. It's also wise to make acceptance and final payment conditional upon the EMR demonstrating that it meets all specifications and passes acceptance tests.

The final thought for this chapter is for you to remember that the EMR is not (yet) authoritatively regulated by the FDA, but many believe it ultimately will be. Unless you get legal advice, you are acting as your own lawyer. This is a specialized area of healthcare law, so we suggest you consult a firm with a specialized healthcare practice.

Crucial Decision

Engage a healthcare IT law firm or do your own contracting and licensing agreement negotiations? Photocopy as needed or download the Scorecard from www.ehrselector.com.

	Topic to Evaluate and Justification
	Does our normal attorney/law firm have the specialized medical expertise to guide us in negotiating our EMR purchase or licensing agreement? If not, who can we use for this specialized contracting?
	Do we need to do "acceptance testing" before we release full payment to the EMR vendor? If so, what should it include?
	Do we need to add an "EMR Stress Test" to our demo requirements, and if so, what should it include?
	Does our medical speciality society or national physician organization guarantee that the EMR systems listed on their sites don't have these problems? Have they checked it out? If not, do we want to expand our search beyond the vendors they have listed?

Indicate which option you chose and briefly note the rationale for the choice. Remember that choices to other Crucial Decisions may force you to return and reconsider these decisions. Don't sacrifice legal requirements for other EMR features. Choose an EMR that provides all the features you need and also creates legally-admissible business records.

Crucial Decision

Engage a healthcare IT law firm or do your own contracting and licensing agreement negotiations? Photocopy as needed or download the Scorecard from www.ehrselector.com.

	Topic to Evaluate and Justification
	How do we assure that a system does not allow the audit log to be circumvented?
	What actions do we need to take to assure that there is a permanent audit trail of everyone who accesses a patient's record, when and why they accessed it; including encounter summaries provided to the patient themselves and encounter summaries provided to specialists we refer the patient to?
	Should all provider roles (nurse, MD, clinical specialist, and so on), have access to the entire patient chart? If not, how is that to be managed?

Indicate which option you chose and briefly note the rationale for the choice. Remember that choices to other Crucial Decisions may force you to return and reconsider these decisions. Don't sacrifice legal requirements for other EMR features. Choose an EMR that provides all the features you need and also creates legally-admissible business records.

CHAPTER 14

Configuration & Deployment

> **Crucial Decision**
> **Can someone in-house support your EMR, or do you need an outside contractor for local support services?**
>
> This chapter also addresses the following questions:
> - How do you create secure, regular, offsite backups?
> - Which wireless network protocol is right for you?
> - How do you prevent/handle loss of power?
> - How do you prevent/handle loss of Internet?
> - How do you prevent/handle hardware failure?

EMR Adventures

At the doctors' lunch room at Hometown General Hospital, several docs have become engaged in talking about EMRs, and several more are listening in.

Dr. Goldstein has been relating what he did to get their new EMR properly installed and configured. "It was a challenge for us, mostly because there were so many details and decisions I didn't anticipate," remarks Dr. Goldstein.

"Like what?" inquires one of the residents, who adds, "I'm finishing up my residency this year, and am planning to start my own practice, so I will have to do this soon too."

"For one thing," replies Dr. Goldstein, "We ended up putting in almost two of everything; for example a wired and a wireless network in every room."

"Why did you do that? Why didn't you just put in one or the other, or at least do some rooms with cables and the others wireless?" the resident asks.

"That was our first thought, but we read this book that encouraged us to consider how we could design the system so that if it failed, it wouldn't take out our whole practice and we could get back up and running as quickly as possible, without having to track down and wait for our practice management repair guy to come and rescue us."

"Yeah, we took the same approach," adds Dr. Karen Bell, "and I'm glad we did because it has saved us twice so far, once when an IP switch failed and took out four exam rooms. We just plugged those network cables in to four unused ports on our other switch and were back up in literally 1-2 minutes."

"How were you able to diagnose it so quickly?"

"Well, when more than one, but not all rooms fail, the IP switch is what they have in common, so Mary – my office manager, who has become something

Successfully Choosing Your EMR: 15 Crucial Decisions. By © Arthur Gasch and Betty Gasch.
Published 2010 by Blackwell Publishing

of a computer geek – looked at our two central switches and saw that they were all plugged in to one of our switches, whose power light was also off. She checked and when it was plugged in, concluded it should have been working but wasn't, so she unplugged the four cables and popped them into the switch below, and sure enough – the network data lights began to flash and all four rooms came right back up."

"Where did she learn to do that?" asks Dr. David Rodriguez.

"Right here at Hometown General," comments Dr. Bell, "the hospital is running bi-weekly computer and network training workshops during lunch and at 5:30 PM, and I sent her over to check them out. She said she was learning a lot so she has continued to attend. And judging from what she was able to do last week, it seems like she is right."

"That's great," injects Dr. Jonas. "My nurse, Stan, has been looking for a course just like that one, but I didn't realize that the hospital was running one, what does it cost?"

"Basically, $10 because it runs during lunchtime and a meal is provided. Other than that, it's free."

"Boy, that's great that the I.T. department is helping like that, I'll let Stan know, I'm sure we can pick up the meal cost if he's willing to give up his lunchtime to attend the course."

"I think Scott, my physician assistant, would be interested also," comments Dr. Glass. "He carries his Blackberry around with him everywhere and seems very interested in our EMR. He runs the backups for us every night now, before he leaves."

Just then Dr. Bell looks up at the clock and comments, "It's 1:15 and I've got office hours in 15 minutes – I've got to go."

"We all do, but this has been interesting," comments Dr. Day, who has also been listening from another table.

"See you all later."

Facing Your Technical Apprehensions

Chapters 14, 15 and 16 address what MSP research shows to be physicians' true objection to implementing EMRs; that is, the sense of having to adopt a new technology that physicians know very little about and fear they cannot manage. We suggest it can be summed up with the statement, "I don't know how to...manage this EMR," "...keep my practice safe," "...find the technical people who I can trust, and so on." It seems like an overwhelming task to address, and so it's been just easier to ignore it all and hope it will go away. Well, it isn't going away.

The "I don't know how to's" can seem overwhelming to busy physicians who are stretched trying to meet the current constraints of practicing medicine and stay current with the latest medical information. Unless you have grown up with computers, or just popped out of a medical school where you learned to use computers, this transition may seem daunting to you. Now that the

"I can't afford an EMR" excuse has been removed from the table, the real objection and stumbling block has finally surfaced. This book will help you face and overcome it! Don't waver. Hospitals are acquiring physician practices again, but look more favorably on those with successful EMRs deployed. In facing the EMR challenge, you don't have to do this all by yourself. Engage the entire staff to focus on the crucial issues. Have them read some books and relevant news sources, speak to your hospital I.T. team, and visit our Web sites. However, caution them to browse in private mode and to check the site's security policy before leaving any personal information there. Don't sign up for anything if there are not iron-clad statements about protecting your privacy.

As you read these next three chapters, you may realize that there is a lot about technology you don't know, but that isn't news. The next three chapters will get you over the technology hump. You'll learn how to configure, deploy and manage EMR technology, and how to set up your system to keep the bad guys out. That's really all you need to accomplish. This chapter sets the stage and reveals the game plan and principles. Remember, you don't need to become a computer expert; think of these chapters as a virtual "driver training course" for understanding medical computer technology.

Consider your first spin through these three chapters as a tour of the neighborhood. We are driving and taking you around your EMR technology property, so that you gain a sense of what it encompasses. It will raise some new questions. That's good. You can discuss them with your EMR support person/team. See if anyone in the office resonates with the discussion. If so, you may have found a computer geek or in-office support person. Use this information to evaluate computer support people to determine if they understand the unique support issues that a medical EMR computer system entails.

Your goal in surveying this chapter is to ultimately become the driver, but not the auto mechanic. Our goal is to help you understand what you are driving, get a sense of how to handle it, learn where the engine is, what type of fuel it runs on, what the electrical system does, where the jack is and how to change a flat tire in a pinch. Your car doesn't always break down next to an auto repair shop and, with EMRs, you won't be able to count on problems occurring when your tech person is physically present in your office.

For what it's worth, this is the next to last big hurdle in the process of successfully choosing your EMR. These sections are a bit long, a bit technical and may seem a bit overwhelming. Read these chapters anyway, and we suggest you read them in sequence. You need to understand the basics of the system configuration in order to formulate a strategy to make it manageable and secure. So does your staff, because it means some behavior changes. If you leave a paper chart lying around, you expose patient data to your staff and violate the patient's privacy. If you leave your computer's back door open then you expose your patients' confidential records to the world. The stakes are higher with automation, but delivery of medical care has always been a high stakes game, hasn't it?

Your Staff Will Reflect Your Attitude

We know one outstanding physician who will not have Internet access in his office. He says, "I'm afraid I don't know enough about computers to protect the electronic records in my office." That's OK, but what's missing is, "but I'm sure I can learn." Unless he includes this last part, he will prejudice his staff. They will re-articulate his negative conclusion back to him – "We don't think computer medical records are safe, we don't know how to manage them," they may say. Would you expect them to say anything else? Don't take such staff reiteration of your fears as confirmation that your employees aren't ready to change. They will be ready to change when you are ready to lead them in that change! Are you ready, is the question.

What a difference it will make if you say, "There are some things I don't understand about computers, but I know I can learn how to work with this new tool, I have confidence we all can. We can do this together, and help each other succeed." Express the second attitude and help your staff overcome their fears through your leadership.

You're not the first to face a technology problem and succeed. What about farmers, who for millennia plowed their fields with horses? Today they use tractors. What about engineers who used to be experts on slide rules? Today, they use scientific calculators – and it's good! Each of these groups made a technology change (and learned some new tricks) because the benefits of the technology outweighed the trouble of learning to use it. And so it will be with the EMR. These chapters are technical and introduce some new terms, but focus on the concepts more than the details.

A Technical Tour of EMRsville

Here is the agenda:

• Understand the logic of why it is good to configure computers and networks with redundancy and a design that supports rapid mitigation;
• Discover if your practice has a budding "technology geek," and if not, begin your search to find a technology "geek for hire;"
• Learn the risks you face from inside and outside of your practice, and how to mitigate them;
• Evaluate what training/orientation services you need to make this technology manageable and even comfortable.

Remember the EMR developer you choose is interested in selling you software, but is also interested in making the system supportable and successful. Likewise, whatever computer and network hardware vendor(s) you pick are not concerned with whether the EMR will run well with the utilities pre-installed on the computers they sell you. Hey, in some cases, you're lucky if you can get hardware tech support to even discuss network configuration. Dell won't. Acer won't. Hewlett Packard will if you get the right technician, but their equipment hasn't proven to be that reliable in our offices.

What You Don't Know About Computer Technology (and More)

Let's start hiking up the learning curve. If you are a reader that fills a role other than technician (receptionist, doctor, nurse, billing person), consider this an orientation discussion of the scope of EMR technology. The discussion will cover some deployment considerations, remediation strategies and the funny lingo surrounding this new technology, take from it what you can. It's really written for the office computer geek because getting your new technology (EMR software, security software, computers and network hardware) set up properly will allow the day-to-day operations to become a simple routine that is quite manageable and straightforward.

Calling All In-House Computer Geeks

If you understand all (or even most of) this chapter on first reading – speak up, you are a potential office geek and you are needed. If no one in the practice understands this information, it's a signal that you need to find a non-resident technology geek. Here are fruitful outside places to look for geeks:

- The person or organization currently supporting your CPM system;
- Someone on the I.T. staff of any of the hospitals you admit patients to;
- An I.T. support specialist you find listed at www.ehrselector.com;
- Someone recommended by a colleague whose EMR has been running smoothly for a year or more;
- Someone from a local college or technical school.

Don't be a pioneer – find someone who is already providing technical support for other practices. If you are an experienced technology guru, our apologies in advance for presenting what may be rather basic (or over simplified) information to you. If not, hopefully you will be able to follow the discussion in these three chapters.

Deployment and Configuration Principles

We promote the notion of duplication and spare parts to achieve two important goals:

- Having a system that can't easily fail completely;
- Minimizing your downtime in the event of a component failure.

Others might approach this topic differently, and save you some front-end cash, but downtime is expensive, disruptive and leads to a bad patient experience so we encourage investing more on the front end in order to address failures quickly, when they occur.

There is always more than one approach. We suggest you keep things simpler until you master the technology management issues. In three to four years you will be upgrading hardware anyway; so save the money for the second time around. MSP has deployed both wired Local Area Networks (LANs) and wireless (WLAN) networks, running a mixture of computers of various hardware vintages, various operating systems and network-enabled devices.

We have beta tested for Microsoft and others and are blessed with three geeks in our small organization. That experiences has shaped this discussion.

The Physiology of EMR Technology

The human body is a useful metaphor for your EMR system. The hands and feet are your worksites (exam rooms, treatment prep areas, reception and so on) where the action occurs. The nerves are akin to the network cables running from these worksites. Your office network IP switch is analogous to the spinal column (where all those nerves/cables come together), and the EMR server and patient data repository is like the brain. If you've chosen a Web-based EMR, then your brain is in the Internet cloud, otherwise it's in your office.

Envision the Internet as a public extension of your private office intranet (in-office network). The system serving your office will have these elements:
- The EMR software on the server located in your office (or elsewhere);
- User computers located at all worksites around your office;
- An intranet (LAN) that connects the worksite computers to the central EMR server in your office or the Internet if you use a Web server.

Protect Your Brain (EMR Fileserver)
The EMR application and all patient "electronic charts" are normally on one computer (the EMR fileserver) as shown in Figure 14.1.

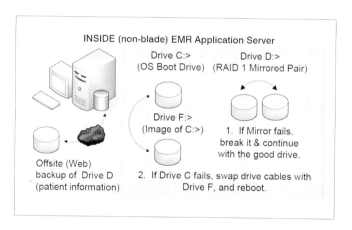

Figure 14.1 Typical EMR Fileserver Computer Configuration

Like the brain inside your skull, physical access to your EMR server site needs to be controlled and normally limited to your EMR office geek and any trusted outside support person. Other staff members won't need (or be granted) access to this EMR server. Your old chart room, a convenient storage area or other lockable office are good places to locate the EMR fileserver. Choose the best implementation of the EMR fileserver for your office situation – a tower computer (as shown), or a blade server (which we will explain shortly) or some "thin" client/server arrangement (also detailed shortly).

Control Sign-on Access

There can be no "guest accounts" on your EMR fileserver, every staff member will operate with "user" level privileges. The geek, the outside maintenance person and the owner of the practice should have a second login with administrative status as well. Even administrator(s) should routinely sign-in using their "user" privilege login; elevating to "administrative" privileges only when this level is needed for some specific reason. Encrypt patient data and locate it only on the EMR fileserver. Never physically download and store patient information anywhere else.

Centralized Clinical Storage

When you need access to a patient's EMR database, invoke the EMR application from any workstation in the office (or connected to it) and let it create a chart-like display for you from the data on the EMR fileserver. Make any updates on the display form and let your EMR worry about how to store that data on your EMR fileserver's database. Think of the EMR program running on the central server as a librarian (or administrative assistant) who retrieves patient "charts" when you need, allows you to work on them, and then re-files them when you are done and have signed off your entries. Your assistant is always there, so you don't need to know the details of the filing system.

RAID-1 Provides Redundant Storage

Patient data is too important to be kept on a single physical disk, so instead it's kept on at least two – in a RAID-1 configuration. RAID stands for Redundant Array of Independent Disks. A RAID-1 array is really two physical hard disks that the operating system treats as one (virtual) disk and assigns only one drive designator to, such as Drive D. Whatever data it writes to Drive D is written to both physical disks. Both these physical drives make up the Drive D (RAID-1) array. Because identical information is being written to two drives, a RAID-1 array is often referred to as a "mirror." The two drives become exact images of each other. You can see the two drives in Figure 14.1 that are referred to by the operating system as one logical drive, in this case Drive D.

RAID-1 mirrors provide extra protection for patient database files being stored on the EMR fileserver, because failure of a single drive leaves a complete and good copy of all data on the other drive that didn't fail. As a user, you don't have to do anything more than purchase the PC server with a RAID-1 array in it, or create one yourself – which is fairly easy to do. A computer with a RAID-1 array will have a minimum of three hard drives; Drive C (the boot drive) and the two physical drives that make up the RAID-1 array.

Vulnerabilities of RAID-1 Arrays

Since both drives are in one computer, drop a book or other heavy object onto the top of that computer and you can crash both disks in your RAID-1 array at the same time, trashing both copies of all patient data. Therefore, make sure your EMR server environment is physically safe. Locate your computer where nothing can fall onto it and where it can't fall off something.

If you are in an earthquake zone, take special precautions. Shock mount the entire computer. A four inch section of dense foam that the computer rests on top of, might do the trick. Of course always make daily offsite backups to somewhere outside of your threat (flood/earthquake, etc.) zone.

If you need to store more information than will conveniently fit on one physical disk in a RAID 1 array, use a RAID 0+1 arrangement. This stripes data to two (or more) RAID drives, and then creates a mirror of each striped drive, increasing the capacity of data that can be stored.

Boot Failure Contingencies

A boot drive failure (while rare) is a serious problem that you must determine how to mitigate. In Figure 14.1, since the EMR fileserver has the data, if the EMR fileserver can't boot, your patients' data isn't readily accessible.

- If the Operating System (OS) files on Drive C fail, the computer won't boot, or if it does, some programs stored on it may not run correctly.
- If the fileserver doesn't boot, it will never be able to load your EMR program, an issue we discuss in the next chapter.

The Blade Server Alternative for Hospitals or Larger Offices

Instead of using conventional PCs available from retailers, larger practices and hospitals might consider blade servers (Figures 14.2, 14.3 and 14.4). The blade power supply rack accepts up to 8 "blade" computers. Each blade computer can be either a workstation or your EMR fileserver. Indeed, there are different types of blade computers with different capabilities as shown in Figure 14.3. Whatever type computer you need, choose the corresponding computer blades and plug them in.

The blade approach keeps all computers together in one, safe, protected place, and thus restricts users' from fiddling with them and perhaps creating a vulnerability that might otherwise go undetected. For the smallest offices, blade servers are more expensive, but as office size grows, they become cost effective. Blade servers also make swapping out a computer as simple as removing a blade and substituting another that you have on hand.

The blade server changes the way you deploy the hardware you need, and the way you manage it, as shown in Figure 14.4. The remote user (shown seated at desk number two) has his keyboard, terminal and mouse and interacts with one of the workstation computer blades in the blade rack. The EMR server blade is located in the same rack.

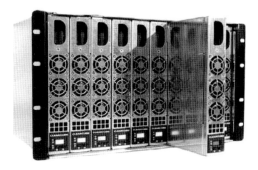

Figure 14.2 Blade Servers Centralize Computer Hardware

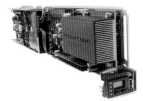

Figure 14.3 Different Blade Computers for Different Applications

The administrator interacts with that (or any) blade from his/her administrative workstation, which could be either in your office or at some remote site.

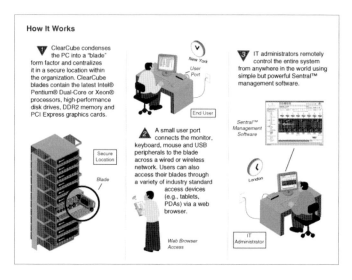

Figure 14.4 Blade Server Utilization in the Healthcare Setting

Since all of the computers are in one rack, the only thing at the user locations are a display, keyboard, mouse and network card that lets the user interact with his/her specific "blade" computer in the computer room, keeping all computer hardware in one place where it's easy to manage.

Windows Server OS Versions

The one EMR fileserver needs to run a true server version of Windows, such as: Windows 2003, Windows 2008 or Windows Home Server. Avoid using a workstation operating system like: Windows XP Pro, Windows Vista anything, or early versions of Windows 7, as these are not true fileservers.

Workstations at the Point of Care

There can be various types of workstation in the exam room or reception area or other points of care.

Thin Client Server Variation

The computer in each care area, where you access the patient's chart while you are interacting with the patient, is your local workstation. A "thin" client approach allows you to run only limited workstations instead of more expensive computers. If you are running Windows Terminal Server or Citrix on your EMR fileserver, you can run terminals at your workstation locations. Check with your EMR developer to see if their system supports a thin-client/ server approach. Not all do.

Thick Client Server Approach

This is the most common approach. It uses a PC (not a terminal), like the one depicted in Figure 14.5. Most small practices choose conventional PCs, laptops or tablet PC at their worksites.

In the case of a Windows-based system, all workstations should run a professional (non-server) version of Microsoft OS at each worksite. Note, any Windows Home or Media Center versions don't qualify, only Windows 2000, XP Pro or Vista Business versions. Professional versions allow the computer to join domains and enhance network services and configurations.

Workstation Form Factors

Workstation computers are available in the following physical form factors:
- Desktop PCs;
- Tower PCs;
- Laptop PCs;
- Tablet PCs w/wo a mobile cart.

Each of these computing platforms has its uses and advantages.

The PC Workstation

The basic PC is depicted in Figure 14.5. We suggest that it have two hard drives (Drive C and Drive D). The second (Drive D) is an exact image of the normal boot Drive C. There should be no patient data on these workstations, but there should be virus and malware scanners, firewalls, the client-side of the EMR application and whatever other application files you need to run concurrently. Most of these are static program files. If Drive C becomes corrupted or unbootable for any reason, Drive D can be swapped with it, to restore the computer so it can be booted. This process is detailed in the next chapter.

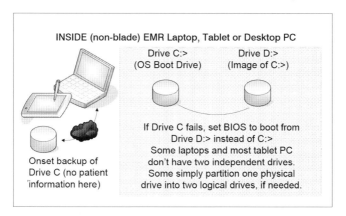

Figure 14.5 Desktop Workstation Configuration

Laptop PCs

Laptops are appealing because they are battery-operated, mobile computers. While most laptops can only be operated for two to three hours before requiring a recharge, the new Dell Latitude E6400 can operate up to 19 hours in some modes before needing a recharge. HP also offers the EliteBook 6930p laptop with an ultra-capacity battery providing up to 24 hours of operating time. If you lean more towards increased performance, and battery operating time is not an issue, laptops intended as desktop replacements with faster clock speeds, more memory and higher-end graphics may appeal to you.

Mobile Cart and Tablet PCs

Many practices prefer mobile PC workstations or even handheld tablet PCs for interacting with patients in exam rooms. Mobile carts, like the one shown in Figure 14.6, can be configured to support a tablet PC, a laptop, or a desktop PC that is running mobile. The arrangement shown is a cart with an LCD display and a desktop PC. Can you find the PC? Look behind the LCD display on the side view – there it is. See how small the computer is compared to the flat panel display? Almost any size LCD can be used, a nice feature now that there are wide-format 23", 24" and even 25" displays available for less than $240.

Desktop PC Used in Mobile Application

The PC in Figure 14.6 is typical of the new smaller, low-power consuming PCs. This particular one is the AC-line operated (no battery) HP dc7900 Ultra Slim model that offers a built-in Intel wireless 802.11a/b/g chipset. This allows it to seamlessly integrate with any one of these three popular, wireless network protocols. The miniature size of the PC makes an extremely small footprint for use on the cart. The PC draws only 135 watts and obtains power from a battery at the bottom of the cart (if the cart isn't plugged in). The versatility of the wireless networking allows a user to see what other networks are in range in your building, since it listens to the three most commonly used, wireless networking protocols – 802.11a/b/g.

Candidate Mobile Carts

Figure 14.6 shows different arrangements for a mobile workspace.

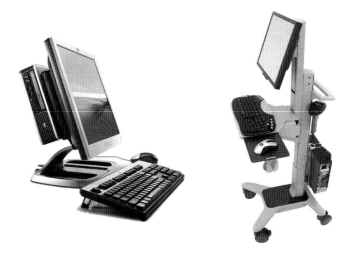

Figure 14.6 HP dc7900 Ultra Slim Computer, LCD & Keyboard (Left); Battery-Operated Neo-Flex™ Mobile WorkSpace by Ergotron (Right).

Mobile carts and AC-powered computer arrangements appeal to many physicians. The mobile workspace could just as easily host a conventional, battery-operated laptop PC, if you prefer that. The cart shown is height adjustable for typing convenience and the Constant Force (CF) patented lift-and-pivot motion technology provides fluid, one-touch adjustment. For more information visit www.ergotron.com.

Mobile cart arrangements are popular because they allow the cart to be pushed close to the patient, and the user height adjustment makes it convenient to chart whether the caregiver is standing or sitting, so that the caregiver can maintain eye contact with the patient during the exam.

(AC) Power to Your Practice

You can't run an EMR without electricity so design (or redesign) your office to become immune to power failures – both short and longer-duration interruptions. Most offices are already protected from short-duration interruptions with Uninterruptible Power Supply (UPS) devices (if you have deployed UPS devices already, skip forward to the Backup Power Generators section). If you haven't added a standby power generator to cover your practice from longer-duration outages, we suggest you do so.

An effective approach requires both:

• A UPS with auto-voltage regulation support at each work area and the file (or Internet) servers/routers, and all network components;

• Standby power for longer-duration interruptions.

If you don't work in a hospital or other facility with emergency power, inexpensive, gas-driven standby generators are now readily available.

Choosing a UPS For Each Computer

First, choose a UPS with auto-line voltage regulation. Use a reliable UPS supplier like American Power Corporation, aka APC (www.apc.com), or Tripp-lite (www.tripplite.com). By installing a backup generator, your UPS operating time can be only 5-10 minutes since your generator will come online in about 30 seconds to a minute.

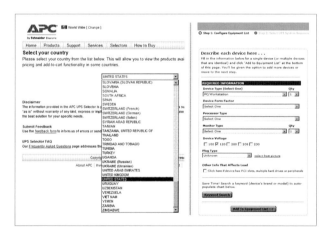

Figure 14.7 Finding the Right UPS for Your Office Computers

Choose the right capacity and reduce it if you also have a backup generator. Each of the major UPS suppliers have calculators on their Web sites, as shown in Figure 14.7. Budget $99–$225 per computer for the UPS devices required. You will need one UPS for every desktop or stationary line-operated PC. Battery-operated computers, of course, don't need these.

Backup Generators

Backup power generators can run using natural gas for however long they are needed, two hours or two weeks. Natural gas-driven generators can be located outside of an office building on a concrete pad and take up little more space than a home air conditioner (Figure 14.8). An automatic transfer switch feeds power into your office whenever the utility power fails or is interrupted for more than a minute.

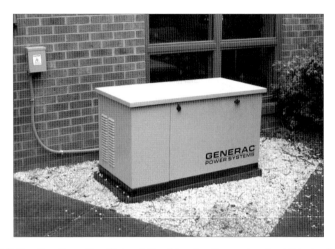

Figure 14.8 Smaller Capacity, Natural Gas Standby Generator for Mid-sized Office

Small backup generators are very practical for solo and small physician practices. Larger capacity units aren't much bigger (Figure 14.9 shows an 18kVA unit). If your EMR is in a hospital, the hospital will already have backup generators and all you have to do is plug in to the emergency power system.

You will still need a UPS to avoid any computer power losses during the transition to emergency power backup generators. Transitions can take up to 30 seconds or longer – during which time AC-powered computers would experience a power loss and crash.

Budget $3-4000 for a licensed commercial electrician, $1-2,000 for the automatic transfer switch and $6-9,000 for the actual gas-driven, backup generator (depending upon its capacity).

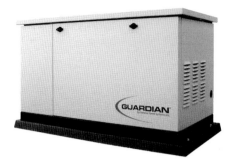

Figure 14.9 Larger Capacity, Natural Gas, Mid-sized Office Standby Generator

Backup Internet Services for Your Office

Uninterruptible Internet service to your office is only mandatory when you are using a remote, Web-based EMR. In all other cases, loss of Internet for a reasonable period of time is no big deal. In in-office deployments, where the Internet isn't essential, choose any broadband supplier that is reliable, available and offers cost-effective service in your area. That might be a cable, telephone or satellite company. Figure 14.10 provides some basic information about commonly-used broadband network suppliers.

Figure 14.10 Comparison of Various Internet Connection Alternatives

ISP Alternative	Speed Issues	Reliability	Service Issues
Dial-up Phone	Not fast enough	Good	2-3 days
ISBN	Not fast enough for more than 1-2 MD offices as a fail-safe alternative	Excellent	2-3 days
DSL	Fast enough for 1-2 MD offices	Excellent	1-2 days
Cable	Good for offices up to 5-6 MDs	Good, but can fail	TV gets service priority over data customers - up to 1 week delay
Fiber Optic (where avail.)	Excellent (2-3 x's cable)	Excellent	1-2 days is typical for Verizon in NJ
T1 Dedicated	Excellent	Excellent	Same day usually
Satellite	Good	Excellent except during storms	Same day usually

One caveat, avoid cellular approaches offered by telephone companies because they are expensive and relatively slow. They might be useful for providing e-mail during Internet outages, but reliability inside buildings (particularly hospitals) is often poor, so they aren't suitable for continuous Internet connections.

Rapid Internet Switch Over

In Web-based ASP approaches, you can make switching from primary to backup Internet connection fast by coordinating in advance the IP addresses on both network routers. This will assure that devices with static IP addresses work when the secondary network comes up. In the U.S., backup Internet connections for a practice will cost ≤ $150/month if you need them.

The Blended (Office-Web server EMR Model)

A blended EMR deployment is an excellent approach because it mitigates Internet failure issues, and may be a little easier to manage than an in-office client/fileserver approach.

A blended EMR model couples a Web server in your office running on your intranet (local area network) to your users' Web browsers, with a Web server operating from across the Internet at your ASP provider's location.

This blended Web server approach takes Internet interruption and several other risk factors out of the support equation. If the Internet is interrupted, the blended system runs the EMR application locally on your in-office, Web server using your own local area network; similar to the way that an in-office EMR client/server would. When the Internet is available, the office Web server "sees" the remote Web-based EMR application server.

Each user's Web browser has two different Web servers it can connect to; one in your office, one at the ASP serving your EMR application over the Internet. Ultimately, patient data files are kept in both places and shadowed – keeping the database servers synchronized. The downside of the blended approach is:
- You have to buy the in-office hardware to run the in-office Web server;
- You have to manage the in-office Web server. That will require a higher computer skill level than in the usual ASP Web server model.

This approach avoids the need for, and cost of, a second Internet connection. You may not have to change to the latest EMR Web-software just because the Internet ASP site has adopted it, as long as the EMR database structures remain compatible on both systems (which is not always the case). Less expensive and powerful computers will work because you are only using their Web browsers and most of the heavy EMR lifting is being done on the Web server. You always have a copy of your own files, and a running EMR Web server (in your office) which gets you out of the middle if your EMR developer and your ASP provider get into some sort of dispute or failure mode.

IP Network Signaling

Earlier we referred to network cables as being like nerves in the body. Using this same metaphor, the actual signals transmitted by the nerves are messages and their control and structure is somewhat like the TCP/IP network protocol. There are two major protocol versions, IPv4 and IPv6 and each will be discussed shortly. IP stands for Internet Protocol, which are a series of addresses that refer to specific nodes on a network. Each node can have a device attached to it. Routers guide a message to the node indicated by its IP address.

For many years all computers have used IPv4 (version 4) addresses, so called because the address is comprised of 4 groups of 3-digit numbers (ranging from 0 to 255). However, as the Internet grew we began to run out of unique address numbers/nodes. This resulted in the new IPv6 addresses, which provide up to 340 trillion addresses, enough for all of the devices and locations humanity currently envisions. Some of your newer computers may be using IPv6 addresses already. You can do an inventory of the addressing being used on your network by using a network audit tool from Spiceworks (found at www.spiceworks.com). IPv6 networks are now being deployed and have new Quality-of-Service (QoS) and security capabilities.

If possible, you should build your entire network on either IPv4 or IPv6; although IPv6 is backwards compatible with IPv4, there are glitches in mixed networks using different versions of the Microsoft Windows operating system. Vista and later versions of Windows are based on IPv6 while Windows XP and earlier versions are based on IPv4, although they also support IPv6 based on patches and service packs.

Building Redundant Networks

Structure your office for redundancy by providing every office worksite with access to two networks – one wired LAN and one wireless WLAN. We will discuss the wired LAN (Local Area Network) strategy for one room. You can then replicate it for all the others. Every worksite should be served by the cabled LAN, not just areas with stationary PCs (Figures 14.11).

- Every room will have a wired LAN, through one of the four available Ethernet ports in each room (available on the 3CNJ1000 switches).
- If the CPU is a mobile laptop or tablet PC, it will normally be served by the wireless WLAN using one of the available 802.11 WLAN protocols.

Figure 14.11 shows one network cable running back to a central switch/wiring cabinet, where your EMR server, Internet server, router and firewall are located. It also shows the 3Com 3CNJ1000, 4-port Ethernet switch at your worksite (exam room, med room, reception). In Figure 14.11, a desktop PC is attached to one of the four available Ethernet ports. A phone is shown attached to another port. If it's a VOIP phone, it attaches to an IP port, whereas if it's a conventional phone, it would be plugged into one of the two phone "feed-through" ports available.

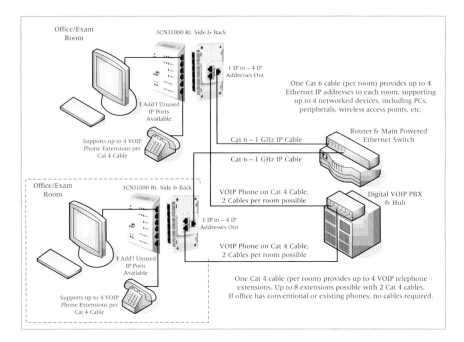

Figure 14.11 LAN & Telephone Integrated Wiring Strategies In Your Office

The same Cat-6 cabling that carries your network cabling that provides Internet service to your PC, can be used to provide Voice Over IP (VOIP) telephone service as well, as shown in Figure 14.11.

If there is only need for a single voice line in each room, you could use a magicJack plugged into one of the computer's USB ports, and a phone plugged into magicJack to provide nationwide, free telephone service. This would be suitable for only a very small practice that could survive with one line per exam room. Most applications would require multi-line phones. A multi-line phone with from 4 to 7 VOIP extensions is simple with the 3CNJ1000 Ethernet switch. Each room then is a duplicate of the typical room shown above. In the simplest configuration, one Cat-6 cable is run. In the most complex configuration, only three cables are required.

The In-Room, 3Com 3CNJ1000 4-Port Switch

The 3CNJ1000 product (in Figure 14.12) offers enormous flexibility and ease of installation. It is small and fits into a standard duplex wall box (the same size as an AC power outlet in your home). It uses pre-wired Cat-6 cables[1], which just plug-in. This alone saves enormous installation time and provides for the reliability of using pre-manufactured cables, rather than fabricating them on site.

---

[1] Cat-6 cable is the 1.0 GHz version of Cat-5 (100 MHz) cable. It is used in Gigabit LANs.

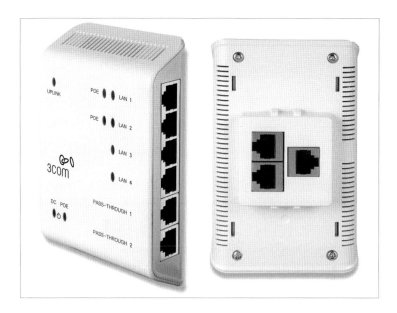

Figure 14.12 3CNJ1000 4-Port, 2 Pass-Through Switch (Front/Right Side & Rear views)

The 3CNJ1000 Ethernet switches require 48V DC power. This is supplied over the Ethernet cable, or if that isn't available, by using a small power adapter that can plug into a nearby AC outlet and into the left side of the 3CNJ1000. If power comes over the LAN cable, it is passed on through the LAN 1 or 2 connectors. Notice the POE (Power Over Ethernet) lights adjacent to the LAN 1 and LAN 2 signal lights. They glow when the switch is receiving power from the Ethernet cable, making power interruptions easy to spot – no light, no power. The Cat-6 cable coming in brings one IP address, but splits it into four different ones, allowing four different network devices to be plugged in and work simultaneously at speeds up to one Gbit/second each. The signal lights by each port flash as data moves through the switch, providing a useful, visual troubleshooting feature. The bottom two RJ45 receptacles are pass-through connections of whatever is plugged into the back of the 3CNJ1000 – usually one or two, Cat-5 phone cables.

• One Cat-5 cable supports four telephone extensions;
• Two Cat-5 cables support seven to eight telephone extensions.

Optional – A Second 3CNJ1000 in a Room
Need more than four IP addresses at one worksite? Use a second switch and get up to seven IP addresses, three on the first switch and four more on the second. Simply patch either Port 1 or 2 on the first switch into the pass-through connector, and out the back of that switch and into the input on the second switch. You can use the second pass-through to route four telephone

extensions to the second switch as well; support two phones at two different locations in the room and have seven IP addresses. Very flexible.

The design of the office overall is simply a replication of the design in this room, so the total installation is easy, fast, clean, simple and inexpensive. The 3CNJ1000 device sells for about $165. Eight worksites, each with one 3CNJ1000, would support 32 different network devices (with up to four in each room).

The Central Switch Size and Deployment Strategy

You can figure out the size of the central switch by counting the number of rooms/locations that need to plug into it. Let's say you have seven worksites (reception, billing, MD office, three exam rooms and a med prep area). Each will have one cable coming to the central switch. At a minimum you need an eight-port switch. So buy two eight-port switches – plugging four cables into one and the other three into the other. Each switch would have three spare ports and four used ports.

Suppose some day four of your rooms suddenly stop working, but not all eight of your rooms. It's likely that they are all plugged into the same switch, which has just failed. But there are four unused ports on the second switch. Simply move the four cables from the bad switch, to the four unused ports on the good switch, and your problem is solved in 30 seconds or less – because the office was designed for rapid failure mitigation using redundancy. Cost of the repair – zero. Initial expense of <$150 on the front end, no appreciable down-time and no need to call the computer repair person at $100 to $125 per hour to come fix anything.

The wired LAN design discussed here is easily scalable. A second MD adds four more ports, so use two 12-port switches (instead of 8-port ones). A third MD adds four more ports, so two 16-port switches would work, and so on. The fourth MD moves you to three 12-port switches and so on. You design it for the contingency of a failure of any one (not two) of the total switches, because the odds of a random failure of two or more switches is low.

All bets are off if the building is struck by lightening or flooded etc., but even those scenarios are manageable. Keep some spare switches unplugged in a closet, where a power surge can't impact them. Replace the bad units with the good ones and you're back up. The guiding principle of laying out your office, is to continually ask the question, "What if this device/component fails, what impact will it have on the office? What can we do in the office design to mitigate the failure and make the recovery fast and cheap?"

Centralized Network Devices

We will now discuss the central switch, the ISP's router, its Dynamic Host Configuration Protocol (DHCP) server and any firewalls. Think of your office network as being similar to a patient's nervous system. Just as all nerves from the extremities funnel through the spine to reach the brain, so all worksite IP cables run to a central switch (like the spine) and are fed into the domain server (or the network router). In this latter case, the network is simple and the router and DHCP server are supplied by the Internet Service Provider (ISP).

If you deploy an in-house EMR that isn't connected to the Internet, your in-office EMR server could provide the DHCP services. The router has the broadband coax or fiber coming into it from outside, and usually has at least four Ethernet ports. These can feed the central IP switches discussed above. Don't use more than two of the four. You know why, right? You want a redundant design that has two spares.

Many routers have integrated Wireless Local Area Networks (WLANs) that support some 802.11 protocol. These are really a two-way radio, which is the ultimate point of convergence for the wireless and wired part of your network. It is possible for the wired part of the router to be bad, but the wireless part of the router to be working perfectly. We have actually had this happen in our offices. In that case the entire office switches over to WLAN (if it's been prepared to do so).

If the Wired Network Fails, Go Wireless

In order to get your stationary PCs running on your wireless network, you will need some wireless network radios for them. The trade-off is initial cost versus speed of repair and staying in operation with minimal disruption of services.

About the Router

If your network extends to the Internet, your ISP will connect you to it through a router that your ISP "gives" you. The router exists to direct data coming into the internal office network from the Internet to the correct IP addresses that asked for it.

Start by signing into the router from your Web browser at http://192.168.1.1 or perhaps 192.168.0.1. You will be greeted with a login name and password prompt. These are the admin and password assigned when the router was shipped (your ISP technician may have changed it to something like "admin" and "password1" but that doesn't offer any security).

You can make the router more secure by changing the user name to something secure such as, Manag3r, and make the password stronger by using something like, "As1ts9". Use capital letters, numbers for letters and phrases to make these recallable but difficult to hack.

"As1ts9" represents "a stitch in time saves nine". The "A" is capitalized, and the "i" is changed to "1". This is a fairly strong password, not one a hacker is likely to guess and an auto attack program will not figure it out before your router begins blocking logon attempts. Write the password down somewhere accessible in case your mind was working better than your memory was six months ago. Once signed in, restrict its hours of operation to your office hours, so the Internet is effectively "closed" when your office is physically closed.

Routers are generally not interchangeable. If you have a Verizon FIOS network for example, at this point in time you have an ActionTek MR424WR Rev. something router, and you are stuck with it – for better or worse. On other ISPs you may have other router choices.

Wireless Networking Integrated with the Router

Since wireless networking is built in to the router, you have restrictions on what WLAN protocols you can choose. Many of the current laptops come with 802.11a, b, g, or n protocols, but ActionTek only supports 802.11 b or g, so you can't use the other, newer protocols unless you disable the wireless functions on your router, and install a separate wireless network subsystem that doesn't depend on your ISP's router. Then you can have anything you want (but at extra expense of course).

Occasionally (about once a quarter) all the devices on our FIOS network fail to communicate or become extremely slow. We then power down the router and force it to reboot and reauthenticate with Verizon, and within two minutes the network works well again for another four to six weeks. Interestingly, when FIOS first came out, the frequency of this was about once a week. Two bios flashes later, the problem seems to have improved.

The forced renegotiation is usually not a problem if you give folks a quick heads up, so they don't try to chart while your router is rebooting. It's not an issue in the office if you have an office-based server, but if you are working with an EMR over the Internet, you will lose connectivity during the two minute reboot and handshake sequence and won't be able to chart at all (briefly).

The DHCP Server – The Network Traffic Cop

Tucked away inside the router, is a program called the DHCP server. The DHCP server works inside of the office to assign non-conflicting IP addresses to each device that wants to be on the network. No two network devices can have the same IP address. If two networked devices try to use the same IP address, they interfere with each other, and may cause the entire network to fail. Some network software will alert you to this. Each network device gets its own IP address when it powers up and its network "checks in" with the DHCP server.

The network router isn't the only device that has a DHCP server program, every computer running a server version of the OS also has one. This includes the EMR fileserver and perhaps an e-mail exchange server (that talks to the Internet). Since there can be only one DHCP server, these others must all be turned off by default. We discuss letting the router's DHCP server be the active one, but you can configure the network differently, if you want to, perhaps for security purposes. Whatever DHCP server is the active one, gives all network cards a unique IP (Internet Protocol) address.

IP4 vs. IP6 Addresses

Networks today have both older IP4 addresses, and newer IP6 addresses. If you have computers that have Windows XP or earlier OS, you are probably using IP4 addressing. If your computers use Vista or Windows 7, they were configured for IP6 addresses. The IP6 is backwards compatible with IP4, but IP4 computers require patches to work on IP6 networks. We discuss the IP4 addressing below, but the same principles apply to IP6.

IP Address Ranges in the Office

When a device appears on the network, it seeks the DHCP server looking for a unique IP address. If it finds the DHCP server, it gets a pre-reserved IP address used only for the in-office network. For IP4, these addresses have forms shown below:
- 192.168.[0,1].[1-255]; or
- 10.10.10.[1-255].

All addresses on the network have the first three numbers in common, and differ only in the fourth number.

Any IP address the DHCP server assigns to a computer or other network device is a dynamic IP address, which means it can be changed at the pleasure of the DHCP server at any time.

Some devices on your network don't ever want their addresses changed by the DHCP server (or anybody else), so they take a fixed IP address (known as a static IP address). The DHCP server excludes the range of predefined, static IP addresses from the pool of IP addresses it can assign, so there is not a conflict between the static and dynamic IP address range.

Any device that needs a fixed address takes a static IP address. Suppose you have a network laser printer, located on the IP address 192.168.1.100. Depending on how other computers' network printer ports are configured, they may point to this static IP printer address. Therefore, if the printer's IP address changes, none of the computer printer ports would be properly configured, and network printing to that printer would fail (until it is fixed).

Allocating Static IP Addresses

Static IP addresses are chosen so as not to overlap with the DHCP server's range of dynamically-assignable IP addresses. To assure this, you log into the router and inform the DHCP server of IP addresses reserved for static use.

Since you are already signed into the router, set the dynamic range of IP addresses to 192.168.1.10 to 192.168.1.30 (leaving room for 20 devices) and your static range might be 192.168.1.100 to 192.168.1.110 (room for 10 more devices). If you want a more secure network, don't have more IP addresses in the range than actually exist on your current network. Also, each switch consumes an IP address. If you have reduced IP addresses to one per device on the network, don't forget to increase this range before you connect a new computer, so there will be an available IP address for it.

Turn all printers' DHCP modes to off and set their IP address manually to an address in the static IP address range. Most printers will print out their network settings, including their IP range. Tape the print out to the printer so that you have it handy. Once configured properly, this shouldn't change suddenly.

Overcoming Changed DNS Addresses

The router is usually the home of the Web URLs that do Domain Name System (DNS) lookups for URLs and changes them into IP addresses. The Domain Name System (DNS) server table is a list of all IP addresses on the Web that relate to Web site names. Think of it as a list of names (John Doe) and street addresses where John lives (123 Main Street, Middletown, NJ). Such a list would tell the post office where to deliver the mail, based on John Doe's address. It works the same way on the Web.

When you type http://www.google.com for example, that is sent off to your ISP's DNS server that resolves it to the IP address: 74.125.127.100. The idea is that the string "google.com" is easier to remember than its true IP address. DNS server updates are all supposed to happen automatically, but if everything suddenly slows down, call your ISP and double check whether the two DNS addresses in the router are still valid. If these numbers change because your ISP moved their DNS sites, but didn't update your router entries – goodbye Internet speed. Comcast was infamous for doing this. Verizon is much better.

We suggest that you keep an office network configuration book and include standard procedures and configuration settings for the entire office, so you have something to refer to later when this has all become fuzzy and you need to troubleshoot your system in a hurry.

Software Generation Incompatibility Issues

Mixing IP4 and IP6 networking (on computers running Windows XP Pro vintage and Windows Vista) can create serious network issues and machine crashes. If you start out from scratch with all computers running Vista or a later Operating System (OS), this won't be a problem. On the other hand, if you have older computers (using IP4 addressing) and mix in a new fileserver (with IP6 addressing) you could be in for some trouble getting your older computers to access the network fileserver located on your newer server.

While IP6 is supposed to be backwards compatible with IP4, we added one Vista Home Premium computer to a network where all other computers were using Windows Professional operating systems and servers, and had numerous network issues and then tried to share a drive on the Vista system share files that could be mounted by older computers running IP4 networks. A three hour-plus service call, where Microsoft's technician took over two of our computers, was required to make them "compatible." No wonder Vista is so unpopular. Be cautious when adding computers with newer operating systems to existing, working networks made up of computers with previous generation operating systems and do it after hours in case of crashes or required reboots during configuration.

Software Version Creep

There is no doubt that each new iteration of the operating system offers some new benefits compared to the last one. Vista offers improved security, but initial versions were buggy. The 64-bit versions were particularly cranky, not accepting unregistered third-party drivers, which cut a lot of hardware configurations out. So most computer suppliers installed the 32-bit versions even on computers with 64-bit processors. What a waste. Many existing application programs didn't work on 64-bit versions of the OS, so upgrading to Vista was doubly expensive.

Your medical office is no place to be experimenting with buggy operating systems. At this point Vista is ready, but Windows 7 is also released to manufacturing. We believe that if you haven't already updated to Vista, you skip it altogether and go to Windows 7 when it is out and shows itself to have no serious bugs.

Firewall Role and Purpose

Your firewall is your second security cop, sitting between your internal network and the Internet. It needs to guard what is coming in and going out, and watch who is sending and receiving information. PC networks (and computers) have thousands of "ports" (addresses) that can be accessed for a variety of purposes. Your firewall keeps those ports closed except for specific ones that need to be open for some reason. Hackers will frequently scan your computer, trying to find an open port that it can use to penetrate your network. Your firewall is the first line of defense in preventing hackers from succeeding.

There are two types of firewalls – hardware ones and software ones. Think of a hardware firewall as a dedicated computer running only a firewall program. A software firewall is a program that runs on one (or all) of the network's existing computers. If possible, install your hardware and firewalls before you go live with your EMR application. This will allow your firewall (set in a learning mode or an interactive mode) time to understand your non-EMR-related network traffic.

Is Network Craziness Due to the Firewall?

If your network is working and suddenly ceases doing so, what changed? Is it some new rule in your firewall? To see, turn it off. Does the problem disappear? If so, you can conclude it's firewall related. If not, turn it back on and look elsewhere. If you have trouble here, know that you are in good company. Tinkering with firewalls and router tables are the two areas where novices run into the most difficulty, and both need to be tinkered with if your office network is to be secure and HIPAA-compliant.

Don't Wait for Hackers, Try Penetrating Your Office

If you find the firewall intimidating, call in your I.T. support person. If you want to see if you have your firewall set up properly, go to Gibson Research

Corp (www.grc.com) and use the programs you find there to try to penetrate your site. If they are successful, they will let you know where your problem is and can "fix" it. Repeat this exercise until you can't penetrate your site. This is a good way of learning about your firewall and also of having some confidence that you have it set up correctly.

If you just can't get the firewall right, call your I.T. support professional. Once you have it configured, use a utility available from Gibson Research Corp (www.grc.com) called Shields Up!! to determine if your firewall can be penetrated.

When Will My Disk Fail, How Close Am I?

Have you ever owned an Inkjet printer? A bit before you actually run out of ink, you begin getting "ink low" messages. Your response is to ask, "Do we have a spare ink cartridge on hand, or do we need to go buy one?" Wouldn't it be nice if there was a similar early warning system for hard disk failures? S.M.A.R.T. (Self-Monitoring, Analysis, and Reporting Technology) was supposed to be that system, but the data isn't really available to you.

Gibson Research Corporation's SpinRite disk utility makes this warning available and checks your disks quite thoroughly. It will cost you more than this book, but it's an excellent tool. It is the only one we are aware of that actually makes the hidden stats from your hard drive controller, available to you as an error trend. You may be surprised at how many write errors there are that have to be fixed by the controller hardware. You will need to run this on weekends when the computer can be dedicated to this test for a couple of days, as it boots from a separate removable media (floppy disk or whatever).

Think of this as part of your new EMR motif, as "wellness care" for hard drives. If you run this once a quarter, you can track the trend in those errors. As the errors trend upward, the disk is beginning to fail. If you have deployed mostly SATA drives (a storage-interface for connecting hard drives and optical drives), you can have a couple on hand to replace bad drives. You can then either wait for a failure, or when the error rate has substantially increased, make an image of the disk and replace it before it fails. Be sure to destructively erase the old drive, particularly if it contained any patient data.

Wireless (WLAN) – Your Alternative Network

The usual wireless network suspects are listed in Figure 14.13, along with some advantages and comments. Most popular networks work at either 2.4 GHz or 5 GHz.

The 2.4 GHz band is unlicensed but still works because everyone uses standardized LAN protocols to avoid conflicts with each other. Here are some of the major WLAN protocols used in that band:

- 802.11b, the oldest, also known as WiFi;
- 802.11g, a newer, faster LAN protocol; and
- 802.11n (the newest, speed champ).

There are also other protocols in this band. One of them is Bluetooth (802.15.3) and another is Zigbee(ADD BAND). Both of these are very slow and were created for other purposes, and therefore aren't listed above. We suggest you work within the protocols listed above in the ISM band or use 802.11a if you decide on the 5 GHz band.

Separating WLAN from Your Router

Your choice may depend upon what networks are already deployed around you, or what your router supports. But you don't have to choose what the router supports, simply turn off its WLAN and install your own wireless network behind the office firewall. You can then choose whatever network protocol is best in your office setting. In fact, if you are in a large office building that is served by one broadband company (Verizon FIOS, e.g.) that supports 802.11b and 802.11g, installing 802.11n or 802.11a might be a smart thing to do. Remember, both the 2.4 and 5 GHz bands could also have some intermittent wireless telephone activity in them. Sniff out what existing network traffic there is before you decide.

Sniffing Out Your Wireless Space

This can be accomplished in a couple of ways. If you have chosen your computer hardware (such as the HP discussed previously) and purchased one that supports all three wireless network protocols (b, g and n), then you can look at what other networks are in range to see what comes up. Whatever doesn't come up may be a good choice.

Figure 14.13 Selected Wireless Infrastructure Alternatives

WLAN Protocol	RF Band GHz	Vintage Year	Speed Mbits/S	Comments
802.11b WiFi Alliance	ISM 2.4	1999	2.5-11	Very widely deployed. Low, may be insecure.
802.11g	ISM 2.4	2003	<54	If configured to sense 02.11b, will slow its data rate to avoid interference.
Bluetooth 2.1+EDR	ISM 2.4	2003	2-3	Use by many phone, keyboards, mouses and other devices.
802.11n	ISM 2.4	2009	160	When finalized will be widely deployed.
802.11a	5	2003	<54	Like 802.11g but at a higher frequency.

Otherwise use a "network sniffer." One popular tool is NetStumbler (available at http://www.netstumbler.com/downloads/). It allows you to detect and identify wireless access points available and operating around you. It can be used for a variety of wireless network troubleshooting purposes, such as:

- Test and verify wireless network functionality;
- Detect other networks potentially interfering with yours;
- Locate and identify rogue access points within your network;
- Help aim and place antenna for maximum wireless coverage.

NetStumbler (or others like it) will allow your installers to figure out what frequency (2.4 GHz or 5 GHz) is least used in your office building and what LAN protocol to use for your wireless network. It will also allow you to periodically check and see if any new networks have sprung up that might be potential interference sources for the one you have set up. See Figure 14.13.

If you use a sniffer and go through the process described, when your network first comes up, it will be interference free. You have no control over when the office next door decides to deploy a network using your same band and WLAN protocol, so take another look every 6-12 months or anytime that wireless network performance becomes flaky.

Portable Computers Come With Wireless Hardware

Almost every laptop and portable tablet computer comes with 802.11b and 802.11g networking. Some of the newer ones offer 802.11n protocol as well. Because 802.11b has been around so long, there are a lot of people using it, including some medical patient monitoring applications – life critical networks in hospitals. In any hospital environment never bring a network in and online without checking first with your hospital I.T. department. They should know what else is running on campus and in what bands, and can help you select, deploy and manage your medical LAN, so that it isn't interfered with or interfere with other wireless networks that are operating, or create a security hole.

At our MSP office, we chose a fiber optic (FIOS) Internet connection (from Verizon) and 1-Gbit fast Ethernet for the internal network to connect our offices to the Internet, and that came with a router that supported either 802.11b or 802.11g. Since "g" was fast enough and readily available on our existing laptops and our router, that's what we chose. FIOS has served us well. We get decent up and download speeds for less than $100 a month. This particular network serves nine computers (a mixture of workstations and servers), two of which are wireless laptops.

WLAN Data Speeds Vary

Returning to Figure 14.13, notice the different WLAN protocol data speeds; some are much slower than others. Even the fastest is slower than a wired network, although 802.11n comes the closest to the wired speed. Listed are the maximum speeds, but WiFi 802.11b devices can run as slow as 2.75 Mbits/second when network load is high. We don't recommend this technology any longer. The 802.11g protocol is newer than 802.11b, and 802.11g devices are a better choice and also readily available. 802.11n is the newest and will therefore have the longest life, and also has the fastest network speeds. There is no conflict nor interaction between any 802.11 protocol used in the 2.4-GHz ISM and 802.11a used in the 5 GHz band.

If you decide to not use the wireless that comes integrated with your router, seek help from your wireless vendor. Aruba or another supplier supports all three protocols (802.11a,b,g) in a single Access Point (AP) and that may be an advantage. The main challenge with wireless WLANs is potential interaction with other wireless networks operating in your building, now or in the future. Therefore, use computers and APs that support as many protocols as possible, in case you need to change protocols later on.

Avoiding Wireless Problems

Wireless networks have some downsides. The top four concerns are:
1 Potential for loss of equipment;
2 Dead spots interfering with transmission of the wireless system;
3 Systems easier to hack if not properly secured; and
4 More expensive than cabled networks.

These potential problems go away if the wireless network (WLAN) is properly designed and deployed. Some EMR developers recommend and support newer 802.11a networks (Figure 14.14). Fairly evenly supported by EMR developers are WiFi (802.11b), high speed (802.11a) WLANs at 5.6 GHz and WiFi with DECT protocol for voice over IP applications. We expect wider support for 802.11n as the standard is finalized and adopted.

Figure 14.14 Wireless Attributes Supported by EMR Developer

Wireless Attribute	% EMR Developers Supporting
802.11g High Speed LAN	62%
802.11n WLAN	49%
802.11b (WiFi) WLAN	39%
802.11b WiFi with Voice over IP	37%
802.11a WLAN at 5 GHz	33%
WiFi w DECT for Voice over IP	30%
Cellular Modem	21%
Bluetooth	19%

Avoid Cellular and Bluetooth (802.15) networks for in-office WLAN between computers. Bluetooth is fine to connect your keyboard and mouse to your computer because that is what it was created to do. Cellular is not always reliable from inside of buildings, has slow data rates, poor quality of service, is expensive for network time and requires dial-up.

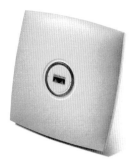

Figure 14.15 Wall or Ceiling-Mountable Wireless Access Point

Avoid Zigbee networks, which are too slow for medical network applications. Wireless access points supporting multiple protocols are now integrated into quite small packages, as shown in Figure 14.15 (Cisco 1131 AP), making them easy to mount and relatively unobtrusive. Similar products are available from Aruba and other network suppliers that offer less expensive products.

Figure 14.16 National Hospital Market Shares of Wireless Vendors

Wireless Network Vendor	National Market Share
Cisco	29%
AT&T	10%
GTE	7%
Verizon	7%
Nortel	4%
Pacific Bell	4%
Sprint	4%
Comstat Communications	2%
Motorola	2%
Ericsson	<2%
Bell Atlantic	1%
Breezecom	1%
IBM	1%
E.F. Johnson	<1%
Lucent/Avaya	<1%
Qualcomm	<1%
Windata	<1%
Others, not listed above	~26%

WLAN technology works equally well for any type of deployment. Newer operating systems (Windows XP, Vista and Windows 7) make wireless networking less troublesome and therefore more attractive for medical use. Which wireless network companies are available is a highly-regional affair. Figure 14.16 shows the 2009 MSP national hospital market share analysis for various wireless vendors. Readers interested in regional data should contact MSP at www.medsp.com for a more detailed report.

Essential Software and Utilities

Once you've purchased your office hardware (computers and networks) and installed and properly configured them, you will need to acquire and install some essential utilities (also see Chapter 16 – Protecting Your Patient Data).

Server Undelete Programs
A common problem is the need to prevent accidental deletion of patient (or other important) data files by a network workstation accessing the EMR application running on a central server. Deleting a file locally does not remove the actual data from the hard drive, but instead deletes the index to it, so that the space it occupies is shown as available to be written over. With local undelete (a trash can), the index is written to an Undelete "folder," so that it could be restored (if the OS has not already written on top of its original contents). Restoring data from this trash can is straightforward (so long as you do it before it is overwritten) as the file or folder can be "restored" to the original location. In computers running Unix or Linux, data recovery usually involves easy commands and scripts.

However, if the file is deleted by a workstation across the network, the server's undelete function is never triggered. Instead of the index being written to the trash can, it is simply erased. Out of the box, Windows provides no protection for this. The trash can only protects programs deleted on the server, and since no one has access to the server, that isn't the way files get deleted – they get deleted from workstations operating across the network.

A server undelete program is an invaluable resource, as it watches files being deleted by workstations across the network, and writes their index information into a network-level "Recovery" folder. In the MSP/Andrew EMR Benchmark, less than one-in-five of the EMR developers had tested their systems against File Scavenger or Executive Software's Server Undelete or similar programs. Be sure you choose one of the available Server Undelete utilities and install it to run silently in the background on your EMR fileserver, so it's there if you ever need it, because sooner or later you will.

Securely Deleting Patient Data
Just as important as keeping patient records secure and protected from accidental deletion, is being sure that when you do need to discard old

computers, the records/data they contain are completely removed from their hard drives. Otherwise, you can inadvertently create a serious and expensive HIPAA violation. This occurs most often when you are upgrading your EMR server that contains patient records and simply delete the files. Deleting patient files is inadequate. If the OS and the patient data are on the same drive, formatting the hard drive removes data, but also removes the operating system. Simply file deleting the patient data files removes the index to the data, but not the data itself. The data can still be easily recovered with the right software tools. This is one reason to keep data on one drive and the operating system on another, rather than using one drive for both. Patient data can then be removed by reformatting the drive containing the patient data or it can be destroyed using a secure file delete program. Many utilities are available to do this. If secure, HIPAA-compliant deletion of patient data is not built into an EMR application, use one of these utility programs.

Daily, On and Off-site Backups

Daily backups of updated files automatically saved off site (as well as on site) are critical and are the last line of defense when the worst happens on site. These off-site backups can be used to restore files in the event of unanticipated hardware failures or if there is an accident on-site (or malicious incident). Set backups to be done automatically using a backup script, but check to see that they have occurred. For all backups it is useful to encrypt the data being stored on the backup media. EMC/Dantz Software offers Retrospect backup software. It's a full-featured, but relatively expensive solution. There are other products with these same capabilities and some may be less expensive than Retrospect.

Summary of Good Network Operating Practices

Following simple procedures can enhance the reliability of your system:
- Suggested power up – power down sequence. It's simple, server is up first – down last. This allows all files to be closed correctly, and allows all network clients to be recognized by the fileserver when each workstation comes up.
- Leave the EMR fileserver always on. Suspend all workstations to standby or to hibernate after hours when the office is closed. Turn off all LCD displays when not in use (the light sources that illuminate them wear out). Recharge any battery-operated, mobile carts overnight so that they will be ready for use the next day.
- Deploy EMR fileserver network undelete software, which allows files that users have deleted over the network from the EMR fileserver to be recovered on the server (detailed in Chapter 16).
- All workstations should have user (not administrative) permissions. There is a tendency, particularly in versions of Windows prior to Vista or Windows 7, to operate the computer with administrative privileges.

- Defragment files on the EMR fileserver every couple of weeks. Defragment the hard drives on all workstations every other week also, but stagger it with the EMR fileserver schedule. For a better defrag, use a better defragger program. Perfect Disk (Raxco) or Diskeeper (Diskeeper) both do a much better job than Windows. Set these to run after your office has closed, and after the nightly backup has occurred (see Chapter 16).
- Run SpinRite monthly on weekends on key computer disks, as this program can take 24 hours or more to complete.
- Download, but don't install, service patches – install them manually.
- Rerun intrusion detection daily and after any network or firewall changes.

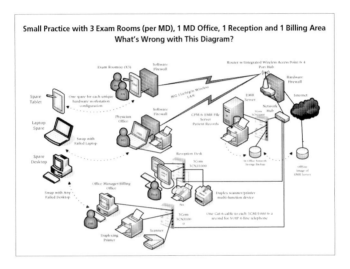

Figure 14.17 Can You Find the Flaws?

Keep every computer behind a firewall. In a pinch, a computer served by a cabled LAN will go wireless and that isn't the time to be fumbling with configuring a firewall to protect it.

Test What You Have Learned

There is a lot of detail in this chapter. Here's a quick way to see if it's sinking in. In Figure 14.17 we show a medical office layout. Take a few minutes to look at the picture. Compare the configuration depicted to the concepts we have been discussing in this chapter. How does it measure up? Would this be an acceptable configuration for a medical office? What, if anything, should be changed? Make a list of any deficiencies you see. Also note what is good about the design. Once you have made your lists, read on.

Office Configuration Strength & Weakness Summary

Overall, this office design departs significantly from the concepts discussed in this chapter. Let's recap some of the major differences. The most glaring weaknesses are:

1 Lack of hard wired and wireless networks run to every worksite. Some locations are served by wireless networks, some by wired, but not both at all.

2 Lack of spare EMR network fileserver computer (in case primary server fails). There is a spare for the laptop and for the user workstation – that's good, but none for where all the patient data is.

3 No UPSs are shown for any of the computers or the router, which means this entire system crashes at the slightest power fluctuation. Even momentary power fluctuations will crash the server and every user workstation.

4 No spare 3Com 3CNJ1000 switches are shown. If one fails, it can't be quickly replaced without a spare. One spare switch could be included for a cost $165.

5 Firewalls adequate for normal operation, but not for contingency operation on all wireless networks.

6 There is no second network switch/hub with half of its ports empty, so if this fails, the entire practice is down until a replacement is located.

7 Nothing indicates that there is emergency power available.

This overall configuration is a seriously flawed design for a medical EMR environment as it has too many deviations from the criteria we have discussed in this chapter. It's not a fault-tolerant or resilient configuration, even though it does have both in-office and off-site software backup. After reading the chapter we bet you spotted all or most of these weaknesses? Good for you.

Wrap Up

There are many details to be addressed in planning for an EMR system installation. We have touched on some of the major hardware and software items and offered general suggestions for you to keep in mind. Some of these have budget implications. The high-redundancy approach is not the least expensive approach, but should help you to stay out of trouble. How this approach can help is the subject of the next chapter. Planning the office strategy is an important part of selecting the EMR and successfully deploying it, for any type of EMR you ultimately choose. It is somewhat simplified if you choose an Web-based EMR solution.

CHAPTER 15

Crisis Planning & Mitigation

Crucial Decision
What must you do to keep from having an "EMR Emergency"?
This chapter also addresses the following questions:
- How long a service loss should you plan for?
- Will you be better served by a wired or wireless network?
- Is Internet access vital to your practice, what if it fails?
- How do you devise a fail-soft hardware strategy?

EMR Adventures

There's an old saying that goes, "stuff happens!" And since it does, you might as well plan for it in advance. Remember our friend, Dr. Oliver Jonas from Chapter 13, Lawyer-Proofing Your EMR? Poor Dr. Jonas, days after the Medicare Compliance Specialist left his office for the final time, the following scenario took place. Dr. Jonas did not plan for life's little surprises, let's see what kind of a mess he's in this time...

"I am certainly glad that the Medicare compliance fiasco is over. Now I can get back to practicing medicine and trying to recover some of that money we borrowed to pay those stiff penalties. Well, we altered our EMR so that problem should never happen again," says Dr. Jonas to his nurse, Stan. "I am scheduled to see Mr. Brown now, he hasn't been doing well of late and I am really counting on our EMR to help me with what has occurred over the past few months with Mr. Brown. His daughter has been keeping track of his medication, his weight and much more on a PHR she has him enrolled in. She brought his PHR in with her, so I will have a lot of data to add to my exam. At least I know it will be properly identified as his data, and not my data. I've learned my lesson on that one! I'll probably need some extra time during the exam."

"Take all the time you need, we purposely scheduled Mr. Brown as the last visit of the day," says Stan.

"Great! I'll head in there now... did the lights just flicker? What the heck? What's happening? Why did the lights just go out? Get a flashlight, will you?"

As Stan feels his way cautiously along the walls and ducks behind the receptionist's desk to retrieve a flashlight, Dr. Jonas takes his penlight from his pocket and heads to the exam room to reassure Mr. Brown and his daughter (and to leave them his penlight). Dr. Jonas gropes his way back to the front

---

Successfully Choosing Your EMR: 15 Crucial Decisions. By © Arthur Gasch and Betty Gasch.
Published 2010 by Blackwell Publishing

desk to determine what happened. The waiting room is dark, although there are some wall-mounted emergency lights in the hallway outside his office. Too bad he didn't install any inside his office. Even though the lights don't go out very often, it would be nice when they did if the patients could at least see to get to the hallway.

Stan says, "Well, I hear sirens, it seems as if someone hit a telephone/communications pole up on the main highway out front. I called the power company. They are running that canned message stating that they are aware of the problem and will be working on it. They anticipate that we will have power in about 4 hours, best guess. We can't work this way, do you want me to help Mr. Brown out?"

"Oh my, I really wanted to examine Mr. Brown and have all of the medications and data from his past visits," frets Dr. Jonas. "Of course, I can do a cursory exam using a flashlight, but he's so upset right now that I'm sure his vital signs will be skewed. Isn't there some way of making the EMR work? I really need that data to make an informed assessment and to change Mr. Brown's medication so that he's more comfortable."

"I'll try to get through to the power company again to see if there is some way of speaking to a live person," says Stan.

"Oh, I wish I had installed that back-up generator when we put this building up," moans Dr. Jonas. "But it was an extra $10,000 and money was tight and well, the power didn't fail very often, so we didn't install it."

Unexpected Events Happen

Well, it seems that Dr. Jonas is in trouble again, but could your practice end up in the same trouble? An auto accident can take a power pole out anywhere.

We aren't sure how many practices have a contingency plan, perhaps most think that if the EMR goes down, they can always revert back to paper charting. Of course you can return to paper, but you may find it a painful experience once you have embraced EMRs and are accustomed to the help they provide you. This would be particularly true if you're trying to work in a dark building where none of the other equipment works either. With a little front-end planning and time investment, you won't have to revert all the way back to paper.

Dr. Jonas is facing a simple, short-term power interruption problem, but there are other emergencies he should be planning for in addition to a power failure. Hazards like fending off hacker attacks are covered in Chapter 16 (Protecting Your Patient Data). Configuring your office so it is resilient and doesn't experience hard failures is the subject of Chapter 14 – Configuration & Deployment. This chapter discusses contingency planning for three specific disasters – (1) loss of power, (2) loss of Internet service and (3) failure of computer or network hardware.

A power interruption can affect any practice, no matter what your choice for EMR implementation; if you don't have power, you are down until it's restored. Battery-operated computers (either laptops or tablets) may allow you to continue for an hour or more, but when their batteries finally discharge, if the power hasn't been restored, your practice is down.

The second issue is loss of Internet connectivity, particularly if a Web-based, SaaS EMR solution is deployed. No Internet, no EMR (unless you chose a "blended" in-office approach). If you deploy an in-office server-based EMR, you can run it even when the Internet is off-line, as long as your office has power.

The third crisis is loss of in-office networking. Planning your hardware configurations as described in the last chapter and having spare parts will provide protection and allow rapid mitigation.

The information that follows will help you deal with EMR emergencies that arise, and will leverage your system design so you can quickly restore normal operations. Hopefully someone in your office with sufficient background to manage such interventions will emerge; but if not, find a reliable outside service organization to assist when problems arise.

Principle One: Have a Current File Backup

The first principle of contingency preparedness is – you will have backups. The second principle is – you will keep a backup copy offsite. If you don't do daily backups, a single event can destroy your practice and adversely impact every employee, partner and patient. Many insurance companies won't pay for any remediation if you don't have an offsite backup.

Check with your insurance company – the time to find out what small print applies is before you have a loss and find that you are not covered. If you are using the ASP, Web-based EMR server model, your ASP is your offsite backup, but in that case, do you have an onsite backup of your patient files? It's a contract issue, it is best to have a lawyer involved.

Daily, Offsite Cloud-Based File Backups

Install a product like Jungle Disk, which mounts a cloud-based storage database as a network file system on your EMR fileserver. It is then a simple matter to have it update the "cloud" version of your patient files (out there somewhere in the Internet sky) with those files that have changed during the course of the day while you were seeing patients. If it starts at 2AM, by office opening, your "cloud" version and your in-office version should be in sync. Be sure to tell your firewall to allow that traffic out, so it isn't blocked as the firewall tries to protect you.

Cloud storage costs about $15/100 Gbytes of storage per month. Think of it like a storage bin for patient files; it's there if you ever need it but otherwise you can pretty much forget it, as long as you pay the monthly storage fee. To find out more about this secure, cloud backup, browse http://www.jungledisk.com/plus.aspx.

Daily In-Office Backups

Couple your offsite backup with your daily, in-office copy of the EMR fileserver using Retrospect (or whatever professional, server backup utility software you like). There are two in-office backups to be performed daily. First, make an exact copy of the RAID-1 mirror drives that contain your patient files. Then, do a daily backup of your server's boot disc (drive C) to another drive, preferably inside your EMR fileserver. Make sure this occurs after the system has all your charts closed, perhaps right after your office closes – everyday. The rest of this contingency discussion assumes you are doing your backup religiously. For Retrospect info, browse http://www.retrospect.com/.

Principle Two: Deploy EMR Fileserver Undelete Program

These we discussed in Chapter 14 – Configuration & Deployment. When a file located on the EMR fileserver is deleted by a workstation across the network, it is gone (erased immediately) and does not go into the server's undelete folder. One program to address this problem is Undelete 2009 Server version. We suggest that you install and use it.

Properly setting network security for users (very few have server administrator rights), and securing the EMR fileserver from all normal users, also provides a measure of protection from intentional file deletion by employees being terminated or whomever. Undelete 2009 isn't foolproof, particularly for anyone with administrator rights, but for the intentional deletion of a subdirectory for example, it's great. We have used this program since 2005 and it has saved important files on a couple of occasions. When a file is accidentally deleted, simply "GoTo" the undelete bin on the server and restore it.

Every user should be encouraged to report when they have deleted something, but since it will reside on the EMR fileserver, the ability to restore such files will be restricted to someone with administrator rights.

Principle Three: Make Sure That Your Practice Has AC Power

Your proneness to power failure depends upon where you live, but everywhere has some vulnerability due to weather, overtaxing of the power grid, or like Dr. Jonas, automobile accidents that can kill power and communication at the same time. The tricky thing about power failures is guessing how long they will last and whether your EMR will survive the outage. The details of preventing a power failure disaster in your office were already covered, but Figure 15.1 is a summary of contingency planning for power failures.

Figure 15.1 Various Approaches to Power Line Backup

Approach	Duration	Install Issues	Costs/Comments
Plan A: Software controllable, desk UPS with voltage display and auto-transformer	5-20 min	Plug it into the wall and plug computer, phone and light devices into the UPS. Simple and quick.	$99 – $200 per device backed up
Office-wide UPS	Variable	Consumes space inside your office and may require inside wiring that can be expensive.	$6,000 – $12,000 depending on capacity
Plan B: Natural gas power generators	Indefinite	Complex: Requires a generator, transfer switch, source of natural gas (or gasoline) and a professional electrician to install everything.	$8,000 – $25,000 depending on capacity

Principle Four: Have a Second, Independent Internet Connection

Internet connections generally come into your office from one of three sources; the sky (over satellite), over a cable of some sort (fiber or coaxial) or over a line from the phone company. Make sure that your primary and backup Internet connections don't share a common failure pathway.

If you are depending on an Internet-based EMR that is provided as an SaaS by an ASP, then Internet is critical to you (unless you have deployed a blended Internet solution). Your contingency plan is to have a second, independent connection to the Internet. Cable, T1 or fiber optic broadband could be your primary pathway, and then satellite could be your secondary choice.

Select Only Methods That Don't Share Common Vulnerabilities

Do cable, fiber or telephone services share any telephone poles anywhere between your facility and their points of origin? If so, choose a different route for your backup Internet connection. Even if they are buried services, if they have a common vulnerability (fires occur in manholes, so do explosions, flooding, and digging through buried cables). Because satellite points a small dish to the sky, it doesn't share any physical media with any other broadband services, which makes it a useful backup Internet connection. In cases where microwave is still available, that is also a secondary choice. In the rare case where other broadband alternatives come to your facility by completely independent means, you could choose cable to backup fiber or whatever.

Your contingency plan is simply to switch from your primary to your backup Internet connection and provider. Resolve any IP address issues and continuing on. That covers all failure on your end of the Internet, but what about failures on the other end of the Internet, at the ASP facility that provides your EMR service?

Internet Contingencies Beyond Your Office

A contingency plan for both short-term and long-term EMR disruptions at the ASP facility are needed in the event of:

- Natural disasters, fires or other events that impact your data center serving your EMR application;
- Hardware failure at your ASP data center that takes your EMR offline;
- Financial or other dispute between the EMR developer and the ASP provider that causes the ASP provider to shut-down the EMR servers;
- Failure or bankruptcy of the EMR developer;
- Failure or bankruptcy of the ASP provider;
- Breach of the ASP site by hackers or any other event that results in loss of your patient data. Who is liable for the HIPAA violations and remediation required? If your licensing agreement language isn't right, you are – even though you did nothing to cause the problem (see Chapter 18);
- Your EMR developer launches their next software version that makes the functionality of your EMR no longer workable for you.

You certainly can't prevent most of these, but you can definitely take actions that will mitigate the impact. Being prepared means having the right licensing agreement with your EMR developers and your ASP provider (if they are two different organizations).

Remote Internet Contingencies Addressed in License Agreement

All of these emergencies are beyond your control and each contingency needs to be specifically addressed in your EMR licensing agreement, including legal remedies if they ever happen. You can find legal firms at www.ehrselector.com that can provide astute legal assistance before you sign your agreement and give away (or don't establish) your legal rights. Figure that your legal services are going to cost anywhere from $5K to $15K and consider it money well spent.

When Your EMR Developer Isn't Your ASP

There is a fair chance that the company that developed the EMR application and sells you the EMR Internet service isn't the company that is providing the actual Internet application to you. In fact, you may not want them to be.

Just because a company can write a good EMR application, doesn't ensure that they have the experience or resources to run a Class A Internet application network. That's why ASPs exist. Consider the qualities of a good ASP:

- Has hardened, hacker-proof Web sites located in two (or more) different areas of the country that are physically secure from natural disasters and have access to the Internet, even during times of national emergency;

- Creates backups and protects the server files (which include your patient records) on a daily basis (if not continuously).

Does that sound like your EMR software developer, in his one office with his 50 people all involved in writing the next release of the EMR application, or selling the existing one?

Mitigating Internet Loss with a Blended In-Office and Web EMR Configuration

Here are two things you can do to mitigate your loss of Internet risk:

- Deploy a blended (in-office Web server and Internet ASP EMR server) system (or forget the Web-based approach and deploy an in-office EMR);
- Have daily, incremental backups of data files written to an independent site on the Web and mount that site with Jungle Disk or an equivalent product.

Principle Five: If it Breaks, Swap it Out

Whether or not you need Internet connectivity to access an EMR application, every EMR needs in-office (intranet) networking connectivity, e.g. a Local Area Network (LAN) to connect your computers and other network devices (printers, scanners, and so on) together. As a provider of care, you are a user of that network. When a network device or a computer fails, this connectivity can be disrupted, bringing your whole office to a standstill.

The general approach to device or network failure contingencies is "Swap-It-Now, Fix-It-Later." The guiding principle is that down time is expensive, so maximizing up-time is the primary objective. The contingency approach depends on these things:

- You build an office configuration that has redundancy and is supportable in the first place. Don't cut corners;
- You can isolate any problem to a particular bad component;
- You have a spare part on hand to swap out the bad component;
- Your support team can fix (or replace) the defective part at a later, more convenient, time.

Keep Spare Parts on Hand

Having spare parts/computers costs you on the front-end, but it saves precious time and expensive emergency service calls, when you have a problem. It's a good trade-off, we believe. What spare parts you need is based upon whether you are dependent on the Internet for your EMR. If you have a Web-based EMR, you will need spares for all of the in-office hardware and network components, including a duplicate router.

What you need is also dependent upon your office configuration. Do you have a conventional computer acting as an EMR server, or one "blade" of a blade server – for example? In one case you need extra computers, in the other, an extra workstation and server blades.

A Sample Spare Components Inventory

Here is a short list of recommended swap components based upon the configuration and deployment strategy explained in Chapter 14. If you have a different configuration, you will need to adjust it for your office and the actual equipment you have. This is a typical list for the office layout described:

- A screwdriver;
- A spare firewall (if yours is hardware);
- A spare router that support wireless networks;
- A spare stationary PC (or blade – if you are using a blade server);
- A spare UPS (Uninterruptible Power Supply);
- A spare server PC (or server blade – if you are using a blade server);
- Two spare hard drives, formatted but empty. Make sure they cover the older IDE drives if you have any and newer SATA drives if you have any;
- A spare LCD/flat panel display;
- A spare PC power supply;
- A spare keyboard and mouse (wired or wireless);
- A 12' (4-meter) Cat-6 Ethernet cable;
- A spare USB cable;
- A spare firewire cable;
- A USB extension cable;
- Some batteries for any wireless devices you use (keyboards/mice);
- A spare wireless access point;
- A spare 48-volt Ethernet (power-over-Ethernet) power inserter;
- A spare 3CNJ1000 Ethernet switch;
- A spare computer fan or two;
- A spare RAID storage card;
- A spare, mobile cart and a wireless computer that can be rolled in and used in any room;
- One spare tablet PC if you are using tablets;
- One spare stationary PC workstation.

That's the short list, and it's obviously not too short. Now that you have the spare parts, you need one more thing – someone in your office to diagnose where the failure is and deploy the spare to replace the defective unit.

Principle Six: Incorporate Duplication Into Your Networks

As discussed in Chapter 14, redundant networks should be accessible from every work location – one wired one and the other wireless. All legs of the Ethernet wired network terminate in each room with the same 3Com 3CNJ1000 switches. The strategy for resolving network issues is therefore:

- Quickly isolate its scope and fix it if possible; otherwise
- Switch to the secondary network and fix it later.

3Com 3CNJ1000 switches offer four independent Ethernet ports in each room but have only one Ethernet cable coming in from the central switch and router location in your office.

Make your default network whichever one is more appropriate to the work done in the room. If it's an exam room with a portable computer, your primary network is the Wireless Local Area Network (WLAN) and your cabled network is your backup. If the location is the billing office, with a stationary PC and printer, the cabled network would be your primary network, because it's more convenient than using a WLAN.

Switching is often as easy as switching off the wireless WLAN and plugging in a 12' long Cat-6 Ethernet cable (into the 3CNJ1000 wall-mounted switch at some convenient location in the room). Then remember not to trip over the cable!

In the case of stationary PC workstations, you will have to make sure they are equipped with a wireless WLAN connection and may have to add this to most standard PCs, which do not normally come with it. One desktop HP PC discussed previously does offer wireless WLAN built in.

Principle Seven: Configure Computers to Have Swappable Boot Drives

Remember the configuration in Chapter 14, in which an extra SATA drive is inside the PC, which has an image created on it of the normal boot (Drive C)? In the event of the failure of that drive, your remediation is quick – swap out the PC with the mobile cart-based PC. Then at your leisure:

- Swap the drive cables between Drive C and its bootable image (i.e. Drive F). Check that the machine is rebooting correctly;
- Fix/replace the old Drive C (now Drive F) and when fixed;
- Make an initial image of the now Drive C;
- After testing it, put it back in service.

The computer that acts as the EMR server is another matter. It will need a minimum of four SATA drives (if it has an internal mirrored pair), or two SATA drives if it is using network-accessible storage arrays.

Control Access to Your EMR Server and Storage

Some computer side panels can be easily removed without tools to expose their drive bays. Some even have drive bays mounted and accessible from the front of the computer, making installation and removal easy and fast. This makes getting to a drive much easier and faster than in the past, allowing a mirrored pair to be broken and the bad drive (in the mirror) to be speedily removed and replaced. This is really a security issue.

Is Your Storage on the Network, Not in the EMR Server?

However, an interesting alternative is to locate your storage in a RAID array that attaches directly to the network, (or you guessed it – two of them). Each night transfer files from the primary storage to the secondary array, so that all patient records updated that day are synchronized on both. If you make the primary a RAID 1 configuration, and an error occurs, you break the mirror and continue with the good drive.

If you make the secondary pair just two normal drives, you can alternate full images of the RAID 1 primary set, to each drive, so you always have the data from yesterday and the day before on the backup set.

There are network controller disk arrays that hold 2 or more drives, starting at around $189. Whatever one you choose, buy two of them as one becomes the spare for the other. Remember one thing, the bigger the drive (storage-wise) the higher its error rate will be (and overall, the shorter its life is likely to be). If you doubt this, run SpinRite a while, log the data and prove it to yourself. Thank goodness for error-correcting-codes! Unless you have a lot of imaging studies, that should keep you in patient records for a while. There are 4 bay, network accessible configurations also. The size you choose would be determined by the size and type of your practice. Disk has become a relatively inexpensive media on a cost/gigabyte basis, but always deploy two.

Principle Eight: Quickly Isolate the Scope of the Problem

Isolating the scope of the problem can often guide you to its source. Computer problems that affect the entire practice all at once, tend to be:
• The server;
• Failure of a network central switch;
• The router;
• The firewall;
• The anti-virus, anti-spam software.
On the other hand, problems that affect only a specific location (or group of locations) in a practice, are more likely to be related to:
• A single PC failure;
• An in-room 3CNJ1000 switch failure;
• A firewall or anti-virus/anti-malware program on a single computer at one location.
Use the scope of the failure to point you to the location of the problem.

Principle Nine: Force the Problem to Move

You can also use the redundancy of the system to your advantage. Carefully make a well-thought-out change in the system configuration, and see if the failure follows the change or remains unchanged by it. For example, if you think one of the four 3CNJ1000 ports is bad, plug your cable into a different port. What happens? If you think the port on the central switch is bad, plug the run to your room into the spare port on the other central switch. What happens? If you think the firewall might be causing a network problem, disable it temporarily. Does that fix the problem? If you think an anti-virus/ anti-malware program is killing Internet access speed (and it can), disable it temporarily. Does the Internet speed return?

The results of such tests will help you find something that affects the difficulty, and then you will know where the problem really is. Swap out that device and see if it fixes the problem.

Principle Ten: Obtain Online Help When You Need It

Realistically, the first few times you troubleshoot anything can be scary, particularly if the problem affects more than one EMR user. That's a good time to have a more experienced person help you through the thought process.

With programs like Gotomeeting, GotoMyPC and others readily available, it's easy to invite your offsite service professional into your office over the Internet. They can even take over your keyboard and mouse and walk through the fix while you watch in awe. This can both expedite the repair and help you go up the learning curve for the next time. Just be sure to lock down the port used once the service assistance session is over.

Principle Eleven: Solving the Network Speed Issues

The first thing you want to determine when you receive complaints that the network is slow, is whether the bottleneck is inside your office or over the Internet. If you have no Internet, the answer is obvious, but if you do (which is most cases), the first step is to measure Internet speed. FIOS is supposed to be fast, particularly for download speed.

Below is a test we ran using Cisco Network Magic network management tool Version 5. Notice in Figure 15.2 that the speed is over 10 Mbits/second, somewhat less than the 16 Mbits/sec that FIOS is supposed to be providing.

A month later, the same software test showed that the download speed was 4 kbits/sec or 1/250th of what it was previously over a "fast" fiber optic network. What changed? Well, over the month we had done the following:
- Upgraded the OS from XP Pro SP2 to XP Pro SP3;
- Switched from ParetoLogic anti-virus to Kaspersky anti-virus;
- Switched from Sunbelt's firewall to Kaspersky firewall, because it was part of their integrated security suite;
- Updated some outdated hardware drivers;
- Updated the ATI video drivers.

Could any of these have contributed to the problem? Definitely, perhaps a change we made inside the network was the bottleneck, even though it appeared to be an Internet issue. Where to start?

Anti-Social, Anti-Virus Programs
What affects Internet speed besides the Internet? All the data moving into and out of the intranet has to move through the router, so that's one area to

look when things slow down. Data also has to make it through the anti-virus, anti-malware programs that are looking for hidden treasures and Trojan Horses that messages might contain, that's another place to look. Long experience and gut instinct told us to look at the anti-virus program first, because they are notorious for causing slow-downs. Some anti-virus developers toy inside the Windows OS kernel to run in protected mode. Microsoft attributes about 90% of blue screens to anti-virus and video driver problems. Besides, we had changed the anti-virus from another program to Kaspersky anti-virus and we had changed nothing on the firewall, which had been running without issues.

So we disabled the Kaspersky anti-virus and ran the same network test again (see Figure 15.2). Sure enough, with Kaspersky disabled, the download speed rocketed back to over 11 Mbits/sec. Kaspersky was the culprit! It had to go. It was replaced with Eset's Nod32, an equally effective anti-virus and Internet suite, but one we have always found to be fast. We then retested to see if Nod32 did any better. The network speed test measured over 11 Mbits/sec. What had first seemed like an Internet problem, was in fact an anti-virus program problem. For those who are leaning towards an Internet-based SaaS ASP EMR service, obtaining network throughput will be critical, because it will appear to make the EMR slow as molasses in January if the anti-virus is acting up.

Interestingly, Kaspersky is better-known than Nod32, but in this particular aspect, it didn't work nearly as well. Brand identity doesn't always mean outstanding product performance in anti-virus programs, or in EMRs.

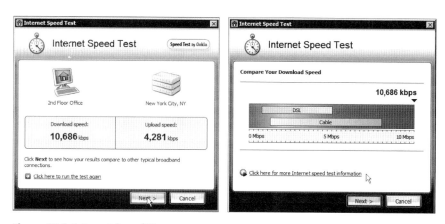

Figure 15.2 Internet Speed Test

It would be helpful if more EMR developers tested all of the available anti-virus/anti-malware programs, and let buyers know which worked well with their products. Without such testing, EMR adopters are left to perform such tests themselves.

If your firewall has been installed and working for some time, there is no reason why it should suddenly fail, unless there is some participating event. Many common programs such as e-mail programs, media players, word processing programs, have flaws that allow them to often be exploited. One way to approach throughput is to look at Internet throughput first, and if the problem is not there, to look inside your office network second.

Internet Download/Upload Speed Tester (bits per second)

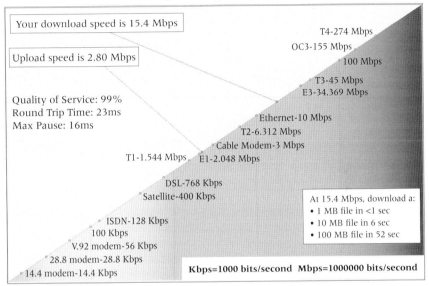

Figure 15.3 Alternate Free Internet Speed Test

There are several network speed tools on the net and some in other tuning products that can help you. A free site that can conduct this test is located at http://www.wugnet.com/myspeed/speedtest.asp. See Figure 15.3. If you make multiple tests, be sure to use the same tool/program to test each time, so the results are truly comparable.

Wrap Up

Rapid mitigation of a problem depends, to some degree, on the ability to anticipate the problem, to identify the resources that would be required to relieve it and to prearrange to have those resources on hand. The general contingency principles addressed in this chapter help you understand how to keep your office EMR running smoothly and how to provide a means of rapid remediation if something fails. We have explained what your office personnel can do to rapidly restore some types of system failures, and how to create the system in such a manner that it is readily serviceable with components already in use or with those found in your recommended spare parts inventory.

A good reference for more in-depth study of this topic is: *Medical Records Disaster Planning: A Health Information Manager's Survival Guide.* By Tom Walsh, et al., published by AHIMA Press (go to www.ahima.org).

CHAPTER 16

Protecting Your Patient Data

> **Crucial Decision**
> **What must you do to protect your patient records from loss or theft and to make them HIPAA-compliant?**
>
> This chapter also addresses the following questions:
> - How do you protect against viruses, malware, keyboard loggers and more?
> - Why do you need to implement firewalls?
> - What computer options need to be activated or deactivated?
> - How can you determine your level of security?
> - Ways you can undermine your own security

EMR Adventures

About six months after installing his EMR, Dr. Goldstein enters his office and is immediately met by Becky Kelly, the office administrator, who blurts out that something is very wrong with their EMRs. She cannot seem to type more than a word or two before the EMR just freezes and will not respond except very sluggishly – she says she doesn't know how the office will be able to see the patients scheduled for that afternoon.

"I have tried all that I can think of – I even rebooted! Nothing seems to help me get the system response back," says Becky.

"Is this affecting all of our workstations or just yours?" asks Dr. Goldstein.

"I don't know," Becky replies. "I got so caught up in wrestling with my own computer that I didn't think to check the other users. I'll do that right now."

"Good thought. Let me see if this thing is affecting my system also," says Dr. Goldstein as he logs in to his own computer. Dr. Goldstein's system seems fine and is not exhibiting the problem. After taking a fast inventory of the other office staff, Becky returns with the good news that other computers don't seem to be affected.

Dr. Goldstein then tells Becky, "Unplug your computer's network cable and shut it down immediately. Start an unscheduled deep virus and malware scan on the server and on your computer. Recheck all our penetration protection and replace your workstation with our spare one. Call Jack Bauer, our system security manager. Ask him to do some benevolent hacking and then stop by and deal with any malware threats. If anybody can make the computer tell us what's changed, he can."

Successfully Choosing Your EMR: 15 Crucial Decisions. By © Arthur Gasch and Betty Gasch.
Published 2010 by Blackwell Publishing

"I guess I could also check our EMR Rapid Remediation check list and see what else I might do," volunteers Becky, "but I knew I needed to disconnect my workstation from the network and did that before I came in to see you."

"That's good, do the check list too," says Dr. Goldstein, "and then grab the spare workstation on the cart in the computer room."

Keep Your Office Safe, Secure and HIPAA-Compliant

Many EMR developers make hardware recommendations, but very few supply in-depth software security and protection recommendations – leaving that to you. And the ARRA (HITECH) legislation has raised the bar for HIPAA compliance, breaches and remediation.

Here is a recommendation to consider. Buy an EMR with all the capability you will ultimately need (in the future) but don't necessarily deploy it all today! Some capabilities may require more expertise to manage than you have when you first deploy your EMR. As medical records become more computerized, patient data can be breached in many places. You can only deal with the risks that emanate from your office EMR system since you will have no control over patient data sitting in many other systems.

Configuring an office-wide system so that it's safe and secure involves a few new software utilities and some additional research on your part. You will need to create proper user roles, security policies and settings on all computers. If you aren't comfortable or don't have the skills, have someone help you. Be encouraged, once your system is properly configured, it will only take routine tests and diligence to keep it safe. Commit to keeping official logs of the actions you have taken to test practice security. This log could be invaluable if you ever find yourself in a lawsuit alleging a data breach from your EMR system.

Breach Threats Are Real

Threats abound from computer hackers, crooks seeking to steal patient identities and financial information, computer viruses and malware, and from human mistakes or curiosity. This is an area where preventing situations is paramount. The best bad event is the one that never happens!

To give you an idea of how widespread the problem of personal information loss is, in 2009 (through June), there have been 109 separate incidents of loss of personal information affecting 9,611,265 Americans. Since 2005, social security numbers, names, addresses, phone numbers, and a variety of other personal data has been breached on 262,606,331 Americans! The largest (in 2009), was the loss of 1,000,000 identities from the Oklahoma Dept. of Human Services, followed by 530,000 medical records lost by the State of Virginia, whose government systems were hacked May 4, 2009. Another

100,000 identities were lost by Peninsula Orthopedic Associates, and the list goes on.[1]

Express Scripts System Breach

The above numbers do not include the most recent breach and extortion of the Express Scripts benefit management system that netted thieves the identities and medication records of over 700,000 American patients. This latest breach raises serious questions about how Meaningful Use (MU) can reduce the risk of such breaches, which are essentially outside of the EMR venue. It's apparent that Express Scripts couldn't guarantee the protection of the confidential patient information entrusted to them, and has little ability to mitigate the damages that occurred to patients whose medication information was taken. *"Only a year after being hacked by computer extortionists, does pharmacy benefits management company Express Scripts acknowledge that hundreds of thousands of network users had their information breached – long after the horse (was) out of the barn. Last November, the company reported that someone had threatened to expose millions of customer prescription records, but was vague about how many. Now the company says that about 700,000 have been notified."*[2] Worse yet, some patients whose data was stolen were approached by the same extortionists.

Unless federal law enforcement demonstrates that it is able to apprehend the perpetrators of such massive HIPAA violations, credibility of electronic prescription transfers and mining of prescription information for insurance purposes is fundamentally called into question. Government has not been aggressive about tracking HIPAA violations in the past, so medical identity thieves have had open season on this low hanging fruit, and apparently Express Scripts was low-hanging. Which other benefit management organization is next?

Data breaches are a significant problem that needs to be solved. The more organizations authorized to tap into electronic transactions, the more vulnerable the average patient's record becomes. The good news is that your practice is not generally a target because you don't have enough data to come after when there are targets like Express Scripts that can net information on a large number of patients in a single breach.

Sometimes Patients Are Their Own Worst Enemies

In some ways, the weakest link in patient record security is the patient, particularly if they (or their kids) frequent the Internet. When Google announced its new Personal Health Record (PHR) service, the attending press asked Google about data security and unauthorized release of confidential information. Google touted the security of their network and commitment

---

[1] Data consolidated from information reported by Privacy Rights Clearinghouse, 3100 – 5th Ave., Suite B, San Diego, CA 92103. Web: www.privacyrights.org. Visit that Web site for individual organizations and details on these breaches.

[2] *Express Scripts: 700,000 Notified After Extortion.* By Robert McMillan. Published Sept. 30, 2009 by Computerworld Security

not to release private information. But the really interesting question at that conference was, "How can Google assure that users' in-home computer systems were as safe and secure as the computers on Google's network?" That was/is the $64,000 question.

Many patients forfeit their own private data and medical records due to ignorance of good security practices and basic home computer security flaws long before most physician EMRs give it up. Most homes are not electronically secure places, particularly if equipped with improperly configured wireless networks. Patients run without firewalls, without anti-virus/malware software, yet blame everyone else when their data is lost and they are themselves the source of the breach.

Have a Medical Record Safety Discussion with Your Patients

Once you deploy your EMR, have a discussion with your patients on their first visit after your EMR goes live. Explain the actions you took to keep their information confidential, and assure them that your practice is secure and that they have no cause for concern. Print a brochure that describes the general measures taken and the diligence being expended to protect patient data. Suggest to your patients that they take some of the same steps to secure their home computers that you are taking in your office. Note that you had this discussion in their chart.

What if You Are Accused of a Breach?

In the unlikely event that you are accused of a breach of patient information, find out if your patient's data existed electronically anywhere else – in the hospital, in another doctor's practice, at their home. Remind the patient of the measures you discussed with them when you adopted your EMR and don't assume because someone accuses you of losing their electronic data, that you are the source of the leak. Rather, help them think through and understand the other, more likely areas of vulnerability.

The Challenge – Keeping the Bad Guys Out

To better understand the software tools you will need, learn more about the threats your office will face. If after reading this chapter you feel uncertain about establishing security, hire a bonded computer support person to do it for you.

Web-based EMRs face a greater risk than office-based EMRs because in Web deployments, all computers in the office are facing outwards, towards the Internet. In-office deployments have only one computer facing outward, all the others can be facing inward, towards the office. In general you want to keep as many computers as possible facing in, and unable to see or been seen from the Internet.

Exchanging e-mail with patients exposes you to greater virus, spoofing and e-mail risks, so don't implement patient e-mail immediately unless you feel comfortable managing a secure e-mail or exchange server. Here is a summary of the major risks to your computers:
- Viruses (many types including rootkit viruses);
- Trojans;
- Keyboard loggers;
- Web browser add-ons and exploits;
- E-mail misappropriation.

Third parties can send out e-mail (spoofed) in your name to others, including your patients. This is particularly dangerous because the person receiving the e-mail may believe they are receiving valid medical advice from you.

Viruses, Spyware and Keyboard Loggers

Viruses are programs that sneak onto your computer and run based on a trigger event by masquerading as (or piggy-backing onto) other programs. If a virus-compromised program is run, the virus or malware runs its own code first (doing whatever it was designed to do) and then finishes by passing control to the host's program code, which performs its normal task – except noticeably slower in some cases. Telltale signs of the presence of a virus are increases in file size, files in the wrong subdirectory and computer sluggishness, even system crashes.

If the file replaced is in the Operating System (OS) kernel, the virus is referred to as a rootkit virus. Rootkit viruses can be challenging to detect and remove since the code replaced is often a critical process that cannot be shut down by the user or the anti-virus scanner. A favorite OS file to corrupt is smss.exe. Do a search for this filename and note all occurrences. Compare file sizes and dates to identify potential infected versions.

Spyware has evolved from viruses and become an even bigger problem in medicine due to HIPAA compliance issues. Some spyware installs by hooking onto computer "services" (that are listed in the Control Panel, under the Administrative Tasks and Services tab). Spyware can also snag hardware interrupts. One type of spyware, called keyboard loggers, "watch" the character strings being generated during data entry to detect personal information being typed, which is then forwarded to a remote computer, unless blocked by a good outbound firewall. A spyware infiltration of a poorly-protected physician office or healthcare organization can be disastrous, but fortunately thieves have so far targeted larger healthcare providers.

Hardware Configuration Resources

Most EMR developers don't configure your EMR system, or charge extra to do so. Figure 16.1 lists some resources to make your system safer.

Figure 16.1 Security Programs and Devices Your Office Needs

Device	Intended Purpose	Configuration Issues	Level
Firewall	Blocks unrequested incoming and outgoing data.	Only open specific ports used by known programs.	Essential
Malware, Spyware & Virus Detection	Detect programs not installed or authorized by user to prevent capture of computer or data by third parties.	Set detection thresholds properly for programs and e-mail applications.	Essential
Network Tracking	Tracks and logs program use of networks.	Define level of tracking required.	Very Helpful
Registry Surveillance	Tracks and logs all programs that modify the registry.	User advisory levels.	Very Helpful
Network Server Undelete	Traps files being deleted on network server remotely by another computer on network.	The size of the undelete storage and the number of versions of a file deleted that can be restored.	Essential to Very Helpful
Encrypted E-mail	Works with post office not to send user ID and hand-shake across the Internet unencrypted.	Level of encryption required and the specific send and receive e-mail port used.	Very Helpful
Router	DHCP assigns IP address and routes data into and out of the network.	Limit IP address range that can be assigned, use MAC ID for known devices, etc.	Very Helpful
Human brain	Common sense decisions and procedures.	Don't circumvent built-in protections.	Essential

Overall Protection Strategy

Protection against all of the above includes defensive software, but also hardware and configuring all computers to minimize office exposure and risk. The overall strategy for initiating and maintaining a safe office has three facets:

1 Configure computers properly for security;
2 Incorporate surveillance into your daily routine and be vigilant;
3 Adopt safe business practices with staff and support partners.

The first step is done once, when each computer (or other system component) is deployed. The other two are on-going activities.

We focused on Microsoft Windows because it has the largest workstation market share. If you are on a Mac or some flavor of Unix, you will have to adapt this discussion to your operating system and computer platform.

The following are useful resources;

- *Network Security for Dummies*, Chey Cobb, Wiley Publishing, 2003;
- *Microsoft Windows Security Resource Kit*, by Ben Smith, et al., Microsoft Press, 2003;
- *Microsoft Windows XP Professional – Administrator's Pocket Consultant*, Second Edition by Wm. Stanek, Microsoft Press, 2005;
- *Anti-Hacker Toolkit*, Mike Shema, McGraw-Hill Osborne, 2006;
- *Windows XP Networking*, Kackie Cohen, Addison Wessley, 2004;
- *Windows XP Hacks*, Preston Gralla, O'Reilly, 2003;
- *Windows XP Annoyances,* Brian Karp, O'Reilly, 2003;
- Tune-up Utilities 2009 (Windows Utility);
- WinPatrol Plus and Task Catcher (BillP Studios);
- The National Institute for Science and Technology (NIST) has worked up security recommendations for various Windows OS versions. The procedures for securing Windows XP are contained in a document located at, http://csrc.nist.gov/itsec/SP800-68r1.pdf. Procedures for Windows Vista and other Windows OS versions can also be found there.

Summary of Computer Configurations

Here are issues that needs to be addressed in your initial configuration:

- **Enable standard file sharing.** Disable simple file sharing;
- **Disable guest user accounts on your system;**
- **Close any obviously open ports.** Your firewall, when properly configured, should accomplish this for you;
- **Disable user-level registry access** and monitor registry changes;
- **Lock down the Windows Installer**, except to administrators;
- **Use an encrypted file system**, if your EMR and Windows (Vista or later) supports this feature;
- **Activate system file protection** so that any OS file changes are restored, keeping computer OS files from being hacked;
- **Disable all inbound telenet services** that could allow an outsider to sign onto your system as a user or system administrator;

- **Deploy a (bidirectional) firewall** between every PC (or browser) and the Internet;
- **Standardize the PC software and firewall configurations**, as much as possible. Firewalls need to block unauthorized traffic in both directions;
- **Deploy anti-virus/malware programs.** Check the impact on processor resources and effectiveness in independent tests. This may be two different programs or one integrated program depending upon the product(s) you select;
- **Deploy network monitoring tools**, which alert you to unsuccessful system penetration attempts. (If you are on a Unix platform, Nessus is a good choice and is located online at www.nessus.org);
- **Run Windows 7 or later versions** of Microsoft's OS for workstations, **and Server 2003 or 2008 versions** on servers. Run the 64-bit version of Windows if your EMR is 64-bit compatible;
- **Limit all Internet access to one computer** and create strong barriers around it (Non-ASP Web EMR users);
- **Shut down Internet access after office hours.** Your router can do this;
- **Forbid Internet surfing, games and downloaded screen-savers.** No personal use of office computers;
- **Configure browsers for high security**, use anti-phishing tools. Don't install Active-X downloads, to keep browsers from being compromised;
- **Use non-standard e-mail names.** Don't use the same pattern (firstname. lastname@myoffice.com and so on) across the whole office, mix it up;
- **Set strong password enforcement policies;**
- **Never use unencrypted (pop3) mailboxes** that send unencrypted user names and passwords across the Internet;
- **Use a robust, two-tier, user-authentication system** that includes a password, plus a biometric or ID badge for initial (login) authentication, thereafter use a badge with a 128-bit alphanumeric code;
- **Use WPA2 security** on all wireless networks (WLANs) for encryption;
- **Authenticate computers using wireless LANs to your office network using their MAC addresses,** as well as their IP addresses & machine names;
- **Keep patient data files encrypted on your server.** Then even if data is breached, it can't be decrypted without your EMR software that has the decryption passcode inside. This helps reduce snooping;
- **Never keep patient data on stationary PCs** (or portable tablets and laptop machines). Keep them only on the EMR fileserver;
- **Securely destroy all files, folders and the recycle bin** on any machines taken out of service, before you discard them. Tune-up 20109 and many other software utilities provide tools to do this;
- **Require a password on backups.** If your working data is encrypted, your backups will be also;
- **Keep your patient records (EMR fileserver) physically safe and secure** in your office, and limit access to it;

- **Deploy a network server undelete program** to protect all of your network files;
- **Install a LoJack- type program in all computers**, which can be activated if the computer is stolen (and reconnected to the Internet);
- **Do not broadcast wireless SSID codes;**
- **Shut down floppy ports and CD/DVD burners.** Establish policies on every computer that limits how it can export information;
- **Set up virtual spoolers.** Equitrac software captures print and copy information with the ability to route print jobs to the most appropriate Multi-Function Printers (MFPs) based on rules such as color vs black & white, or page size or user authentication. Authorized users can unlock the MFP and release print jobs from an Equitrac virtual queue from any MFP on the your office network. This is critical for HIPAA compliance, but often overlooked;
- **Shut off all remote assistance services** on all computers. The in-house person and bonded support person are the only two who should have overrides (see Figure 16.2)

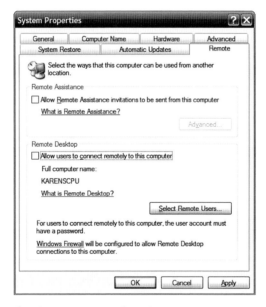

Figure 16.2 Control to Stop Remote Desktop Access

- **Establish passwords for all anti-virus, malware, firewall, and policy software** so that configuration changes require the password. This prevents malware from running or disabling these behind your back;
- **Intelligently limit user (and power user) rights** through the data they actually need to see;
- **Never use ad-hoc wireless networking;**
- **Use shorter screensaver time-outs, and use proximity badges** that blank (or unblank) an EMR when you move away from (or returns to) the

computer. When you return, simply swipe your badge to unblank the screen. Different users should be required to sign in separately, and any open EMR screen from your session should be closed automatically and not visible to any other user;

- **Use secure single-point sign-on.** Sentillion Tap-2 technology offers such capabilities on Cerner, Eclipsys, Epic, McKesson and some other EMRs;
- **Encrypt and secure all password** lists in a vault;
- **Always connect securely to the Internet** (using https:// URLs);
- **Shoot the Messenger.** Many spam attacks exploit the Windows Messenger service. To prevent this the messenger service should be disabled. Use the free "Shoot the Messenger" program from Gibson's Web site;
- **Disable the Universal Plug & Play Service.** A free utility program that can do this is available at www.grc.com (The Gibson Web site). It can also be changed from within Windows. See Figure 16.3;

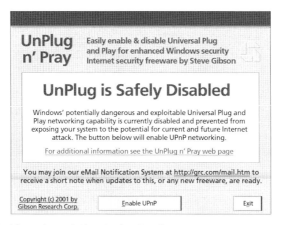

Figure 16.3 Disable Universal Plug & Play Service

- **Create frequent restore points.** Whenever a new program is installed, or you are alerted that registry changes are pending, make a snapshot of the computer configuration. Here's how: Start->Accessories->System Tools->Systems Restore->Create a Restore Point. Name the current configuration or use today's date as the name. Later you can use the "Restore my computer to an earlier time" menu choice, to RESET to any previous (known good) configuration;
- **Deploy more secure computers.** Pick computers with 64-bit processors and install a 64-bit operating system. Don't run 32-bit OS on a 64-bit CPU. Gibson Research's free SecurAble tool will check your CPU and report back to you (see Figure 16.4). Two advantages of this approach are: the CPU handles data in bigger chunks (and is thus faster), and all drivers on 64-bit versions of Windows must be certified by Microsoft. We see this as an advantage. Run on Windows 7, as it enforce running in non-administrative

mode, which definitely helps security. It is OK to run a 32-bit operating system on either a 64-bit processor or a 32-bit processor, in fact it's done all the time, because some applications haven't migrated to 64-bit versions.

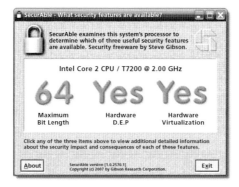

Figure 16.4 SecurAble Shows Capabilities of CPU Chips

- **Choose domains, not workgroups.** This means all Windows XP Pro workstations, no Windows Media Center or XP (or Vista) Home versions. While Windows supports both workgroups and domain-based organization, the domain approach is more secure and therefore recommended. You also must have at least one computer that is a true server version and can therefore act as the domain controller;
- **Dual medical-user authentication.** In order to access your EMR, you must first be authenticated by the workstation being used. That is usually done by entering a user name and password on the workstation. The EMR may then require further information to authenticate you as the user. This might be a machine-readable badge or even some form of biometric ID. Note: with any form of biometric ID there also needs to be a means of liveness verification; e.g. verification that there is a person who is sending the signal and not just a pattern previously recorded, which is intended to spoof the biometric ID sensor. That might be as simple as sensing a finger pulse. Biometric devices with liveness detection are more expensive, so plan to spend about $300 per computer for such devices. Facial recognition systems are also available. Hardware suppliers like Asus and others are increasingly integrating these into their computer systems, under names such as Smart Logon. The goal is to make security tight without it becoming a burden to users. In a domain, all the users and all the computers are known to the domain server. When a user signs on to any network computer, that user's profile is made available to them on whatever computer they are using. This roaming profile includes any policies/restrictions and permissions that apply to the user;
- **Implement proximity screensaver activation.** Each user wears an RFID or other proximity badge. When the badge moves away from the

computer, the screen is blanked. When it (the person) returns, the screen is unblanked and the EMR application is displayed. If you want this functionality, order it separately;

- **Assure that EMR audit logs are enabled.** Keep printed copies of them.

Incorporate Surveillance

Once you have your computers and network system properly configured, the next step is to remain watchful. This doesn't have to take long and can be delegated, but it's important. Here are basic policies you should follow that will keep you out of trouble:

- **Never authenticate the EMR application for another user**, nor let them input data under your login. Whatever they add is likely to be attributed to you, which can create an audit trail and liability issues downstream, as it was to Dr. Jonas. Look for systems that do not circumvent such information (or don't record it in the first place), as this blurs who made entries and when they were made. It also puts the credibility of the EMR as a legal business record at stake;
- **Always sign off records, and log out of your EMR.** Signing a chart generally doesn't restrict you from going back into and appending a correction, or an addition to it, after the fact. Some EMRs let you change entered data or change data using outside database tools while an audit log is disabled. This is a very bad approach. To flush out this issue, ask your EMR vendor, "How can I make changes to the chart while the audit log is disabled?" If his EMR can do this, scratch further consideration of it;
- **Keep all anti-virus and anti-malware signatures current.** Set them to update automatically every 3-6 hours, every day;
- **Create a machine configuration backup** before making any backups. Your first two backups should be after the OS is properly installed and operating, and after the EMR is installed and properly operating (after completion of acceptance testing). Make additional backups and take configuration snapshots before any major changes going forward;
- **Check all PCs with tools that Microsoft or your other OS vendor provides**, including Baseline Security Analyzer and Malicious Software Removal tool. Run these weekly and log the results;
- **Hack yourself.** Test both in-bound and out-bound defenses daily and document your inability to be penetrated or for data to escape;
- **Be professionally hacked** monthly or quarterly. Record all results;
- **Monitor any attempts to change the registry or key policy setting;**
- **Use a network management and reporting tool** to track the time on and off for every application running on every workstation in the network. Look at your logs daily to spot any workstation to find e-mail programs running at odd times, or a browser (for an in-office deployment) running all the time. These could be clues to employee misuse or possible penetration

of your system. Look at the destination IP address these programs are communicating with and identify the sites being connected to;

- **Use bonded, support personnel;**
- **Execute HIPAA business-partner agreements** with all partners;
- **Establish a clear, written policy on patient record confidentiality breaches and enforce it.** For a first-time or minor violation, dock salary; for a second or major infraction terminate the individual.

No one barrier listed above will protect your practice by itself, but the combination should be effective. Often personnel can be the weakest link, so talk with your staff about the importance of security and explain what not to do (like personal Web-surfing) that would compromise security or create security holes.

That's pretty much it. The good news is that once these computer configuration issues are addressed, there are only a few surveillance items that will require your on-going maintenance and attention.

In reading the bullet points, if your reaction is, "I don't know how to do most of these things," hire a consultant or qualified service technician. There are also some utilities that may be helpful. Tune-up 2010 and WinPatrol Plus are both useful. Windows provides a Group Policy console. To open it, click Start, click Run, type Gpedit.msc and then click OK. Take a look at the security section. Most choices can be enabled or disabled there, and some have helpful explanation screens. If you need additional help, check with your hospital's I.T. department, if they are willing to lend you assistance.

Build Your Weapons Arsenal

Now that you are aware of the risks and have configured the computers in your office to be less vulnerable, let's focus on the actual weapons of your defense and how to choose and use them effectively. In choosing your weapons, you'll want products with these three characteristics:

1 They are not burdensome and don't bog down CPU resources;
2 They are effective against their threat target;
3 They are the least expensive products that meet the first two criteria.

To roughly determine the overall load on the CPU and your Internet transfer speed, run some tests. Expect the download to be much faster than the upload speed. Figure 16.5 provides an example of an Internet speed test using Shield Deluxe 2009. Http://ndt.iupui.lga01.measurement-lab.org:7123/ is another option; as is – www.speedtest.net. Pick a city near you to obtain the most accurate results.

```
TCP/Web 100 Network Diagnostic Tool v5.5 4a
click START to begin

** Starting test 1 of 1 **
Connected to: ndt.iupui.lga01.measurement-lab.org – Using IPv4 address
Checking for Middleboxes...................................Done
checking for firewalls....................................Done
running 10s outbound test (client-to-server [C2S])...........4.64Mb/s
running 10s inbound test (server-to-client [S2C])..............20.69Mb/s
The slowest link in the end-to-end path is a 10 Mbps Ethernet subnet
Information [S2C]: Packet queuing detected

click START to re-test
```

	START	Statistics	More Details...	Report Problem	Options

Figure 16.5 Internet speed test results after Shield Deluxe 2009 deployment

Here are some tools for determining upload/download speeds:
- http://performance.toast.net/default.asp for free;
- http://www.wugnet.com/myspeed/speedtest.asp;
- http://www.abeltronica.com/velocimetro/pt/?idioma=uk.

Measuring ping response, jitter and dropped packets is also recommended. Go to www.pingtest.net for a fast measurement. Run these tests with and without each component – your firewall, your anti-virus/malware program – running. Use task manager's networking tab (Ctrl-Shift-Esc) to assess networking traffic for all processes and track CPU time consumed. If it's fairly clear that it's not affecting Internet speed, next determine what impact it's having on CPU resources.

Windows Task Manager

File   Options   View   Shut Down   Help

Applications | Processes | Performance | Networking | Users

Image Name	User Name	CPU	CPU Time	Mem Usage	Base Pri	I/O Writes
System Idle Process	SYSTEM	88	28:34:59	28 K	N/A	0
vsserv.exe	SYSTEM	09	2:45:59	36,200 K	Normal	10,332,904
InDesign.exe	Arthur Gasch	00	0:28:40	68,800 K	Normal	48,713
System	SYSTEM	01	0:18:12	44 K	Normal	8,289
g2mlauncher.exe	Arthur Gasch	00	0:11:02	13,200 K	Normal	32
Acer.Empowering.F...	Arthur Gasch	00	0:10:51	33,096 K	Normal	8
services.exe	SYSTEM	00	0:08:24	3,424 K	Normal	1,537
uiscan.exe	Arthur Gasch	00	0:07:42	23,100 K	Normal	21,512
dopus.exe	Arthur Gasch	00	0:03:41	25,456 K	Normal	1,136
iexplore.exe	Arthur Gasch	00	0:03:05	167,464 K	Normal	3,012

Figure 16.6 Anti-virus Program Impact on System Resources

As Figure 16.6 shows, the anti-virus program (vsserv.exe) is consuming more CPU time than any other process, but the impact from inside InDesign (or other programs running) was variable. Test both the impact of anti-virus programs on Internet speed and computer processor resources, as shown in Figures 16.5 and 16.6. We already had a firewall deployed, so this combination was a rather good one, since the system was still responsive. In your case, that would be your EMR (and perhaps also your CPM) running on the same computer server and associated network workstations along with all the firewall and anti-virus/malware applications.

If the CPU resources had been higher or large applications (like the InDesign program or Microsoft Office or your EMR) had been sluggish, then you would look for an anti-virus/malware program that consumed less of the CPU's processing power.

Anti-virus/malware Software to Combat Viruses

Favorite places that viruses, malware and spyware programs can install themselves include:

- In the PC system memory;
- On the master boot record of a PC, so they start when the computer reboots;
- Actually in the operating system kernel itself (rootkit viruses).

Some anti-malware programs monitor who has captured the keyboard interrupt and also search for rootkit viruses. Make sure you choose an anti-spyware/malware program that checks both issues. If you are using a Word Expander to expedite typing, as we discussed in previous chapters, it will probably be detected and is benign, but any others should be noted and investigated.

Results from the MSP/Andrew EMR Benchmark revealed that 41 percent of EMR developers felt testing was critically significant, while another 25 percent viewed it as somewhat significant. However, about one-third stated that the problems weren't significant. Smart EMR developers help their users fend off virus and malware problems. One large EMR developer related that their support staff were spending increasing amounts of time assisting physician office users in ridding their computers of malware, viruses, and other problems because the physician office did not have adequate anti-virus/malware or firewall protection in place.

EMR developers are paying for EMR security problems either way – up front by helping their clients avoid these problems with informed recommendations about what products work, or later when frustrated EMR users call EMR help desks because their EMRs seem to be responding slowly.

Best-Known Products are Not Always the Best Performers

Figure 16.7 shows that the two most often tested anti-virus software products are the two best known – McAfee and Norton. Yet in independent tests, other products perform better. PC Magazine rated Shield Deluxe 2009 as an A+ program. PC Magazine reviewers noted that Shield Deluxe 2009 was up and running in very little time, and they were also impressed with the Shield Deluxe 2009 customer service. The reviewers remarked, *"The Shield Deluxe offers both virus and spyware protection in one, requires low system resources and is among the most competitively priced products on the market today."*[3]

Figure 16.7 Anti-virus Software Tested by EMR Developers

Anti-virus Software	Fully Tested
McAfee	33%
Norton	31%
PC-cillin	12%
e Trust EZ	8%
F-Secure	5%
ESET NOD32	5%
Kaspersky	4%
Other	2%

Shield Deluxe was followed by Webroot 6.0 and BitDefender with B+ ratings. PC Magazine had the following to say about Webroot 6.0, *"Webroot Anti-virus with Anti-spyware 6.0 is a well-developed anti-virus application. It offers users comprehensive anti-virus protection and a wide range of features that are usually only found in the higher-priced Internet security suites."*[4] In addition, PC magazine was able to access the company's service easily and without any further cost.

Concerning BitDefender, PC Magazine noted, *"BitDefender Anti-virus 2009 was all that we expected it to be. Although installation did take a little longer than we anticipated it was not overly burdensome. It provides enough options to satisfy advanced users while at the same time is simple enough that it can be used right after install with no configuration required. As far as its ability to protect, it did manage to catch numerous threats on our computer and prevented several more from even making it onto our PC."*[5]

The review of PC-cillin stated that it had a *"superior user interface, but it had poor heuristics performance and its ability to detect threats other than easily identifiable ones was limited."*[6] That could be a nice way of saying it doesn't work very well and maybe you should avoid it based on their tests.

PC Magazine's review of F-Secure anti-virus found just the opposite, that the product had excellent performance and security news alerts, though the

---

[3] *Software Reviews*. Published 2009 by PC Magazine Online

[4] Ibid

[5] Ibid

[6] A rule of thumb, simplification, or educated guess that reduces or limits the search for solutions in domains that are difficult and poorly understood. Unlike algorithms, heuristics do not guarantee optimal or even feasible solutions and are often used with no theoretical guarantee. Source – Dictionary.com, http://dictionary.reference.com/.

magazine said that the interface could be more helpful. But F-Secure lacks brand identity among anti-virus software applications.

Kaspersky, according to PC Magazine, had strong heuristics and virus detection, and quick outbreak-response times, but a weakness in interface design. Having used Kaspersky Internet Security 2009, we also felt it had a huge negative impact on our Internet network transfer times, particularly uploads. We have seen problems with McAfee and Kaspersky on our own systems that were significant enough that we ceased using these products and switched to others that were more accurate and imposed less CPU overhead, but haven't ever been reported by magazines that carried their ads.

Caveats About Ad Driven Magazine Reviews

The difficulty with any test results reported by computer magazines is that the same publications take advertising dollars from anti-virus vendors.

A crucial component of any anti-spyware product is the definition database utilized by the application. This database contains the identifying characteristics of each spyware application. The definition database must be accurate and comprehensive in order for the application to recognize, capture and remove all the spyware. Equally important is the timely updating of the database containing spyware-signatures.

EMR Developer Spyware Anti-Virus Compatibility Testing

When we asked EMR developers if they test and know the anti-spyware programs that their EMR software is compatible with, there was some fairly even distribution of testing among Spybot's Search and Destroy, McAfee's Anti-Spyware, Lavasoft's and Microsoft's software. Yet brands we found that work better (ParetoLogic, Sunbelt's VIPRE or ESET's NOD32) had been overlooked by EMR developers. Figure 16.8 illustrates that only 10 to 15 percent of the EMR developers test even a few of the current anti-spyware software available.

Figure 16.8 EMR Testing Against Well-Known Anti-spyware Programs

Spyware Software	Fully Tested	Partial Test	Not Tested
Spybot Search & Destroy	31%	9%	60%
Lavasoft/Microsoft	28%	11%	62%
McAfee Anti-spyware	28%	11%	61%
Webroot Spyware	24%	13%	63%
Microsoft Beta 1	21%	10%	69%
CA Pest Patrol	13%	7%	80%
ParetoLogic Anti-Virus	7%	6%	87%
Trend Micro Anti-spyware	6%	9%	86%

ParetoLogic's Anti-Spyware application, apart from finding more problems than some competitive products, finished its scans more quickly (and did not bring system performance to a crawl while the scan process was active). Constant mutations and variations of existing spyware code and the proliferation of new spyware demands that you keep anti-spyware definition databases updated. Newer versions of all these products have been introduced since this survey and our testing, so check with EMR developers about what they currently test, but don't be reluctant to choose a highly-rated, non-tested product. Links to several anti-virus/anti-malware products are listed at http://www.ehrselector.com/ehrselector/EMRToolkit/ASP/EHRhackersoftware.asp.

To fully protect your patient records, you cannot presume that messages from inside your own organization's network, particularly a multi-office setting or Regional Health Information Organization (RHIO) or campus-wide network, are secure and have not already been penetrated with malware. Rather, presume that the network could have been penetrated already. This means that firewalls employed cannot be simple filters of threats from outside the network only, as some versions of Microsoft's firewall are. Firewalls must also filter messages and content from inside the network trying to reach computers outside of your office.

Firewalls – Stop Stealth Data Flow In/Out of Practices

Rogue code is smuggled in, sensitive data is smuggled out; that's the intruder's game. The firewall restricts what comes and goes, limiting it to information you have sent or requested. They can also prevent unauthorized Internet users from accessing private networks. If you have any connection to the Internet, either intermittent (dial-up) or continuous, firewalls to shield both wired and wireless LANs, are essential.

Some firewalls focus on blocking unwanted data coming into your office network by causing accessible CPU ports to be silent and unresponsive to outside ping and other queries. That way the person on the outside has no idea whether the computer ports are open or closed. Mostly they are closed, but a few ports may remain open in stealth mode, for a specific purpose, such as your communicating from your home or the hospital to your office PC.

If the wireless LAN is integrated with the router, then we suggest that all computers using your wireless network (which could be any worksite in your office) need to be behind firewalls. If you are submitting your billing electronically, rather than as paper-based bills, you probably have already deployed firewalls.

Choosing Your Firewall
Keeping firewalls deployed without frustrating users depends on making them user-friendly and easy to configure. We found the ZoneAlarm Pro (not the freeware version) firewall a bit easier to configure on our systems than the Sunbelt or ESET firewalls.

Ask your EMR vendor which of the firewalls they have tested their EMR software with, and any ports or custom settings that may be required for their EMR application to work properly in the "trusted zone" on your office intranet. If all else is the same, give preference to firewall vendors that offer live support over those that just offer e-mail response within 24 hours. Listed below are some common firewall or security suite products. These are rated online at: www.2009softwarereviews.net[7];

- Not rated – AVG Internet Security 8;
- Rated B+   BitDefender;
- Not Rated – Comodo (external link goes to Comodo forum);
- Rated B – Computer Associates Personal Firewall;
- Rated C+ – ESET Smart Security;
- Not Rated – F-Secure Internet Security 2007;
- Not Rated – Kaspersky Internet Security 2009;
- Rated B – McAfee 9.0 (2007);
- Rated B – Norton 2009;
- Not Rated – Norton 360;
- Not Rated – Panda;
- Not Tested – Sunbelt Kerio Personal Firewall;
- Not Rated –Trend Micro PC-cillin;
- Not Rated – VCOM NetDefense Version 7;
- Not Rated – Windows XP Service Pack 2 Firewall;
- Not Rated – Windows Live OneCare;
- Not Rated – ZoneAlarm (very similar to eTrust Personal Firewall).

The MSP/Andrew EMR Benchmark found that ZoneAlarm followed by Black Ice and Computer Associates (CA) firewalls are the most tested by EMR developers. Then came F-Secure (8 percent) and "others."

Educating Your Firewall

In educating your firewall about your EMR and other programs you have installed on your computers, some firewalls scan the computer to inventory installed programs, and then set up initial settings for them, based on a database they have. ZoneAlarm is one that offers to do this inventory. Firewalls have learning modes or at least "user interactive" modes, where they either assume what's going on is OK (and make rules to accommodate it) or they ask you for confirmation the first time things are loaded. Here's the strategy.

1 Teach your firewall your office network first;
2 Teach your firewall the sites of business partners who have signed HIPAA agreements or known-safe software updates sites second;
3 Treat the rest of the world as not trusted.

When you are "training" your firewall about your office network, stay off of the Internet. Firewalls refer to this safe office space as your "trusted network,"

---

[7] Ratings change as new versions are introduced. Check the Web site for the current ratings. Those listed were taken in July 2009.

because presumably there are no enemy computers inside your office working against your security. Hopefully, that is true. Intentionally run all the programs installed on your computer so that the firewall sees and records the port activity from your EMR and any other "safe" applications.

Run any multimedia programs that might require User Datagram Protocol (UDP) ports, not just Transmission Control Protocol (TCP) ports. Help your firewall learn by specifying trusted zone IP addresses or IP ranges that cover all computers and printers on your internal (trusted) network but be sure that only the address range covered by your DHCP server is declared safe to your firewall.

Also include printers and other devices that have dedicated (static) IP addresses. The DHCP server will be located inside your router or running the computer acting as your domain server. Don't enable a DHCP (server) on more than one device. Do enable DHCP listening on all devices that you don't want to assign static IP addresses to.

If you are using multiple firewalls, harmonize their rules and exceptions once one of them is configured properly. It does little good for one firewall to block something that another will allow through. Firewall rules are tricky so once you have them correct, replicate the configurations across all firewalls. Standardizing on a single firewall brand may help you accomplish configuration standardization more easily.

Browsing the Untrusted Internet Outer Zone

The space outside of your office network is the untrusted Internet "bad lands" or Outer Zone (OZ). When a program tries to access the Internet for the first time, a firewall pops up a window asking the user if that is OK on this occasion or permanently. Your firewall can learn about that also. Teach your firewall the safer parts of the Internet first by going to known-safe sites like: your EMR vendor, your CPM vendor, Google or Microsoft and so on. Go to www.microsoft.com for a Windows Update. Register each of the additional Microsoft sites you are taken to. By browsing such sites you are teaching your firewall the good parts of the overall Internet. Let it make those rules permanent.

Finally, you are ready to venture out to any other untrusted Internet sites (the Internet "OZ"). You can monitor the OZ with various network utilities. AirMagnet's Laptop Analyzer and WildPacket's OmniPeak are excellent but expensive ones.

MSP's Firewall Experience

Based upon the popularity of various firewalls, we personally compared ZoneAlarm to two newcomers – Sunbelt and ESET firewalls. All three insert themselves into the Windows firewall socket; allowing your operating system to warn you whenever a firewall is not activated to protect you.

The ZoneAlarm (ZA) auto-notification mode sensed programs being blocked better than the Sunbelt Firewall (SF) and when told to 'allow program', ZA did a better job of allowing program access without further interruption.

The Sunbelt Firewall (SF) choked on allowing access to our customer relations manager software (Sage's Act!) even after we told it to allow that program. Act! wouldn't load from the server across the network while the SF was enabled, but immediately ran when it was disabled. This behavior suggested that a port needed to be open that wasn't. Unfortunately, the SF firewall didn't communicate what port was being blocked, so short of calling the application vendor to figure it out, there was no simple way to fix/open it. How quickly and how well a firewall "learns" what to allow when it's installed after other programs that are already working is important. In order for Act! to work, we ultimately found it necessary to open specific TCP or UDP ports manually.

If you already have a dedicated, enterprise virus/malware product, you may want to purchase a firewall separately. The results of our limited firewall evaluation are summarized in Figure 16.9 (using a 1-5 scale, where 1 = low performance and 5 = excellent performance).

Figure 16.9 Firewall Software Evaluation

Capability	ZoneAlarm	Sunbelt	Windows
Ease of Installation	4.5	4	5
Coverage of Incoming & Outgoing Risks	Yes	Yes	No
Ease of Configuring Current Applications	5	4	3
Ability to Learn & Use	4.5	4	5
Integration with Virus & Malware	4.5	4	3
Product Cost (Workstations)	$39.95	$19.95	Free
Recommendation Order	1st	2nd	Not

TopTenREVIEWS Firewall Tests

Others have also tested ZoneAlarm. In 2009, the TopTenREVIEWS Web site found that the ZoneAlarm Pro 7.0 kept computers safe from hackers, viruses, unwanted pop-ups and adware. TopTen commented, *"ZoneAlarm Pro has strengthened their anti–spyware feature and continued development and enhancement of their identity theft protection."*[8] ZoneAlarm received TopTenREVIEW's top rating for each of the following criteria:

- Feature set;
- Ease of use;
- Ease of installation;
- Reliability;
- Help/support.

---

[8] All reviews of firewalls included were taken from http://personal-firewall-software-review.toptenreviews.com/

TopTenREVIEWS found eConceal Firewall Pro *"to be missing some of options that would be expected,"* but then said that it was a great product and that for average users, less might be more."[9] The same Web site rated Outpost Firewall Pro, Norman Personal Firewall, Webroot Desktop Firewall and Injoy Firewall as good but each one had an area in which the editor's review found a problem. By the way, part of the review is a price comparison. You can bet that your EMR developer has not tested his product against all of these firewalls, so he may provide little help to you in making a final firewall vendor choice.

No matter who sets it up or which firewall you choose, someone has to test that it is working as expected. An untested firewall is false security. The setup will be slightly different for EMRs deployed in-office, than for EMRs that reach across the Internet to an ASP that is hosting your EMR.

Block Most Internet Access from In-Office Deployed EMRs

If you have chosen an in-office EMR deployment approach, since e-mail can be obtained from an exchange server, there's no need for every computer in your office to communicate directly with the Internet. Rather, let one computer handle all Internet access and act as a data repository. That computer should not "see" any of the other computers on your network, but can have a file-share (drive) that is visible to all. That way, all data and security patches downloaded from Microsoft can be deployed to all other office computers by your system administrator. This approach puts one computer at risk and allows you to disable access from the others to the Internet, including from your EMR fileserver. Use a second (different) server to host your EMR repository. It can act as your domain controller. These machines can sit next to each other physically in a secure area.

E-mail Challenges

E-mail is becoming more and more troublesome, particularly for medical professionals. If your patients receive a penis enlargement ad, or an erectile dysfunction pill ad apparently sent from your e-mail address, could that be troublesome, embarrassing and seem unprofessional? You bet. Well, that is not an unlikely occurrence if you are on the Internet on almost any mail server.

There can be two sources of the problem. First, your office system may have been penetrated and you have a malware program sending out this garbage in your name to your mailing list. If your mailing list has the names of all your patients, then they are being sent e-mail in your name. However, if you have followed the suggestions of this chapter, have appropriate security in place and none of your staff are surfing the Internet on office computers, then one (or more) of your patients' computers most likely have been compromised.

No matter whose computer has been compromised, there isn't too much you can do about this. How can you tell which has occurred? If lots of your patients are complaining to you about such messages, or worse yet, calling you

---

[9] Ibid

to discuss the "medical advice" they are receiving with your e-mail address on it, then your office system may have been infected. If so, you need to run full scans with two or three different anti-virus and anti-malware scanners to find which computer is the culprit, and fix it.

If it's only one or a few patients, then their computers are probably the source of the problem, and your name just happened to be one in their e-mail address book. They may not be aware of their system being compromised. You might suggest they run some other virus scanners than their usual ones (or install an anti-virus scanner). It is often hard to get rid of such infections. We recommend ESET's NOD32 anti-virus for this purpose. It also helps to keep Window's current by installing all service packs and recommended patches

Don't hear us wrong. There is secure e-mail, and there are ways of minimizing the potential for your e-mail address to be compromised, but turning on patient e-mail correspondence isn't the first thing you want to do when you get your new EMR system. Wait 6 to 12 months, after everything else is running fine and you feel capable of managing your system, then think through how to launch patient e-mail communications in a way that will protect your personal e-mail address and professional reputation. Typical SMTP e-mail servers are simply not safe.

If you are using browsers connected to an EMR served over the Web by an ASP, you cannot adopt this more secure approach. In that case, every computer will "see" and have Internet exposure and every one must have browser options set correctly and be behind their own firewalls. The SaaS, ASP Web-based EMR approach significantly increases Internet exposure of your office and therefore risk.

Testing That New Firewall Against Outbound & Inbound Traffic

After training is done, set your firewall to its normal mode and then subject it to some testing to be sure it's functioning properly.

That means two things:

1 Nothing bad gets in;

2 Anything bad inside can "phone home."

Any rogue program that can get out of your system onto the Internet can send any data it can access, to someone outside of your practice.

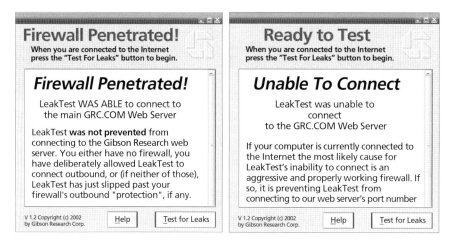

Figure 16.10 Tests of the Windows (left) and ESET (right) Firewalls

We tested the Windows XP-Pro version firewall on one of our machines, (shown in Figure 16.10 on the left) and it failed the test, allowing data to escape. Replacing Windows firewall with the ESET's firewall solved the problem, as shown in Figure 16.10 on the right. Blocking outgoing traffic is important and was a critical flaw in Windows' firewall until Vista, which is why security-minded physicians used other firewalls.

All ports should be in stealth mode, unresponsive to pings or other attempts to discover their status. Shields Up!! can test this, as shown in Figure 16.11.

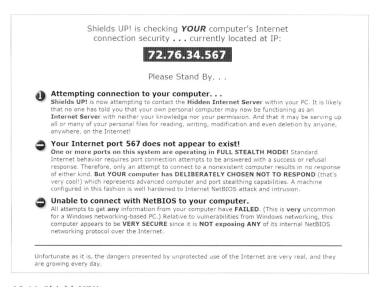

Figure 16.11 ShieldsUP!! port test on a computer

Gibson Research provides these and other testing tools at www.grc.com. Figure 16.12 shows a test of the first 1,024 computer ports A good test shows every port address as green (gray below). If the cell were blue, it would have indicated a problem.

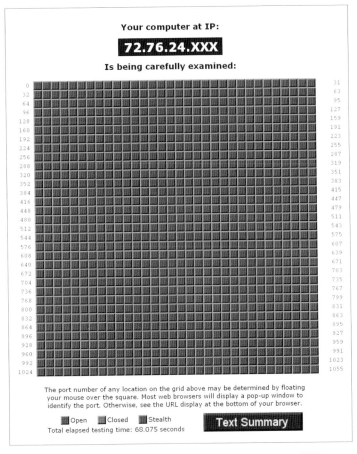

Figure 16.12 Report Showing Results Probing 1,024 PC Ports on a CPU

To document your security, captured the summary report (see Figure 16.13) for your security logbook, showing the results of the test conducted. Keep a logbook of these results. It will take less than one minute-per-day to conduct these tests.

GRC Port Authority Report created on UTC: 2009-07-16 AT 16:38:10

Results from scan of ports: 0-1056

        0 Ports Open
        0 Ports Closed
    1056 Ports Stealth

    1056 Ports Tested

ALL PORTS tested were found to be: STEALTH.

TruStealth: PASSED   – ALL tested ports were STEALTH,
                     – NO unsolicited packets were received,
                     – NO Ping reply (ICMP Echo) was received.

Figure 16.13 Summary Report of Computer Ports Test Finds No Vulnerabilities

Your logbook becomes part of the evidence documenting that you are serious about keeping your system safe and HIPAA-compliant.

The Gibson Research tools we discussed allow you to test your defenses and mitigate any vulnerabilities before you are hacked for real. It helps you assure that your computer network isn't vulnerable. At the end of the day, your self-verification documentation can be used (if it exists), to show diligence and watchfulness if your practice is ever accused of leaking confidential data.

As a final test, contract with a benevolent intrusion company to also probe your security defenses. They may be more creative than the Gibson Research tests you have run. If they also give you a clean bill of health, you can be fairly confident that your system is secure.

Automatic Intrusion Detection and Remediation

Automatic Intrusion Detection (AID) monitoring is becoming more common in bundled security suites, particularly the more expensive, enterprise-level ones. AID software alerts you in real-time to penetration attempts and other network irregularities associated with attacks. Your firewall may have this, but if not, it's available from as a standalone application from third-parties.

In the MSP/Andrew EMR Benchmark, EMR developers are asked whether they provide continuous intrusion detection in their systems or recommend third-party intrusion detection and logging utility software for use with their EMR systems. Only 14 percent of the EMR developers do intrusion detecting. About 22 percent said that they had not addressed this issue as yet. Most didn't even answer the question, which you might take as an implicit "no."

AID software should accommodate automatic responses, because some attacks are computer driven and occur rapidly. When an intruder attempted to breach MSP's Web site security in 2006, they launched more than two dozen attacks in less than six seconds, something that no human could have done manually. This underscores that hackers are increasingly using automation to enhance their attacks. In fact, the best malware attacks now have delays built-in, so as not to alert and trigger AID responses – so hackers adapt too.

Securing Your Wireless Network (WLAN)

With a cabled network, an intruder needs to have physical access to your network, but with a wireless one, someone can potentially access it from outside of your office, elsewhere in the building, or in some cases, even from outside of the office building in a parking lot or on the road. No matter which wireless network you choose, there are things you have to do to make sure it is secure and will remain so. Here is a quick WLAN security check-off list.

- Change the network administrator username and password on the wireless access point or router that hosts your WLAN. Make the password robust but memorable;
- Turn off SSID (Service Set IDentifier) broadcasting and make connection dependent upon the MAC (Media Access Control) ID, and list into the AP/router only the MAC ID of other devices you own. Unless a hacker spoofs one of your MAC addresses, their network cards will have a MAC ID that isn't in your list, limiting their ability to connect, no matter what they try;
- Turn security ON and change to WPA2 or 802.11x security. Never use WEP security (on 802.11b networks), as it is not truly secure or HIPAA-compliant, because it can be easily defeated;
- Shut down your wireless network during non-office hours. By blocking access from it to the Internet, the WLAN is more secure when you are not working in the office. When you are in the office, make sure all wireless devices are ON, so their IP and MAC addresses are in use. That makes it harder for a hacker to spoof them to the router and DHCP controller;
- Load and run a software firewall on every computer using a WLAN to prevent unauthorized network traffic from entering or leaving your network.

These changes are relatively easy and painless to make, but you can leverage your hospital's I.T. staff, or even your CPM maintenance guy to help set up your network. Making the changes recommended above will take about 10 minutes (if you do an inventory of all of the MAC IDs in advance). Finally, your network administrator or someone should monitor your WLAN periodically or use NetSniffer (or equivalent) mentioned earlier. There are many others also.

Take Control – Borrow from the Classroom

Computers in a medical office share some of the same needs as computers in a classroom. Once properly configured, they need to stay that way. Faronics makes several products that help in both settings, as described below:

- Standardizing the user environment is critical for medical offices, particularly those that have patient kiosks. Computers need to be configured to meet security and HIPAA standards, and then frozen so that they can't be inadvertently changed. Many of the configuration changes discussed require setting Group Policies. However, WINSelect can be used as stand-alone or as an easy-to-use alternative to Group Policy Objects (GPOs). It delivers some features and capabilities not offered by GPOs to create, customize or lockdown computers. We mention it because it may help you more easily configure your system, even if you are not familiar with how to use Group Policies or lack an Active Directory network structure. Many of the common GPO customizations such as modifying start button functionality, enforcing Windows Explorer restrictions, and limiting right-click functionality, are provided by WINSelect. WINSelect does not require the administrator to have a high level of technical knowledge, making it helpful for use in the small medical office environment.

- Once computers are properly configured using WINSelect, another Faronics' product, Deep Freeze, can make computer configurations indestructible. Any changes made to the computer – regardless of whether they are accidental or malicious – are not permanent. Deep Freeze provides immediate immunity to configuration drift, accidental system misconfiguration, malicious software activity, and incidental system degradation. Users have a consistent computer experience, which reduces questions to the office support person. Deep Freeze offers flexible scheduling options that enable your office geek to easily create automated update and maintenance periods. Schedule Deep Freeze to allow system and virus definition updates to occur from predefined times – either with the Deep Freeze Enterprise Console or using your preferred third-party desktop management solution.

- Anti-Executable is another helpful tool in maintaining a secure environment and enforcing the policy that users don't add new applications to the PCs. Anti-Executable allows only approved applications to run on a computer or server. Any other programs – whether they are unwanted, unlicensed, or simply unnecessary – are blocked from ever executing. Your computer support person is freed from having to try to track whether new applications are being added. Anti-Executable makes applying Windows and third-party updates easier because on-demand or scheduled maintenance modes allow for application updates and additions with automatic white list population.

These three utilities may be just what the doctor ordered to configure your computers for maximum security without having to call in a systems expert, and they are very reasonably priced (under $100). In combination, they allow you to get the configuration right, freeze it and prevent any additional software applications from being installed and run on your system.

When to Diagnose and Fix Problems

Finding and fixing computer problems can be a time-consuming endeavor that you don't want to mess with in the middle of your busy day when you need to see patients (not sick computers). That's where your computer support manager comes in. Just like Jack Bauer in the opening vignette, your support person should be an expert at "interrogating computer systems to see if they harbor any hidden code or evil intentions, and if found, in taking them out".

Available Software and Hardware Resources

Here are some more sophisticated tools that larger organizations utilize to secure and manage their systems:

- Neuber Security Task Manager and Network Task Manager
- Data leak protection;
- Enterprise firewall;
- Forensics tools;
- Intrusion detection systems;
- Messaging security;
- Network access control;
- Network auditing and compliance;
- Network intrusion prevention systems;
- Secure Web gateways;
- Security information management;
- Unified threat management.

The list below provides some options to consider.

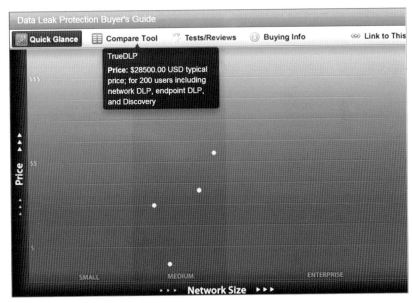

Figure 16.14 NetworkWorld's Product Locator/Buyer's Guide

If you want to deploy any of these products, you'll find a Web-based Buyer's Guide at NetworkWorld (shown in Figure 16.14) that lets you choose any tool category (in this case data leak protection tools) and shows you a graph of the functionality versus the price of the software. If you hover

over any one of the points on the graph, it reveals the vendor, product name and price. In this case, the lowest cost software available was $50/ year. This Web site is a great way to quickly find software (and hardware) tools without searching all over the Internet. The online location is: http://www.networkworld.com/buyersguides/.

How Defensible is Your Audit Trail?

Your EMR should log every Continuity of Care (CCR), or other export of or access to, your patient data (including the date, time, person who accessed/ created it), in its non-bypassable audit trail. This should include how it was delivered to the other party, who that party was and what security was involved.

   If your EMR doesn't provide that record, you will not be able to show that you controlled your files at all, nor who had access to them, nor what the content was when they were exported. When you provide the patient with an encounter summary at the end of his or her visit, it should be logged by your EMR. Know the audit trail in your EMR and depend on it.

Enlist Your Staff In Keeping Your Office Secure

The weakest link in keeping your system secure is your staff. Once you have computers and Internet access, you have the potential for any employee to compromise your security. Opening a bad e-mail, browsing a bad site, it doesn't take much to allow malware into your network. A strict policy of no non-business browsing or Internet use is critical. The policy must be enforced to be effective. Spector CNE is a product that creates an audit trail of all conversations, browsing, e-mails and instant messages, capturing exact details of what is done from every workstation. It can put teeth into your policy. You will have to decide whether that works for you or not. See www.spectorCNE.com for more information. We have not tested this program and are not aware of how it may interact with other programs and you may have to exempt it from your virus and malware detection and scanning programs since auditing every terminal and activity is exactly what it is intended to do. If you decide to use it, let your staff know that all of their activities on office computers are being logged. That in itself is a strong deterrent. Establish a policy for how violations will be handled and then stick to it.

   Most office personnel don't understand how dangerous the Internet really is and are oblivious to such things as Web bugs and clickjacking and how these can be misused to take control of computer systems. Space precludes discussing these in detail but we refer readers to Jim Rapoza's article *Powerless over Clickjacking*, in the October 6th, 2008 issue of eWeek magazine as an excellent reference. Once your staff realizes that what seems like harmless Internet activities can in fact open security holes, they are more likely to understand the need for security policies.

Whitelisting

Whitelisting programs is another way of assuring security. The idea is to make a list of all trusted programs and then banish any other application from accessing the Internet. It is complementary to anti-virus and anti-malware programs, which watch programs that are running for signs of infection or corruption.

Several good whitelisting programs are now available. One recently released was Bit9's Parity Whitelist, now at version 4.1. It was also detailed in the October 6, 2008 issue of eWeek magazine (see page 34) and explains the process and program features of whitelisting. Readers may find this issue on the Web at www.eweek.com or by contacting the publisher.

Authentication

Knowing who is signed onto your system may seem logical but if your system is ever hacked, someone outside will be impersonating someone in your office. A biometric identifier such as a fingerprint can be difficult to spoof, particularly remotely. Fingerprint scanners aren't expensive but some are difficult to use and unreliable. How you "register" your initial fingerprint is important if you want reliable results and is a topic addressed in the May 2006 issue of PC World, in Andrew Brandt's article entitled *Protect your Data System With a FingerPrint Reader*.

Use of biometric authentication can be one part of your two-part, level 4 authentication that will be required by DEA for electronic prescription of controlled substances, so it is worth thinking about as part of your basic configuration. It will also stifle remote hackers trying to log into your system, even if they have your password they won't have your fingerprint.

Data Encryption

Newer versions of Windows OS allow for OS-level encryption of data in individual files and for entire folders (and sub-folders). You should discuss this with your EMR supplier to determine compatibility with their software. This support was added to the OS in some versions of Vista and continued in Windows 7. When data is encrypted by the OS it's called – Encrypting File System (EFS). It is a good reason to adopt Windows 7 for your EMR application once your EMR developer (and your office hardware) fully supports it.

Using EFS provides security of stored data without having to use third-party add-on software utilities and because it's embedded in the OS kernel it should be more secure, as long as you keep your encryption certificate keys secure. Encryption, like compression, is an attribute of files set on the Properties Tab. Windows does not allow files and folders to be both compressed and encrypted and we would not recommend data compression at all for EMR files. With the low price of storage media, it is hard to see the need for compression any longer. For a good description of the creation and tending of Encrypting

File Systems, see the article *Secure Files and Folders By Using EFS in Vista* in the December, 2008 issue of PC Magazine.

Wrap Up

It takes a combination of tools (and the skills to use them) to keep your medical office network safe, secure and running efficiently. It also takes planning and guidance to anticipate and prepare for the various attempted penetrations and other hazards that offices face today. How do you feel about that?

The MSP/Andrew EMR Benchmark documented the degree to which the majority of today's EMR developers explored these issues and were prepared to help physicians with orientation, training and deployment of the necessary tools. It also documented to what degree software you need has been tested and will run harmoniously with currently-available EMR solutions. If you need more help than they can provide, try your hospital CIO or the person who will be maintaining your EMR.

EMR developers need to begin doing a more thorough job of testing security software for compatibility with their EMR(s), and also take the lead in bringing physicians up to speed about security functions. As a physician purchaser of a developer's EMR, request assistance and include developer promises in your sales agreement. After you locate several EMRs that meet your functional needs, give extra consideration to any EMR developer(s) that agree to provide on-site security configuration assistance.

Don't be too quick to launch patient portals or even e-mail initially. According to reports from Symantec, one in every 617 spam messages contains malicious code. One in every 170 e-mails contains a virus, and one in every 220 is a phishing attack.[10] Save yourself and your staff grief and aggravation – don't go there initially. Get everything else up and running first and then obtain some good advice on portals and e-mail before you launch into that uncharted territory. Choose an EMR that supports both CPOE e-prescription and patient portals, so that you can deploy them in the future without changing EMRs or migrating electronic patient charts.

We believe that many problems attributed to EMR products may in fact be virus and malware problems that have penetrated poorly-designed systems, or due to anti-virus and firewall products that slow down computer systems by hogging processor resources and lead to computer instabilities and crashes.

There is an old saying, "People don't do what you expect, they do what you inspect!" CMS and Price Waterhouse Coopers will be performing HIPAA compliance audits at larger hospitals and hospitals that have been the source of policy complaints. They will be looking for both privacy and security weaknesses as well as violations. How widespread such audits will be is something that only time will tell. The effort is in its infancy, and there is not nearly enough manpower to audit individual physician offices.

---

[10] *The Growing E-mail Security Challenge*. By B. Prince. Published April 21, 2008, by e-Week

Keep an eye on the EMR/EHR/PHR Discussion Forum hosted at www. ehrselector.com. It has a variety of threads hosted by well-qualified experts. Reading the threads is open to all. Contributing requires registration. The purpose of the forum is to help you be successful and to share experiences.

There are real legal issues involved with security violations and breaches, so be careful that your licensing agreement doesn't excuse your EMR developer and ASP provider from any liability in the event of a breach. See Chapter 13 – Lawyer-Proofing Your EMR for assistance and Chapter 18 – Negotiating the Agreement.

Crucial Decision

What must you do to protect your patient records from loss or theft and make them HIPAA-compliant? Photocopy as needed or download from www.ehrselector.com

Security Issues	Developer Recommends	MSP Suggestion	Your Decision
Obtain legal advice for purchase agreement		Obtain legal services	
Mandate acceptance testing before system payment		Specify items that are to be tested	
Require EMR developer assistance in security configuration of all systems		Yes, even if it costs extra	
Virus & malware detection software deployed		See text	
Firewall deployed		See text	
Firewall rules standardized across all firewalls		Yes	
Periodic intrusion testing		Outside vendor - at least quarterly	
Secure shredders		TuneUp Utilities 2010 or equivalent	
Server undelete		Undelete Server & Professional, or WinUndelete	
Audit trail is always enabled and can't be circumvented		Yes	
Network configuration		Establish a domain	
Computer OS (if Microsoft) for workstations		XP Pro, Vista Business or Windows 7	
Server and router location		Secured location (controlled access) away from patients and staff	
Web-based ASP EMR solution		Secured browsers and software firewalls on every PC	
In-office EMR configuration		All 'inward facing' computers except one server on Internet	

Security is everyone's issue. This Scorecard helps you think about steps to protect your computers and your patients' information. Threats to computers evolve and become more insidious, so security measures have to be re-evaluated frequently and then tested in your office.

CHAPTER 17

What You Can Expect to Spend

> **Crucial Decision**
> **What will you spend transforming your practice from paper to an EMR system?**
> This chapter also addresses the following questions:
> - How can you create a preliminary budget?
> - Is the Stark program a good fit for you in adopting an EMR?
> - What are the details of the ARRA stimulus for adopting EMRs?

EMR Adventures

The doctor's lounge at Hometown General Hospital is a busy place today with a number of physicians engaged in a lively discussion of how to afford the EMRs that are being strongly encouraged by so many.

Dr. Karen Bell has just finished saying that she is taking her time and following a process in her decision of what and how to implement her EMR but that she is still concerned about the costs. "I know that the relaxation of Stark regulations allow Hometown General's I.T. department to help me, but I am not certain of the strings that are attached with that approach."

Dr. Goldstein responds, "Our practice opted not to go that route because the EMR that the hospital wanted us to adopt did not fit our needs and was one of the most expensive ones. We would have been stuck paying the software maintenance fees, about 25% per year. But I am interested to know whether we qualify for the new government incentives under ARRA, even though we have already adopted our EMR."

"I think you do qualify, at least as I understand ARRA," responds Dr. Glass. "I think as long as your system meets a requirement the government calls Meaningful Use, you qualify."

"Meaningful Use – is that a feature of an EMR? I don't think our EMR has that feature, does it Brian?" asks Dr. Rodriguez.

"No, it's not a feature, I think Meaningful Use is something that an EMR will help to prove so that a practice can receive higher payments from Medicare and Medicaid," responds Dr. Bell.

Dr. Jonas adds his wisdom to the conversation by saying, "Well, these reimbursement benefits are all fine, but I encourage you, Dr. Bell, to come up with a budget to determine how much you can spend on your EMR, that

Successfully Choosing Your EMR: 15 Crucial Decisions. By © Arthur Gasch and Betty Gasch.
Published 2010 by Blackwell Publishing

is the wise thing to do. And I can tell you more areas to watch out for if you are interested. Believe me, I have been burned by my EMR a number of times because I did not include some items or wasn't aware of features I needed to activate. I wouldn't go back to a paper-based practice, but because the EMR is a new way of practicing medicine, there are certain things you need to know."

"I would appreciate anything you can tell me," says Dr. Bell. "I don't want to be a fool about EMRs. I will do a budget and I'll call you later to see when you are free to have a meeting to hear your wisdom, if that is alright with you, Dr. Jonas."

Doctors Rodriguez, Goldstein and Glass ask if they can be included in this meeting to learn from Dr. Jonas as well. "Sure," replies Dr. Jonas. "You may as well all learn from my mistakes – that way, we'll all practice safer medicine."

Cost – The Crucial Bottom Line

Isn't it great that Dr. Jonas wants to share his wisdom? We don't know how real-world this is, but life's trials often make us wiser. If you have not adopted your EMR and you know practices that have, approach the decision makers and seek their counsel. This chapter offers some insight concerning Stark regulations and also the new ARRA legislation. Like Dr. Jonas' advice to Dr. Bell, we hope that you, too, will consider making a budget to determine what you can afford as you finalize your EMR plans.

What an EMR system will cost exactly is hard to answer until you lock down the functionality you want and decide how you will deploy your system (either the ASP or the in-office approach). This chapter includes cost items to consider for each EMR deployment type and a general budget breakdown; from there, your specific preferences will give you a bottom-line figure for your EMR. We'll start out with some general thoughts on EMR costs.

Overall EMR System Costs

A Health Affairs article published a few years ago stated that the average cost of an EMR is $43,000 per MD[1]. That means some EMRs are less expensive and some are more expensive on a cost/physician basis compared to the figure reported by Health Affairs. This cost estimate reflects predominately larger physician group practices, in some cases very large group practices or integrated networks, as the buyer groups. The cost for a smaller group practice can be much less expensive than that.

Life-Cycle Costs Can Double Purchase Costs
The purchase cost of an EMR is not the only, or even the most significant, cost of ownership to consider for an EMR. The annual EMR software maintenance

---

[1] *Medical Groups' Adoption of Electronic Health Records and Information Systems*. By David Gans, et al. Published Sept/Oct. 2005, Vol. 24, pp. 1323–1333, by Health Affairs

fees range from 18 to 22 percent of the list price of your EMR. The exception to this are the costs associated with the Web-based, Application Service Provider (ASP) model, which includes software maintenance fees in the basic access fee/physician (or provider).

That means if a client/server (in-office) system is in place for 4-5 years, the software maintenance costs will equal or surpass its initial purchase costs. Put another way, the life-cycle costs of ownership for an EMR would be about $86K per MD over a five-year period given the mix of EMR developers in the market today. This is yet another reason to get in early on the ARRA reimbursement funding (detailed later in this chapter). EMRs are inevitable and you may as well receive some of Uncle Sam's money.

Establish a Preliminary Budget

There is no one size/one type EMR that works for every practice. Part of your decision of what EMR to deploy will be determining what each EMR will cost, both initially and over the first couple of years you have it. It is sensible to figure out what you need to budget for both the ASP and the in-office approach to EMRs.

Let's assume you are willing to spend "X" dollars on your new EMR. How should "X" be divided among the different expense categories? The amounts in some categories will be quite different for the ASP and the in-office EMR deployments (hardware versus software categories, for example).

Begin by budgeting the in-office approach and split your budget/estimate up four ways. Allocate one-fourth for software, one-fourth for hardware, one-fourth for pre-deployment training, EMR evaluation, professional advice (like legal advice for the contracts and paper chart record conversion), and one-fourth for post-deployment staff orientation and initial customization. Then break down each of these categories into subcategories.

When you have all of your categories and subcategories listed, begin pricing the items in each, and build your budget from the bottom up (like an accountant would). Identify any items that remain unknown in your budget and add them to your training list. See what your consolidated budget figure is approaching. If the total is becoming too high, look at the individual items that are driving up the costs and consider ways to reduce them.

For ASP deployments, you can use your in-office budget numbers and then subtract ~$3,000 off of the hardware section because you won't require a server (unless you think you want a blended deployment). For the in-office approach, your upfront capital expenditures will be higher; for the Web-based method, your on-going infrastructure costs, such as primary (and secondary) networks to stay connected to the Web-based server, will be higher.

The next sections cover some of the items and details of the categories and subcategories for your budget.

Software

EMR Licensing/Purchase Costs

Your EMR software ballpark cost is anywhere from $400/month/MD for ASP EMRs to $43K/MD for larger, multi-specialty, multi-practice group practices using the in-office deployment. Now that is quite a price span, isn't it? Remember, hardware costs are on top of that.

At the lower end of those costs, an EMR is not as difficult to consider but the higher end costs are probably out of sight for some smaller practices. The good news is that if you are a solo practitioner up to a small, single specialty practice with 10-15 physicians, your software costs can be under $15K per MD if purchased, or $1,000/month/MD if you choose an Application Service Provider (ASP) model.

Software Utility Costs

There will also be software costs to provide the firewall, anti-virus, anti-spyware, server undelete, server backup and network management software utilities that will need to be deployed to keep your office network properly configured, hacker-free and HIPAA-compliant. Even in Web-based implementations, most of these utilities will be required because the computer that your Web browser is running on must block keyboard loggers, not be infected with viruses or malware and be HIPAA-compliant.

On-going Maintenance Costs

The cost of on-going support is much higher for software-based EMR products than for medical devices that are also software-based products. By way of comparison, a typical medical device may have a maintenance cost for hardware and software of 8-12 percent per year. Yet a software-only product (like an EMR) vendor may charge customers 16-20 percent per year for support that does not include hardware or hardware maintenance. There is really no good reason for this other than the fees are paying for continued development of the vendor's software.

As long as support/application maintenance fees continue to be paid, you can bet that EMR and CPM vendors will continue to charge them. Perhaps as competition heats up and the number of deals increase, the fees will drop based on market pressure. Larger installed bases of customers will also help, as the development costs have no relationship to the number of clients who license the software.

Generally, the larger established vendors are often the offenders in this area, a factor to be considered if your hospital is offering you an EMR through the relaxed Stark regulations (detailed shortly). If you end up with a large vendor's system and a lot of features that you do not need, you will still be responsible for the maintenance fees every year. Very few vendors break out these costs or allow their clients the ability to opt in or out of specific support elements.

Hardware

Computers and Carts
The cost of hardware depends on the decision you make about installing an EMR in your office versus using a Web-based, ASP model EMR. Installing an EMR in your office has higher front-end hardware costs, which also means ongoing hardware maintenance costs. The ASP model means network costs go up over time.

The use of tablets versus laptops (or desktops) will impact your cost, as will the use of wireless versus wired networks. In a number of the chapters of this book, we have pointed out details of the items that would impact total hardware costs.

Standby Power Costs
Budget $10K for the cost of the backup power generator you will need, as an estimate. Add any building permits required for the power generator, check with your local municipality for these numbers.

Telephone System Costs
What about telephones? Will you integrate them into the 3CNJ1000 devices or leave them as you have them now? Leaving them costs nothing, and you always have the capacity in the 3CNJ1000s to implement voice over IP telephones when you are ready or there is some compelling reason to do so.

Practice Renovations

Based on previous chapters, you may have decided to do some renovations to your exam rooms, your waiting area (if you embraced the notion of patient kiosks) and perhaps to your old chart room. For our purposes, we presume that you have quotes for renovations. Remember to include any purchased or custom-built furniture that will be needed for the kiosk and any other areas being transformed.

System Installation Costs
The wired networking will cost you $225 per room of which $165 is for the 3CNJ1000, $5 for each of the duplex drywall boxes and the remainder is for the cable that is typically required to run back to the central switch/hub/router. If you want a second 3CNJ1000 in the room on an opposite wall, add another $165. Double this room cost to account for the electrician labor involved to install it, or do it yourself and save some money, if you have the expertise and time.

The central switches could be another $300-500 or more if you have a larger practice. The Ethernet power inserter is about $40. The router is included in the Internet access fee you are paying. Figure $145 per computer for an Uninterruptible Power Supply (UPS), with one in each room where there is a stationary computer, one for the server, one for the network switch/hub and Ethernet power inserter (which all might be served by one UPS if they are near each other).

Wireless Network Costs

This varies depending on the size of your office and the number of auxiliary Access Points (APs) that will be required. In a small office, the AP in the router and perhaps one more may suffice. In a larger office you will need a site survey. Figure less than $1,000 for a small office, and obtain a quote from your network vendor for a larger one. Lean toward commercial and not consumer-grade wireless devices.

Training and Consulting Costs

It is prudent to budget for training needs and you may want to involve various consultants in your EMR selection and contracting process. There are companies that represent all of the consultant categories listed below, located at www.ehrselector.com, at least for most of the U.S.

Training Needs

See Chapter 18 for training details and to obtain a general idea of what training is typically included in an EMR developer's price as well as areas where the developer may be flexible. You can stretch your budget by using an approach like "Train the Trainer" for example, but we encourage you to spend as much time and money on training as you can afford. The MSP ESP Web portal has a list of training resources and also training consultants who can develop or arrange training experiences for your staff.

Legal Advice

Every practice needs some legal assistance in approaching EMR (or CPM) deployment. The contracts you sign to acquire or license your EMR provide the only leverage you have after the sale of holding your EMR vendor to the commitments that it makes to you during the selling of the system. Get it right in the contracts and avoid a lot of misunderstanding in the future.

   Remember, many EMR vendors will be changing corporate identities over the next 5-10 years. The ones that don't obtain market traction will fail, others will grow and attract the attention of larger companies. Also, many mid-sized EMR vendors are seeking to grow large enough to be acquired. In such cases, the verbal representation of the personnel who originally sold you the EMR, or even the policies they have been supporting you under, are all likely to change when the larger company acquires them – unless you have the requirements in writing. Having clauses in the contract that make the actual source code available to your practice (only in the event of failure) can be key, as written correctly, these will survive when the new owner takes possession of your previously small and responsive former vendor.

Budget $5,000 to $7,500 if you are a small practice and have done your homework. Budget $10,000 to $15,000 if you are a larger practice. Legal fees for ASP solutions may be a bit more than for in-office deployments. The more ground work your practice can do to expedite the legal process, the less it will cost you.

EMR Consulting Advice

The cost of these services depends a lot on the stature of the EMR consultant. Well-known consultants will cost more than consultants just starting out. It is best to contact a number of consultants and ask for a quote. Be ready to explain the services you need so that they can determine how much time will be involved. Doing your homework will reduce your overall consulting fees.

Cost Accounting Consulting

Since you obviously have books already, you may wonder why you need any accounting consulting. Maybe you don't. But if your books and your CPM system revenues rarely match, and you are operating out of two different sets of cash flow documents, you could be in some difficulty if you are ever audited. Your workflow summary is a good excuse to look at your practice from a cost-accounting perspective, on an encounter-by-encounter basis. Engage a firm that has a medical accounting practice specialty.

Technical Consulting

You may need to hire a permanent, probably part-time, Information Technology (I.T.) person. You may not need any more than a half day to a day every other week once you are up and running. Be sure this person is bonded and interview candidates until you are certain that you can trust him or her with access to your sensitive patient data.

Don't Know Yet List

Your Don't Know Yet list revolves around the questions you don't have the answers to (yet). By the time you read this chapter (assuming you have worked your way through the rest of the book), your Don't Know Yet list could be quite short. The Scorecards you took the time to fill in at the end of each chapter can be used to focus you to areas that you will need to think through in your budget. Here is a list of what you may still need to determine:
- What operating system is best for an in-office deployment?
- Where will the EMR be physically deployed in your current office space and what preparation will that area need?
- How will the system be backed up and secured?
- How will data from all of the charts of your active patients get into the EMR database initially?
- If you use chart scanning, whose charts will be scanned and when?

- Will the scanning be done up front and in bulk or be done just-in-time after EMR deployment?
- Will office staff do this or will a scanning service organization be needed?
- Once scanned, what will become of the paper charts?
- How can the chart space vacated be reused more effectively in the practice? Could it become another/new exam room(s) for example?

This isn't a complete list. It is simply a short list to stimulate your thinking; for those practices that did their homework, simply look at your Scorecards.

Whatever questions you find that you don't have answers for becomes your exploration list. Your EMR Project Manager has the task of finding out what resources, materials, seminars are available to address and resolve these unanswered questions. Whatever list emerges, evaluate the importance of each item/requirement. Is an item a 'Must Have' or a 'Like to Have' item? Does it have to be part of the initial roll out of the EMR or can it taken live later? Whatever you can't find a resource to resolve, means you may need to find an external consultant to resolve. Finally, what is it worth or what is the impact of not having the feature at all?

Enter Uncle Sam

The next few paragraphs are specific to the reimbursement and cost situation in the U.S. market. The Stark Safe Harbor legislation provides alternative funding for EMR adoption. You should consult your healthcare lawyer for details. While we can't cover all of the Stark legislation's details, what follows are some highlights.

This legislation has no Meaningful Use certification requirements and does not apply if you have already adopted an EMR. The legislation allows hospital I.T. personnel to become involved with physician groups adopting EMRs, and allows hospitals to donate the majority of the cost of purchasing EMRs, so long as such EMRs are currently CCHIT-certified. Stark allows hospitals to purchase a group subscription to EMR selection resources on behalf of their physicians. Hospitals may provide I.T. support services to practices lacking I.T. personnel. They may also extend hardware group purchasing umbrellas, conduct training, provide support and so on. That's the good news, but you need to be very careful before accepting a hospital-recommended EMR under the Stark legislation.

Here's an example of how the Stark Safe Harbor might work. If you find an EMR solution that costs $62K at list, Stark would allow your hospital to pay $44K, so that you only pay $18K out of your own pocket. But the software maintenance fee could be somewhere between $11K and $16.3K per year, which you must also pay directly each year after the system is installed. This example could turn out to be an expensive bargain.

Most Hospitals Cool on Stark

Most hospitals have not rushed to pay for their attending physicians' EMR deployments. Only about one-third of hospitals are even in a financial position to consider it. Many hospitals use the Stark legislation to offer EMRs that are hospital legacy I.T. system vendors because they already have interfaces to their (sometimes proprietary) lab, pharmacy, PACS, radiology, cardiology or other diagnostic systems installed in the hospital. That is only an advantage if the EMR proposed also fits your practice workflow. Sacrificing office productivity to obtain hospital interfaces, is a bad trade off.

Legacy Hospital Vendors Support for Practice Specialties

Which I.T. vendors come to mind for hospital diagnostic or clinical areas? You probably think of CliniComp, Surgical Information Systems, McKesson, Cerner, GE Healthcare, Siemens, Epic, Picis, Philips, Misys, Meditech, iMDSoft, Eclipsys and others. Some of these companies don't offer EMRs for smaller physician offices, but others do. The legacy I.T. vendors that offer EMRs are not among the least expensive systems, but a more important issue is the support for practice specialties.

Physicians practice in more than 46 different medical and surgical specialties. Which of these legacy I.T. systems supports all of those specialties? In fact, the MSP EHR Selector includes 46 different specialties so we'll use it to answer that question.

On the MSP EHR Selector there is an "All Specialties" global profile you can use to assert all 46 criteria in one mouse click. A second mouse click compares these specialties to "All Vendors" and returns a list of two – Pulse Systems and PatientOS, an open system VistA EMR. Legacy hospital vendor GE supports only two-thirds of these physician specialties while McKesson and Cerner support only about 45 percent of them. The answer to the question is that none of the legacy I.T. vendors supports all 46 physician specialties. That does not detract from the EMR systems offered by legacy hospital vendors as their physician office EMRs support some specialties very well, just not all 46 of them.

If you are a physician specializing in allergy, geriatrics, hematology, infectious disease, neonatal, infertility, nuclear medicine, pathology, behavioral/mental health, dentistry or plastic surgery and you can only choose EMRs offered by legacy I.T. vendors, you aren't likely to end up with an EMR that matches your needs very well. Your hospital CIO doesn't typically have time to investigate the 200+ EMR products available in the market, but he/she knows that the EMRs for physician offices offered by the hospital I.T. vendors will interface with the same vendor's hospital diagnostic systems. The safest and simplest approach to ensure integration is for the CIO to offer these legacy EMRs to their physicians. The CIO does not appreciate the negative impact the legacy approach may have on physician office workflow and budget.

Dealing With Lab and Pharmacy Interface Issues

In this day of interoperability and national standards, why is interfacing with lab, pharmacy and imaging systems a valid issue? For the past 10 years at the HIMSS and RSNA conferences, all of the legacy I.T. vendors have participated in the IHE pavilion, demonstrating their DICOM and HL7 standard interfaces among radiology and imaging systems. So if the EMR you buy for your office supports DICOM and HL7 standards, shouldn't it interface to the hospital radiology and imaging systems?

EMR demonstrations are important for verification of just such issues. Put together a list of the data you need and the standards required to provide this data in your RFP and in any purchasing or licensing agreement that ensues. Make it a condition of EMR system acceptance that your EMR must interface to whatever hospital systems you decide are important to you before release of your final payment. Have your healthcare lawyer include the language, and clarify any extra cost associated with these interfaces. Often, the costs are negotiable as the interfaces already exist. Use EMR demonstrations to prove that the interfaces work.

That is not to say that simply supporting the same interfaces makes data transfer and true interoperability happen. Over the years, interfacing has been a sometimes thorny issue, which is why the demonstrations proving the interoperability are important.

Collaborate With Your Hospital In Supporting Standards

The best approach to interoperability is standards support, not proprietary interfaces. Bigger healthcare systems (and IDNs) own several hospitals that may each have different I.T. vendors and installed systems. The healthcare system may have invested substantial funds in interfacing these diverse systems but that is not your problem, nor do you want to let it become a burden to your office workflow efficiency.

Steer clear of hospitals offering Stark assistance that propose adoption of one particular EMR by the entire medical staff. It will not work well for everyone. Suggest instead that the hospital purchase a group subscription for all attending physicians to the MSP EHR Selector.[2] Ask your hospital to support modern standards like ELINCS (LOINC) and others, as a vehicle for exchanging lab and other data with your practice; then choose an EMR that supports those standards. Let the CIO generate the list of standards that hospital legacy I.T. systems support and then use them as a guide when choosing your EMR.

Your hospital could even arrange a mini-IHE Connectathon in which all EMR developers would bring a live system and demonstrate that their solutions actually exchange data with your hospital's systems. That is the

---

[2] In checking this with the law firm of LeClairRyan, we are informed that the Stark Safe Harbor provisions allow this as part of the hospital assisting your practice in choosing an EMR. The cost of a group subscription to the MSP EHR Selector is minimal.

type of collaboration that makes everyone's life easier and flushes out all the incompatibility before attending physicians have committed to specific EMRs.

ARRA (HITECH) Legislation Augments Stark Incentives

The American Recovery and Reinvestment Act (ARRA) legislation was signed into law on February 17, 2009 by President Obama. The healthcare I.T. component of the bill is the HITECH (Health Information Technology for Economic and Clinical Health) Act, which appropriates almost $50 billion to encourage healthcare organizations and physician group practices to adopt EMRs. HITECH gives physicians a direct way of obtaining money from Uncle Sam to reimburse EMR deployment costs, independent of the Stark Safe Harbor legislation.

ARRA complements the Stark Safe Harbor exemptions passed by Congress a couple years ago, at least in some instances. Some physicians will be able to collect under each program. To take advantage of Stark, you cannot have an EMR or CPOE system now in place, but ARRA doesn't make that stipulation. In both cases you must purchase an EMR that has current CCHIT-Certification. For ARRA, your EMR must also be certified as achieving Meaningful Use.

Recall the example cited of the $62K EMR system where the hospital had agreed to pay $44K of the cost under the Stark Safe Harbor program. You can receive an additional $44K in reimbursement from CMS to offset your initial purchase of $18K (your Stark contribution) and to offset the $16K per year of software maintenance fees for almost the first four years of the time you own your system. While this is a sweet deal, estimates are that only one-third of hospitals are in a position to move ahead with Stark and unfortunately, some of these hospitals are pursuing the "we will pay for it if you buy what we tell you" approach to offering EMRs to their physicians.

Physicians need to remain tuned in to ARRA as EMR reimbursement by Uncle Sam is inherently tied to Meaningful Use (MU), and the summary advice for MU issued through fall 2009 doesn't define MU at specific levels. You will want to obtain legal help to include MU-compliance clauses in all contracts or license agreements with EMR developers.

Medicaid and Medicare Details

ARRA money is available to physicians involved with Medicare and Medicaid patients. Physicians whose practices are composed of over 30 percent Medicaid patients can be reimbursed up to $63,500 over 5 years. Pediatricians whose practices are composed of over 20 percent Medicaid patients are eligible to be reimbursed the same amount. The government has issued a formula that will provide reimbursement to Medicaid physicians by multiplying 85 percent of amounts from $25,000 in the first year of EMR deployment, up to $10,000 in years two to five.

For physician groups that accept Medicare patients, the reimbursement is $44,000 over 5 years, with decreasing amounts reimbursable over the years.

The ARRA reimbursement money applies to software, hardware, installation and training purposes.

Timing is everything because the later you get into the program, the less your reimbursement from the government will be. If you have adopted an EMR and can show Meaningful Use by November 2011 or 2012, you can receive up to $18K per physician for the first year in addition to normal CMS payments. If you wait until 2013 however, the first year reimbursement drops to just $12K, a $6K loss just because you are "late" in adopting and achieving MU. Worse yet, your future reimbursement also drops so that the total reimbursed through 2016 would be only $39K, rather than $44K.

Get in a year later, in 2014, and total reimbursement is only $24K, which is $20K less than if you were in by 2011 or 2012. Figure 17.1 illustrates the breakdown of reimbursement for Medicare practices.

Figure 17.1 Staggered Reimbursement for EMR under ARRA (HITECH) Bill

Year EMR Deployed	Reimbursement by Year & Amount						
	2011	2012	2013	2014	2015	2016	TOTAL
2011	$18,000	$12,000	$8,000	$4,000	$2,000	$0	$44,000
2012	$0	$18,000	$12,000	$8,000	$4,000	$2,000	$44,000
2013	$0	$0	$15,000	$12,000	$8,000	$4,000	$39,000
2014	$0	$0	$0	$12,000	$8,000	$4,000	$24,000
2015 +	$0	$0	$0	$0	$0	$0	$0

Washington Delays Adoption

To receive reimbursement for deployment costs, any EMR must support MU functionality and be certified as achieving it. Meaningful Use is not directly a measure of EMR functionality, rather it's a measure of achieving some outcomes that depend on EMR functionality.

Because MU clarification was delayed beyond December 2009, the entire EMR industry stagnated. What was intended to be a great stimulus program ended up hurting smaller EMR developers in 2009. Including an undefined term like MU in the ARRA legislation, and then taking 10 months to define it, is an example of problems that occur when important legislation is rushed through Congress.

Today, EMR purchases by individual group practices in the 6-25 doctor range are dramatically slower than before ARRA and won't accelerate until Q1 2010 at the earliest. If MU doesn't ultimately specify something that can be accomplished with existing EMR products, the entire program could fail.

What to Do While You Wait for MU

Start immediately to evaluate EMRs and get a head start on the selection and deployment process. The earlier you start, the more resources will be available to help you. Once everyone starts, resources like consultants, document scanning companies and legal services will be hard to find. Be proactive:

- Do your needs analysis;
- Do your workflow analysis;
- Determine your deployment approach (ASP versus in-office);
- Do a comparison of vendors for basic EMR functionality;
- Do your office modifications;
- Do your existing chart conversions. Use a format like Adobe Acrobat that can be assimilated by the EMR you ultimately choose;
- Run your internal Ethernet wiring;
- Evaluate EMR hardware and choose computing platforms: laptops, tablets, PC's on carts, and so on.

You will find indicators on the MSP EHR Selector to help you choose features that support achieving MU functionality. These can be printed out and attached to your RFP. You should also require them to be demonstrated as part of your system acceptance testing (if your purchasing or licensing agreement is properly written). Getting this preliminary work done as you are choosing your EMR can accelerate deployment and move you to the front of the EMR reimbursement line. From March 2010, you have only nine months to plan, choose and deploy your EMR if you want to be in the first group to receive 2011 EMR reimbursements.

Wrap Up

There are a lot of hidden or extra costs in deploying an EMR and these costs can fluctuate depending on your hardware decisions, how you handle paper chart conversion, what office renovation you choose to do, your network installation costs, any personnel training costs, the addition of emergency power generators, the costs of legal and consulting services and so on. The money to adopt and deploy EMRs isn't available up front from the government, so you may need to arrange a loan or leasing for some components of your EMR. The MSP ESP Web portal (www.ehrselector.com) is building a list of some financial and leasing institutions that are willing to provide you with financial assistance. Use this chapter's Scorecard to organize your budget for such EMR expenses.

Crucial Decision

What will you spend transforming your practice from paper to EMR?
Photocopy as needed or download Scorecard from www.ehrselector.com

INITIAL COSTS

Hardware

Item	Number	Cost per	Total Cost
PC's			
Laptops			
Handheld Tablets			
Microphones for SR			
Carts for Computers			
UPS			

Software

Item	Number	Cost per	Total Cost
EMR App. Software			
Firewall			
Anti-virus			
Anti-spyware			
Server Undelete			

This is a Crucial Decision to begin your budget. Reference previous chapters' Scorecards to focus as to what to include.

Crucial Decision

What will you spend transforming your practice from paper to EMR?
Photocopy as needed or download Scorecard from www.ehrselector.com

Server Backup			
Network Management Software			

Other Upfront Costs

Item	Number	Cost per	Total Cost
License Cost or Initial Deposit (ASP)			
Wiring/Rewiring			
Office Modification			
Legal Fees			
Consultant Fees			
Training Costs			
Chart Scanning Costs			
EMR Software Acquisition Costs (if purchased)			

This is a Crucial Decision to begin your budget. Reference previous chapters' Scorecards to focus as to what to include.

Crucial Decision
What will you spend transforming your practice from paper to EMR?
Photocopy as needed or download Scorecard from www.ehrselector.com

Other			

ON-GOING COSTS

Internet Access Costs (per/mo.)			
ASP Software Maint. Fees (per/mo.)			
I.T. Personnel Assistance Fees			

Anything Else We Need to Budget

This is a Crucial Decision to begin your budget. Reference previous chapters' Scorecards to focus as to what to include.

CHAPTER 18

Negotiating the Agreement

Crucial Decision

Do you need legal assistance to get your EMR contract right? If so, where do you find EMR-specific legal assistance?

This chapter also addresses the following questions:

- Which terms are negotiable in the purchase/license agreement?
- How negotiable are these terms?

Negotiation Control

The initial Purchasing/Licensing Agreement is critical to everything that comes after you make your final EMR product decision. As some of the EMR Adventures throughout the book have illustrated, future options and liabilities of several practices were impacted by the fine print that was not included in their initial purchasing or licensing agreement with their EMR developer. Before signing any agreement, you are the one in the driver's seat and therefore in control. However, after you sign, the negotiated terms dictate future actions.

Obtain Experienced Legal Assistance

Legal information is so important that MSP has included Legal Alert™ links in its EMR/EHR Selector's™ Help Screens. Law firms that deal with typical business matters for your office probably won't be aware of special issues that relate to EMR product licensing or purchasing. Don't pay them to learn at your expense. Obtain your legal assistance from a firm with expertise in EMR. If you are using the MSP EHR Selector (www.ehrselector.com), the Legal Alert Help Screens have introduced you to one such law firm[1] with expertise in EMR (and other) healthcare contracting.

Keep Your Best Interest in Mind and Contract

We have identified and examined some of the legal problems associated with adopting an EMR, most of which are not mentioned by EMR developers, by CCHIT, or by other EMR advocate groups. We have also covered the

---

[1] Because EMR is a new and specialized technology, not all law firms have detailed expertise in this area – be careful to find one that does.

Successfully Choosing Your EMR: 15 Crucial Decisions. By © Arthur Gasch and Betty Gasch.
Published 2010 by Blackwell Publishing

importance of limiting EMR risks, and for you to address these issues in all purchasing, licensing and maintenance agreements you sign. The goal is a balanced agreement that both you and your EMR developer can live with, but one that protects your rights and limits the risks associated with your EMR.

Don't blindly sign any purchasing/licensing agreement presented to you assuming your best interests have been taken into account. Many terms that could protect your interests may have been omitted or removed. This is not because the developers are bad people; but rather, because they have lawyers who have written their agreement to protect their best interests, not yours. In this regard, generally, the larger the EMR developer, the less favorable the sales terms may be (with some exceptions).

Be Willing to Walk Away

There are always two sales to be consummated in any EMR deal. The first is made when the EMR developer convinces you to purchase his EMR. The second occurs when you sell the EMR developer on the fact that the price is too high or the terms are not right. Each sale involves concessions by both sides, so that all parties can live with the deal struck and believe the other gave something to consummate the transaction.

The EMR developer has something to offer, but won't necessarily do so unless you (or your lawyers) encourage him in that direction. Presumably, there was more than one finalist EMR on your list and it is wise to be prepared to walk away from the deal if your first choice is too inflexible in providing term concessions. Think of this like a marriage. It costs a lot to go through a divorce; it doesn't cost you anything to avoid a bad marriage in the first place.

It Begins With Your RFI, Followed By Your RFP

The starting point in your negotiation is your Request for Information (RFI). This is where you ask EMR developers to provide information about their products. From that information you learn in general terms what each developer is proposing. After demos and closer evaluation, you will ultimately create a Request for Proposal (RFP). It should be an unambiguous, clearly-written description of the functional requirements the EMR has to meet in order to satisfy your needs, as it will become the basis of both your contract/licensing document that contains your testing and acceptance criteria. The functional requirements have to be black and white statements that have yes or no, did or did not meet, answers. General requirement statements are worthless, even troublesome if they lead to arguments (if lawyers are involved, they also become expensive). If you use a detailed EHR Selector tool, the list of features asserted can become the basis for your RFI and RFP documentation. In some cases you can jump right to an RFP, since the EMR developer has already asserted they have the feature by listing it on the EHR Selector tool.

The RFP is where you survey what each EMR developer can provide, and the purchasing (or licensing) agreement is where you specify exactly what must be provided. Much of the response from the EMR developer to your RFP is what you will turn around (and elaborate on) in your purchasing agreement. Don't make the mistake of assuming that because the RFP indicated that an item was available, you don't need to specify it in the purchasing or licensing agreement. You need to be very specific in your RFP because that will become the governing document for the purchasing/licensing transaction.

List Detailed Functional Requirements

Consider the statement, "Needs to provide e-prescription functionality." Is that a well thought out functional specification? No! Every vendor will say they provide that and point to one specific function their system performs to "prove" it. There are 14 other specific requirements that make up e-prescription. List every one of these e-prescribing features that you want in your RFP so that you can see what functionality each EMR developer offers you. Meaningful Use (after the June 16, 2009 clarifications) required only drug-drug, drug-allergy and drug-formulary checks for e-prescribing. But consider specifying more functionality, including drug-lab value flags (if hepatic or renal function is impaired), and drug-age checks to catch adult doses prescribed for children, and medication history summaries from the patient's pharmacies that are online via Surescripts/RxHub as the basis for medication compliance discussions with the patient. Also consider automatic loading of the patient's formulary from his/her third party payer, or electronic transmission via standards of medication orders directly to the patient's pharmacy for all non-controlled substances.

None of the above requirements are specified under MU, so if you want them, you will need to enumerate them specifically in any purchasing or licensing agreements. If you are using the MSP EHR Selector, attach a printout of its functional requirements to your RFP. If you enter these criteria and obtain a list of EMR developers, only vendors supporting the criteria will be returned. This is where the detailed criteria the MSP EHR Selector provides can be useful to you.

Making a list of detailed functional requirements can be tedious, particularly expressing them in terms that are technical when you are not a technical person. To assist you, HL7 has created a standard set of functional criteria for EMRs called the EHR-S FM spec, and its now ANSI approved. It contains some 130 major functions and 1,000 sub-criteria that are called conformance criteria. These include functions like medication history, problem lists, orders, decision support, privacy, security, audit trail and more.

These HL7 EHR-S FM specs are specific enough to be unambiguous, and therefore useful in a RFP document. Unfortunately, even though it was adopted in 2007, few EMRs meet the criteria of the standard. If you choose to use the standard, it will be a tedious task to go through with the EMR vendors you are considering.

The HL7 EHR-S FM (specs) cover not only physician offices, but several other care areas, including:
- Emergency Departments;
- Child Health;
- Long-term Care/Skilled Nursing Facilities;
- Behavioral Health;
- Regulated Clinical Research;
- Vital Statistics Reporting.

The standard is available as a series of PDF files.

> "The HL7 EHR-S Functional Model defines a standardized model of the functions that may be present in EHR Systems. From the outset, a clear distinction between the EHR as a singular entity and systems that operate on the EHR – i.e., EHR Systems is critical. Section 1.1.3 describes the basis and foundation for the HL7 definition of an EHR System. Notably, the EHR-S-FM (Functional Model) does not address whether the EHR-S is a system-of-systems or a single system providing the functions required by the users. This standard makes no distinction regarding implementation – the EHR-S described in a functional profile may be a single system or a system of systems."[2]

The standard also includes a section on Records Management & Evidentiary Support in all these care settings. The availability of this standard simplifies the process of specifying EMR functionality in RFPs and legal contracts. Go to their Web site (www.hl7.org) or search the NIST Web site (www.nist.gov/index.html) for more information.

Specify Future Requirements in Today's Agreement

Also specify that all future Meaningful Use (MU) requirements will be implemented in any system you are buying today. Indeed, without MU requirements, your purchase is not reimbursable. That's a $43K hit, so specify that the EMR developer, at his own expense, will develop and deploy all EMR Meaningful Use requirements by October 2010.

Locate Specific Requirements

A good place to obtain a starting list of EMR functions is at a Web-based EMR selection site. In evaluating such sites, you will want one that allows you to drill down to specific functional statements, and doesn't just present general statements like the e-prescription example. There are only a few such sites that offer drill down criteria (see Appendix III for one that does).

Build Functional Requirements from this Book

As you have read this book hopefully you have been noting your decisions and specific requirements to be included in the contracting documents on the chapter Scorecards. Some of these relate to the EMR product itself, but

---

[2] *Electronic Health Record - System Functional Model.* Published Feb. 2007 by HL7 EHR, TC

others relate to training, installation, acceptance testing, data updates, site management and a host of other important issues.

Negotiate at the Right Time

It always helps to know a developer's sales year. Do they run on a calendar year or a fiscal year? If a fiscal year, when does it end? This is important because many companies have sales targets they need to meet and which you can use to your advantage. There are three good times to purchase or license an EMR. The first is at the end of a month, which will often afford you a good deal. The second is as the end of the quarter approaches where you will often get a better deal. However, the best deal comes as the end of the year approaches (unless the vendor has had a very good year, and is interested in holding off some orders so his next year's first quarter will be strong).

Avoid Bad Offers

Sometimes a developer will offer you a "special deal" on one of his EMR product lines (if he has more than one). But is the special deal good for you? What EMR product is involved? Is it the developer's "go ahead" product, one that will have continued development for at least the next 5-10 years? Or, is this a product line for which the developer has no (or little) new development planned (a non-go ahead product)? There are no good deals on non-go ahead products.

Data from existing systems is usually very difficult to migrate from one EMR to another (newer) one – even if they both support standards. Encounter summaries may be migrated, but they often lack the full data context of the medical record (database). Remember, the patient's chart is a database file, not a lot of images of documents and pages. The organization of that file differs from system to system, so while a summary of any encounter may transfer, the actual data behind it may not.

You don't want to be stuck with an obsolete EMR, one in which you've entered a lot of information, only to discover you are unable to transfer it to a new EMR that the company is actually supporting and developing. Look critically at Allscripts/Misys, McKesson, Cerner and other vendors that have two or three different EMR products. They won't all succeed and the customers of products that don't are not going to be happy.

Lock Down the Details in the RFP

Include a request for a 5-year support agreement as part of your RFP. This will ensure that each EMR developer is speaking to you about the same package of services. Otherwise, there is no way to make a true apples-to-apples comparison of system costs. When 5-year support is bundled into an RFP, EMR developers know the information they provide will be used to compare them to their competitors, making the company more likely to cut their margin on service so as not to appear higher in price and potentially risk the deal.

Define Usability

Most RFPs publicly available at the end of 2008, whether from medical specialty organizations or the government, did an inadequate job of specifying important issues according to R. Schumacher's 2008 review of over 50 available RFPs[3], all of which are listed in appendix I of his white paper referenced in the footnote below. Given the information in this book's chapters on workflow inventory and optimization, and EMR system customization, be sure you include the conclusions from your inventory in your RFP. This provides a basis of agreement between your practice and the EMR supplier as to what constitutes a usable system. This is important because being released from purchasing or licensing agreements will be difficult if you haven't defined the terms and requirements carefully in your RFP legal agreement.

Support Through Training and Education

As a point of reference, a typical medical hardware device (ECG machine, ventilator or monitor) may have a maintenance cost for hardware and software of 8-12 percent per year or less. Yet a software only product (EMR system) vendor may charge 16-26 percent per year for support that does not even include the hardware components of the system. There is a lot of room here for negotiation.

Include specifics such as software bug fixes, new and improved application upgrade and enhancement costs, staff training (retraining) costs, emergency repair costs, troubleshooting assistance, and other costs in your RFP. In many cases however, software support costs may not include all of these items. Some vendors will quote these separate from their normal software maintenance, particularly if they are offering a bargain-priced EMR and are themselves a smaller EMR developer.

Solidify Document Scanning Costs

Include the need for the EMR developer to list how/what the cost is of converting your paper charts to electronic format. Often, conversion of existing paper-based records is not included in the EMR price, unless you specifically request that and it is acknowledged in the proposal you receive. Once again, in order to be able to compare apples-to-apples, all of your final candidate EMR vendors must quote the same services.

Obtain Custom Device Interfaces

If you have medical diagnostic devices that provide data about your patients, you are probably used to taking a paper report and attaching it to the patient's paper chart. This isn't going to work in your electronic approach.

The best approach electronically is to have the data from these diagnostic devices (ECG machines, stress testing devices, endoscopes, pulmonary

---

[3] *How to Select an Electronic HealthRecord System that Healthcare Professionals can Use.*
 By R. Schumacher, et al. White Paper published February 2009 by User Centric

function devices, etc.) come directly into your EMR in a structured way. That requires that an interface exists between the device and your EMR's database. You need to specify the device(s) to be interfaced, the device suppliers and model numbers, in your RFP and then have each EMR developer indicate whether they have an interface for each device; and if not, what the cost and timetable would be to create such an interface. EMR developers with more interfaces to the devices you have, offer a stronger proposal – all other factors being equal. Unfortunately, all other factors normally aren't equal, and so it becomes a matter of weighing the strengths and weaknesses of what each vendor can offer.

Define Interfaces to Your CPM Interfaces

Assuming that you aren't purchasing an EMR from your CPM vendor, you need to determine in the RFP whether any interface exists to your current CPM system, and if so, what data can be exchanged in both directions. Include details about the CPM vendor, software and specific release that needs to be interfaced, and ask each EMR developer that has an interface to list what data flows into and out of your CPM.

Secure Future Increases in Maintenance and Other Fees

All charges, particularly those of an on-going nature, should be itemized and listed by the EMR developer in their response to your RFP, so that these charges can have increases capped in the final sales agreement. The agreement should also provide the user specific remedies if increases in maintenance and support fees exceed these increase caps during the first 5 years after your system is deployed.

Purchasing/Licensing Agreement Summary

All of the items included in your RFP are relevant in your actual purchasing or licensing agreement. You are well served if you enter the purchasing/ licensing negotiations having a second, acceptable EMR as a fallback choice in the event that your primary EMR vendor is not willing to compromise or meet your business needs. A potential loss of a deal to a competitor (that also meets your needs) can encourage an EMR vendor to remain flexible at this last stage of acquisition. When the final purchasing/licensing agreement is being addressed, both parties have too much at stake to be unresponsive in working out a deal amicably.

Remember, whatever EMR developer you choose is the one you will have to live with until you do this again, so it is wise to make the deal that your EMR developer can afford to live with as well. You are ultimately looking for a partner and for an on-going relationship. However, partnerships are formed when both parties have their needs met and when there is a mutual respect.

The following list includes some of the areas in the purchasing/licensing agreement that are negotiable.

- The jurisdiction where the contract is enforced (your state laws or the EMR developer's state laws);
- Default consequences;
- Liability concessions for defects in the product;
- Business interruption damages in the event that the interruption is due to an EMR failure or an ASP server interruption or other factor that is directly attributable to your EMR developer (or his designated ASP partner);
- A cap on increases in yearly maintenance fees, which if exceeded, releases you from the contract;
- Provisions in the contract for "acceptance testing & verification" and for a full refund if the EMR fails the acceptance testing.

Other areas to specify to your EMR developer before deployment:

- First payment due after successful completion of acceptance testing;
- Specific regulations and industry standards with which your EMR system must be fully compatible. Include an exit clause if the system is not compliant with these regulations or industry standards;
- Require 100 percent support of HIPAA, including all HIPAA-required electronic transmissions;
- Protection if the vendor's ASP system allows a breach of confidentiality and HIPAA violation, and you are named in a lawsuit. Does your contract force you to indemnify your EMR supplier, and even defend him if the breach is his fault?
- EMR developer warrants that the EMR software will be modified to meet future MU requirements effective from the time you purchase until the end of 2014 (when payment incentives no longer apply);
- Restricts who can access your patient records and how your consent must be obtained in advance from your EMR developer or their ASP (if the EMR is hosted by a third party);
- Include interfaces to other computer systems that are currently deployed in your office (or hospital department) or will be purchased and deployed before the final phase of the EMR deployment;
- Source code to be held in escrow and made available in the event of EMR vendor failure or acquisition by a competitor or under other circumstances;
- EMR vendor warrants that all software is free of viruses, Trojans or malware;
- Allows you to contest and withhold unstated expenses and charges not specified in the purchasing/licensing agreement;
- If you will be adopting an ASP, Web-based EMR solution, make sure that contesting unspecified charges not in the licensing agreement does not allow the EMR developer to withhold services from you;
- Sales support, staff training, and other items you want in the contract.

This is by no means an exhaustive list of areas to consider when thinking about your final sales contract. You need to be sure to include all phases in the initial purchase contract language and to attach a full description of how your system is to ultimately function. Without such terms in your initial purchase agreement, you can end up paying extra for components when they are needed for the second or third phase of your implementation.

You can also expect to pay more for an in-depth level of post sales support, either as an increase in the basic maintenance fee, or at least on a per-incident basis every time you use one of the additions to service/support that you specify. The latter would be preferable, as per-incident should hopefully occur less frequently than having to pay for bundled service/support.

To find initial details of what to include in purchasing/licensing agreements, some physicians look to boilerplate legal agreements (from physician organizations for example), or to agreements created by the now defunct DOQ-IT program. We don't think these types of documents serve physicians well. For one thing, too much variation in requirements from EMRs that are deployed in your office to EMRs provided as a service over the Internet occurs. Also, there are too many legal issues such agreements are silent about or do not fully address. Most boilerplate legal agreements are not in-depth enough, particularly considering how varied the laws are from state to state.

A boilerplate purchasing/licensing agreement crafted by a third party is not enough to protect your rights; you can start there but you must refine it extensively and add your EMR specifics to ensure that you are fully covered. A good contract should be designed to provide remedies if your system does not perform as specified. Note the key word is specified. Be sure to specify performance in detail.

If you somehow arrived in this chapter but haven't read Chapter 13, Lawyer-Proofing Your EMR, you may want to go back and read it – it's an eye-opener. Many EMRs create legally-flawed documentation, including those offered by the largest and best-known vendors. A medical law firm experienced in EMRs will know all the terms and places to push, the areas you probably don't know. Expect this to cost you from $5K to $15K depending on the size of your system, where it will be deployed (in your office or on the Web) and how open or rigid your EMR developer is in changing their standard agreements to accommodate you.

MSP/Andrew EMR Benchmark Norms

To help you understand areas where you can negotiate a better deal, it's helpful to know what the "norms" are across the industry. The MSP/Andrew EMR Benchmark provides just such information. We present some of the specifics from that data in the remainder of this chapter.

Training Support

The majority (87 percent) of EMR developers provide their own support to physicians/users with 3 percent charging more for this feature. Very few (8 percent) use third parties, and a few more use a combination of the primary developer and another organization to provide support.

Training/Help Desk Support Details to Consider

In spite of assertions that "we use our own staff to support your EMR," you should explore where that staff is, what is their native language, whether they are direct employees, and their technical and clinical backgrounds. Don't overlook such factors in your EMR developer selection process. The larger an EMR developer and its installed base, the more likely you will be to find foreign-run call centers providing first level system support.

Service Support

Very few EMR developers have their own, national field support organizations, and even the larger EMR developers that may have local service people may not have people who are totally familiar with their EMR product. This is because the EMR could be a specialized and small part of their overall electronics business. How qualified is an MRI or X-ray or medical device service or support person to work on EMR systems at all, much less their fine points? Is EMR software support the primary technology that the support organization was created for?

In some cases, you may receive more relevant, expeditious and higher quality support from a smaller or mid-sized EMR vendor that has their developers or direct tech support/clinical training personnel handle their call desk.

Remote Access Simplifies Support

New Active-X and Citrix technology are making remote troubleshooting of computer systems a practical reality. With this technology, a remote service or support technician can install an Active-X application on your computer that allows them to take control from their remote location. They can then run through the troubleshooting steps much faster than if they direct you through them and are able to view the results immediately. This should accelerate the diagnosis of any problems and speed their resolution. Check to see if the support desk of your candidate EMR developers employ such technology, and if there is an extra charge for accessing it.

Our research shows that 80 percent of EMR developers offer remote technology for troubleshooting. Of the 80 percent, just 3 percent state that it is an extra cost option and 8 percent say that it is available from a third party. Since just about every EMR developer claims to have the ability to offer this service, be sure to include the requirement that they actually do so in your purchasing agreement, and specify whether or not you pay extra. The answer is "or not," since 4 out of 5 companies provide it at no extra cost – so why would you pay for it?

How Quickly Customer Support is Available

Support next week for a problem right now is not support! Support on Monday for a failure on Friday is not adequate for most care settings. Most EMR developers state that they offer service 7 days a week, however their hours on the weekends are often limited (See Figure 18.1). The EMR developers listed varied hours and amounts of service times. The next largest group offered 24 hours, 7 days a week followed by business hours Monday through Friday and a few less listed business hours in the time zone in which they operated. The fewest answered that their hours are 8AM Eastern to 7PM Pacific time. Most of the support help locations are listed as being in the United States, but there are some developers that use foreign/off-shore technical help locations. If that is the case, you will want to speak to these people before you purchase the EMR. Language barriers can exist even though they speak English.

Figure 18.1 Help Desk Support Hours

Level of Help Available	% of Vendors Offering
8AM-5PM Eastern through Pacific Time Zones	8%
Business Hours in EMR's Time Zone	14%
Business Hours Mon-Fri in Your Time Zone	15%
Help Available 24-Hours/Day Non-Weekends	28%
Help Available 24-Hours/Day 7 Days/Week	28%

Specifying your support requirements is an area in which you can save money. The key is not to require 24/7 EMR support if it's not necessary. However, if 24/7 support and availability is required, expect to pay extra for it. Most EMRs deployed in physician offices do not require 24/7 support because the office is not open 24/7. Usually 14-hour support that is available 6 days a week is sufficient to solve application problems that might happen during operational office hours.

It is important that support be generally available when you are not seeing patients in your offices or making rounds, as well as when office managers or other local support personnel are available to work with an EMR developer's help desk. Saturday is a great time to solve problems for a medical office that needs to be open for business on a Monday through Friday basis.

When 24/7 Support is Essential

If the EMR developer's client is a hospital, then 24/7 support is essential. EMR developers that serve these inpatient settings (CliniComp, Picis, Philips, GE, Wellsoft and others) generally do offer 24/7 support. Particularly with 24/7 support, it is critical to find out where the help desk is located and with whom you will be speaking (see Figure 18.2).

Figure 18.2 Help Desk Technical Support Located

Help Desk – Primary Location	% of Vendors Offering
U.S. Only	80%
Part U.S. and Part Off-shore	15%
Canada Only	3%
Part Canada and Part Non-Canada	1.5%
Non-U.S. and Non-Canada	0.5%

Support Via the EMR Developer's Web Site

Some EMR developers offer technical assistance via their Web sites. Figure 18.3 shows that most often help is in the form of Web assistance with a frequently asked question section. Some EMR developers also offer a "live-chat" capability where users would be able to e-mail questions to the developer's technicians and their answers would be returned live, creating an on-line dialogue.

Figure 18.3 EMR/Web Support Offered (Multi Answers Allowed)

Feature	Yes, Now	Yes, in the Future
Online/Web Assist with FAQ Section	79%	4%
Online/Web Assist with Live Chat Section	31%	29%
Users Can Submit Questions Online/Web	57%	7%
Auto Reply Message after Question Sent	30%	

Over half of all EMR developers offer question submission through their Web sites, but less than half send an auto reply response to indicate that your e-mail question was received.

Training Issues

A new EMR system will require orientation and training. Do you want training support bundled into the price of your EMR system or unbundled?

Amount of Training Included in EMR Cost

The amount of training provided varies widely (see Figure 18.4).

Figure 18.4 Amount of 'No-Cost' Training Offered On-Site

Training Offered	% of Vendors Offering
<8 hours	45%
8-16 hours	8%
16-24 hours	4%
24-32 hours	8%
>32 hours	35%

Training Material and Support Provided

Training content is shown in Figure 18.5. Some vendors provide other training services. Some vendors have on-going training integrated into the EMR, which is very desirable for orienting new or temporary staff members.

Figure 18.5 Training Material – Support Provided (Multiple Answers Allowed)

Material	% of Vendors Offering
Manual	86%
GUI Reference Guide	59%
Help in EMR itself	58%
System Admin/Back Up Guides	44%
CD/Web Video	38%
Hardware/Network Instruction	28%
Self Paced Learning	19%
Questions to Technician via Web	82%
Web Assist with FAQ	79%
Live Chat with Technician	31%

Most of the EMR developers provide a user's manual for their EMRs. About 60 percent offer either a quick reference command or GUI (Graphical User Interface) guide or enable help via the EMR itself. Less than half of the EMR developers offer system administration and back up guides, CD or Web training videos, hardware and network instruction or self-paced learning.

Most EMR developers offer users the option to submit questions through their Web site. Web assistance is offered through contact with the company's support technicians or by utilizing a Frequently Asked Questions (FAQ) section. Unless the support response is instantaneous (which it often is not), this is an inefficient way to obtain a satisfying response. Less than one third of the developers offer Web support that includes a chat live feature where users and company support technicians are able to interact by typing questions and receiving answers in real time.

Point aside, don't look just to your EMR vendor for training. In addition to system-specific training, there are EMR training consulting companies that offer the basics of medical computer technology, sometimes as Web-based self-study courses that staff members can take whenever it's convenient for them. However, this should not be from your office as you will want to keep office computer use of the Internet to a minimum.

Training Locations

EMR system training is most often stated as being offered at all sites by the developers, indicating that many of them are flexible and available to meet individual customer's preferences. 5 times as many developers charge for additional training at the customer's site than developers that offer the training for no fee at the customer's site. If the customer is willing to travel to the developer's site for training, the developer is still 2 times more likely to charge for the training than not charge. As Figure 18.6 shows, there are significant differences in the amount of "free" support offered. However, developers that offer more free support are among those with higher system purchase prices.

Figure 18.6 EMR Training Available Where?

Where EMR Training is Provided	% of Vendors Offering
EMR Company Site @ No Cost	5%
EMR Company Site for Additional Fee	11%
Customer's Site @ No Cost	7%
Customer's Site for Additional Fee	36%
Any Site Customer Prefers	41%

If your EMR developer is one of the 11 percent that wants to charge to come and train your staff, you can use this as a good bargaining chip. Ask the EMR developer to pay your staff's way to be trained at his facility. When he balks at that, offer to accept the developer's trainer to come to your site, at the developer's expense for free training.

Cost for Follow-Up Maintenance

Figure 18.7 shows the details of how developers have chosen to offer follow-up contract support. Almost half (47 percent) of the developers charge between 19 and 25 percent. An additional 25 percent charge between 15 and 18 percent of the cost of the initial software license price or purchase cost.

Figure 18.7 EMR Contract Support Cost (During First 12 months)

% Cost of EMR List Price Contract	% of Vendors Offering
0% Free (included)	15%
<6%	6%
<10%	1%
Between 10-14%	6%
Between 15-18%	25%
Between 19-25%	47%

The "free" support is typical of EMR developers offering Web-based ASP models, as the figure is bundled into your monthly price and cannot be separated. Of the remaining EMR developers, notice that nearly three-quarters require monthly maintenance fees that on a yearly basis amount to somewhere between 15 to 25 percent of the cost of the initial purchase LIST price (not discounted price). This means you are buying your system all over again every 4-6.5 years. When that fee starts may be negotiable – either immediately, or at the end of the first 12 months? Obviously, at the end of the first 12 months is better for you financially. This may or may not be negotiable with any specific EMR developer.

Client User Groups

There is a wide variation in the willingness of EMR developers to support client user groups, probably because many EMR developers have recently entered the market and may not yet have a sizeable installed base, which allows user groups to be self-supporting. Of those EMR developers that do offer a user group, Figure 18.8 provides some support activity details. (Note, not all EMR developers have user group support or encourage them.)

Figure 18.8 User Group Details

Company-Sponsored Physician User Group	% of Vendors Supporting
User-Group Elected Officers Receive Honorarium	7%
Customer Pays Their Way to User Group Meetings	59%
User Group Fees NOT Included in Maintenance Fee	32%
User Group Fees Are Bundled into Maintenance Fee	2%

The EMR developers hosting user groups often include detailed product training classes, new product overviews and other topics of general interest. They are good sources for customized templates created by other physicians in your specialty. If an EMR developer does not have a user group, inquire about their plans to establish one.

Wrap Up

Space prohibits a full discussion of contract terms. In addition to the norms that the various figures in this chapter provided, there are many additional issues that will need to be clarified in your contract negotiations. We definitely recommend involving qualified, EMR-specific, healthcare legal firms in helping you negotiate any vendor agreements and ensuring the important terms are right. Some EMR developers will barely negotiate terms, if at all. This may be a sign that you might want to reconsider them as a long-term partner and supplier (all other things being equal – if there is a viable alternative supplier).

   If you don't have, or know of, any legal firms that are experienced in EMR-specific, healthcare matters and litigation in your area, check with the qualified attorneys listed on the www.ehrselector.com Web site. Securing the right direction on the front end is a whole lot less expensive than taking remedial action when something goes wrong after all contracts are negotiated. Users of the MSP EHR Selector will find "LA" denoting Legal Alert tags, indicating that there is relevant legal information in the item's Help screen.

EMR Developers & Their Products

EMR Developer Survey Listing

> This appendix contains a list of EMR developers that responded to a request for product information, which is summarized in a table. There is also an expanded list of contact information for EMR developers.

This appendix includes contact and other information on EMR developers. There is a feature table showing the basic characteristics of EMR products from developers that responded to a request for information. There is also a list that includes only the contact information for a larger cross section of EMR developers. These two tables do not include all EMR developers because we omitted companies if their contact information was not readily available, as well as those that did not respond to our request for information.

The feature table was compiled from responses to an e-mail that the authors sent to EMR developers. The companies listed are those that responded by the publication deadline. It is best to use the data from this table as a rough indication of any developer's capabilities and to independently verify the most current EMR functionality directly with the developer. There is a list of EMR developers posted on the www.ehrselector.com Web site that may be more complete than either of those included in this appendix.

Successfully Choosing Your EMR: 15 Crucial Decisions. By © Arthur Gasch and Betty Gasch.
Published 2010 by Blackwell Publishing

Figure A1.1 EMR Developers Responding to Request for Information

EMR Name	EMR Current Version	2008 CCHIT	Offers Full EMR Capabilities	Offers Chart Conversion Services	Claims Embedded User Workflow Engine	Supports In-Office Kiosk	Supports Opt. Patient Portal	Combined EMR & Practice Management	Upgradable to FULL EMR	Product is EMR-Lite Only	Problem List From Unstructured Data	E&M Quick Coder Integrated	CPT Codes	ICD-10-CM	ICD-9-CM Billing	Vendor Proprietary Front-End Vocabulary	SNOMED CT Ontology/Terminology	MEDCIN Front-end Vocabulary	Rx-Rx, Allergy Checks	Vendor Maintained, Proprietary	First Databank, Gold, Multum, etc.	Any PC Web Browser	a Unix/Linux/FreeBSD OS	a Macintosh OS	a Windows OS	Document Scan w/OCR	Document Scan, No OCR	Handwriting with Templates	Handwriting Recognition	Freeform Typing Unstructured	Dictation, SR w/NLP Structured	Dictation, SR w/o NLP	Template with Pick Lists	RxNorm	LOINC reporting	DICOM	CCD / CCR	HL7 Messaging	Office, Client/Server	Another, Unlisted - Indicate	Webserver, In-Office Plus Remote	Webserver, ASP In Office	Web, ASP, Remote Server
ABELSoft		X	X	X				X			X	X	X	X	X		X		X			X			X	X	X		X			X	X		X	X		X	X		X		X
AllMeds	5	X	X		X	X	X	X			X	X	X		X		X	X	X			X			X		X		X			X	X	X	X		X	X			X		X
Amazing Charts		X	X		X	X	X	X			X	X	X		X						X		X	X	X		X	X	X	X	X	X	X	X	X		X	X					X
American Medical Software		X	X		X	X	X	X			X		X		X				X						X		X		X			X	X	X		X		X	X				
BetterHealth Record	6		X						X				X	X	X										X	X	X											X	X		X		X
Catalis Accelerator	4.4		X		X	X	X	X			X	X	X	X	X	X	X	X			X				X	X	X	X	X	X	X	X	X		X	X	X	X	X		X		X
Cerner		X	X	X		X	X	X			X		X		X		X	X	X		X	X	X		X	X	X	X	X	X	X	X	X					X	X				X
ChartCare EMR	v6.5		X			X	X						X		X							X			X	X	X						X		X	X		X					
Clicks application generator	10				X			X					X	X	X	X		X			X	X	X	X	X		X			X		X	X				X	X	X		X		
ComChart			X										X		X																												
DavLong Bus. Solutions Medinformatix	9.4c7		X	X		X	X	X		X		X	X		X		X				X		X		X		X		X	X		X	X			X	X	X	X		X		X
Daw Systems ScriptSure	7.0		X	X	X	X	X		X	X			X	X	X	X	X	X				X			X	X			X	X			X	X		X	X	X			X		
DoctorsPartner	7.65	X	X		X	X	X	X				X	X		X						X				X		X						X	X				X	X	X	X	X	X
DocuTAP	4.5	X	X	X	X	X	X	X					X		X						X				X		X			X			X					X	X	X		X	X
DOX Podiatry	2.8.12		X	X	X	X	X	X				X	X		X					X		X			X	X	X	X		X		X	X	X			X	X	X	X	X		X

Feature	EasyChart	Elysium	e-MDs	EMRWorks	FlexMedical	Galen Corporation	GEMMS	GE Healthcare	gMed	gloStream gloEMR	Greenway Medical	Health Probe	HemiData MD-Journal	Infinite Software MD-Reports	iSalus Healthcare OfficeEMR	McKesson	MDoffice
EMR Current Version	18.2	9	9.3	5.5						5.0		8.0.0.301	4.2.2	9i	09/10		6.9.7.2
2008 CCHIT	×	×					×	×		×	×			×	×	?	
Offers Full EMR Capabilities	×	×	×	×	×	×	×	×	×	×	×	×		×	×	×	×
Offers Chart Conversion Services								×						×	×		×
Claims Embedded User Workflow Engine		×			×		×			×				×	×		
Supports In-Office Kiosk		×						×	×					×	×		
Supports Opt. Patient Portal		×				×	×	×	×			×			×	×	×
Combined EMR & Practice Management		×	×	×	×	×	×	×		×	×				×	×	×
Upgradable to FULL EMR													×			×	×
Product is EMR-Lite Only	×																
Problem List From Unstructured Data		×					×	×	×		×				×		
E&M Quick Coder Integrated		×		×		×	×	×	×	×					×	×	×
CPT Codes	×	×	×	×	×	×	×	×	×	×				×		×	×
ICD-10-CM	×	×		×	×	×				×	×						
ICD-9-CM Billing	×	×	×	×	×	×		×	×	×				×		×	×
Vendor Proprietary Front-End Vocabulary												×					×
SNOMED CT Ontology/Terminology		×												×	×	×	×
MEDCIN Front-end Vocabulary		×															
Rx-Rx, Allergy Checks		×			×	×	×	×		×					×		
Vendor Maintained, Proprietary	×											×					
First Databank, Gold, Multum, etc.	×		×	×						×			×	×			×
Any PC Web Browser	×	×				×	×	×		×		×				×	
a Unix/Linux/FreeBSD OS												×					
a Macintosh OS												×			×		
a Windows OS	×		×	×	×	×	×	×	×	×		×	×	×	×	×	×
Document Scan w/OCR	×	×				×	×	×	×						×		
Document Scan, No OCR		×		×	×	×	×	×		×		×	×	×	×	×	×
Handwriting with Templates								×		×		×			×		×
Handwriting Recognition			×	×	×				×	×					×		
Freeform Typing Unstructured	×		×	×				×		×		×	×	×	×		×
Dictation, SR w/NLP Structured								×	×								
Dictation, SR w/o NLP		×	×	×	×	×		×		×	×	×	×	×	×	×	
Template with Pick Lists	×	×	×	×	×	×	×	×	×	×	×	×		×	×	×	×
RxNorm		×						×		×				×	×	×	×
LOINC reporting	×	×					×	×	×	×				×	×	×	×
DICOM	×	×	×			×		×	×	×				×	×	×	×
CCD / CCR	×	×				×		×	×	×				×			
HL7 Messaging	×	×	×	×	×	×	×	×	×				×	×		×	×
Office, Client/Server	×	×	×	×	×	×		×	×	×			×			×	×
Another, Unlisted - Indicate																×	×
Webserver, In-Office Plus Remote		×								×		×					
Webserver, ASP In Office													×	×			
Web, ASP Remote Server	×	×		×				×		×			×		×	×	×

EMR Name	EMR Current Version	2008 CCHIT	Offers Full EMR Capabilities	Offers Chart Conversion Services	Claims Embedded User Workflow Engine	Supports In-Office Kiosk	Supports Opt. Patient Portal	Combined EMR & Practice Management	Upgradable to FULL EMR	Product is EMR-Lite Only	Problem List From Unstructured Data	E&M Quick Coder Integrated	CPT Codes	ICD-10-CM	ICD-9-CM Billing	Vendor Proprietary Front-End Vocabulary	SNOMED CT Ontology/Terminology	MEDCIN Front-end Vocabulary	Rx-Rx, Allergy Checks	Vendor Maintained, Proprietary	First Databank, Gold, Multum, etc.	Any PC Web Browser	a Unix/Linux/FreeBSD OS	a Macintosh OS	a Windows OS	Document Scan w/OCR	Document Scan, No OCR	Handwriting with Templates	Handwriting Recognition	Freeform Typing Unstructured	Dictation, SR w/NLP Structured	Dictation, SR w/o NLP	Template with Pick Lists	RxNorm	LOINC reporting	DICOM	CCD / CCR	HL7 Messaging	Office, Client/Server	Another, Unlisted - Indicate	Webserver, In-Office Plus Remote	Webserver, ASP In Office	Web, ASP Remote Server
MD-Navigator	5.0		×	×	×			×				×	×	×	×		×		×		×	×		×	×	×	×	×	×	×	×	×	×		×	×	×	×					×
MED3000			×								×	×	×		×		×	×				×			×	×	×					×	×		×	×		×					×
MedLink Total Office	3.1	×	×		×	×	×	×				×	×		×		×				×				×		×		×	×		×	×	×				×	×				
NexTech		×	×	×	×	×	×	×				×	×	×	×						×	×		×	×		×	×		×		×				×	×	×	×		×	×	
NextGen EHR	5.5.28	×	×			×	×	×	×	×			×		×						×				×		×	×		×	×	×	×		×		×	×	×			×	×
Noteworthy NetPracticeEHRweb	7.0	×	×	×	×	×	×	×				×	×	×	×	×					×	×		×	×	×	×	×	×	×	×	×				×	×	×		×	×	×
OmniMD	Omn-iMD8X		×			×	×	×					×	×	×	×	×	×			×	×			×	×						×	×			×	×	×		×		×
Optimus EMR System		×	×										×								×				×							×					×			×	×	×
Opus Healthcare OpusClinicalSuite	6.3	×	×	×	×	×	×						×		×						×		×		×	×	×			×			×		×		×	×		×	×	×
Orion Health	2.3	?	×						×				×		×		×		×						×		×						×		×	×					×	×
PatientOS		?	×								×		×	×	×		×		×			×	×		×		×			×		×		×	×	×	×	×	×			×
PracticeOne,		?	×					×					×		×		×		×	×			×	×	×		×			×		×			×		×			×		×
PracticeFusion			×		×		×	×				×	×		×	×				×					×		×	×	×	×	×	×	×	×			×	×				×
Praxis Electronic Medical Record	4	×	×	×	×	×	×	×				×	×	×	×	×								×	×	×	×	×	×	×	×	×				×	×	×	×		×		
Pulse Systems			×	×	×	×	×	×				×	×	×	×	×		×	×						×	×	×		×		×	×	×	×	×	×	×	×	×		×		
RelWare Enterprise	2.0		×	×	×			×					×	×	×	×		×	×			×				×	×	×			×		×	×	×	×	×	×	×				×

Feature	Sigmund Software	STAT! Systems Q.D. Clinical EMR	Spring Medical SpringCharts EHR	SSIMED EMRge	SuiteMed	SuiteMed IMS	TheraManager	Waiting Room Solutions EMR & Practice Management System	VersaSuite	Wellsoft EDIS
EMR Current Version	3.4X	6.1	9.5	7.0	12.0.5	2009		4.0	8.0	v11
2008 CCHIT					X					X
Offers Full EMR Capabilities	X	X	X	X	X	X		X	X	X
Offers Chart Conversion Services	X	X			X	X		X		
Claims Embedded User Workflow Engine	X	X	X		X			X	X	
Supports In-Office Kiosk		X			X	X		X		
Supports Opt. Patient Portal				X	X			X		
Combined EMR & Practice Management	X			X	X	X		X	X	
Upgradable to FULL EMR										
Product is EMR-Lite Only										
Problem List From Unstructured Data										
E&M Quick Coder Integrated		X	X	X	X			X	X	X
CPT Codes	X	X	X	X	X	X		X	X	X
ICD-10-CM	X	X	X					X		X
ICD-9-CM Billing	X	X	X	X	X	X		X	X	X
Vendor Proprietary Front-End Vocabulary		X						X		
SNOMED CT Ontology/Terminology					X			X	X	
MEDCIN Front-end Vocabulary			X		X			X	X	
Rx-Rx, Allergy Checks										
Vendor Maintained, Proprietary	X	X	X							
First Databank, Gold, Multum, etc.		X		X	X	X		X	X	X
Any PC Web Browser	X	X						X		
a Unix/Linux/FreeBSD OS		X	X							X
a Macintosh OS		X	X							
a Windows OS	X	X	X	X	X	X		X	X	X
Document Scan w/OCR		X							X	
Document Scan, No OCR	X	X	X		X	X		X		X
Handwriting with Templates		X	X		X	X		X		
Handwriting Recognition		X	X		X	X		X		
Freeform Typing Unstructured	X	X	X	X	X	X		X	X	X
Dictation, SR w/NLP Structured		X						X		
Dictation, SR w/o NLP	X	X	X		X	X				
Template with Pick Lists	X	X	X	X	X			X	X	X
RxNorm		X			X			X	X	X
LOINC reporting			X					X	X	
DICOM			X					X	X	
CCD / CCR			X	X	X			X	X	X
HL7 Messaging	X	X	X	X	X			X	X	X
Office, Client/Server	X	X	X	X	X	X			X	X
Another - Unlisted - Indicate		X				X				
Webserver, In-Office Plus Remote	X	X			X	X				
Webserver, ASP In Office	X	X			X	X				
Web, ASP Remote Server	X	X		X	X	X		X		

Figure A1.2 EHR Vendor Contact Information

3M Health Information Systems
Loan D. Gordon
800-440-7119
lgordon@7medical.com
www.7medical.com

4Medica
Ravi Sharma
310-348-4100
rsharma@4medica.com
www.4medica.com/

ABELSoft
Kelly McKay
800-263-5104
www.abelsoft.com

Absolute Medical Software Systems
Sales Manager
877-763-3729
Sales@absolutemedicalsoftwaresystems.com
www.absolutemedicalsoftwaresystems.com

Accumedic Computer Systems
Jacob Shemesh
803-796-7980
jacob@accumedic.com
www.accumedic.com

ACOM Solutions
Gregory Church
866-286-5315
RAPIDinfo@acomemr.com
www.acomhealth.com

Acrendo Software
Barney McComas
800-403-2330
info@acrendo.com
www.acrendo.com

activeMD.com
1-866-401-1068
Notelogix.com

Addison Health Systems
Greg Winterkamp
800-496-2001
admin@writepad.com
www.writepad.com

ADL Data Systems
Wayne Jobe
800-965-7475
waynej@adldata.com
www.adldata.com

Advanced Data Systems
Marc Klar
800-899-4237
marc.klar@adsc.com
www.adsc.com

AdvancedMD
800-825-0224
info@advancedmd.com
www.advancedmd.com

AdvantaChart
866) 999-3232
team@advantachart.com
www.advantachart.com

AllMeds
William Rust
888-343-6337
brust@allmeds.com
www.allmeds.com

Allscripts
Lee Shapiro
800-654-0889
www.allscripts.com

Alma Information Systems
281-488-7016
www.speech-pro.com

AltaPoint Data Systems
Douglas Lyman
888-258-2552
douglas@altapoint.com
www.altapoint.com

Alteer Corp.
949-789-0500
info@alteer.com
www.alteer.com

Altos Solutions
Samuel Jones
650-559-6040
sjones@AltosSolutions.com
www.altossolutions.com

Amazing Charts
Kathleen Repoli
866-382-5932
sales@amazingcharts.com
www.amazingcharts.com

American HealthNet
www.americanhealthnet.com

American Medical Software
Robert Bridgeman
800-423-8836
rbridgman@americanmedical.com
www.americanmedical.com

Amkai
1-866-265-2434
www.amkai.com

Anasazi Software
Mike Morris
sales@anasazisoftware.com
www.anasazisoftware.com

Aprima/iMedica
Randy Schiff
866-960-6890
rschiff@aprimaEHR.com
www.imedica.com

Askesis Development Group
David Ryland
412-803-2400
info@askesis.com
www.askesis.com

Assist Med
888-774-7717
sales@assistmed.com
www.assistmed.com

Athenahealth
Jonathan Bush
888-652-8200
athena@athenahealth.com
www.athenahealth.com

AutomationMed
Jack Goldstein
401-919-5222
jdgoldstein@automationmed.com
www.automationmed.com

AutoMedicWorks
Bill Johnson
bill@automedicworks.com
www.automedicworks.com

Avid Anesthesiology Solutions
Jack Mayo
770-495-8005
jackmayo@avid-anesthesiology.com
www.avid-anesthesiology.com

Axolotl Corp.
Raymond W- Scott
888-296-5685
rscott@axolotl.com
www.axolotl.com

Benchmark Systems
Roger Green
800-779-0902
frontdesk@benchmark-systems.com
www.benchmark-systems.com

BetterHealth record
Jack Kemery
610-696-3656
info@bhgusa.com
www.bhgusa.com

BlueWare
231-779-0224
info@blueware.net
www.blueware.us

Bottomline Technologies (Formerly Optio
Software)
Marcus Hughes
800-243-2528
info@bottomline.com
www.bottomline.com

Brunmed
Michael Milne
866-812-8669
mmilne@brunmed.com
www.brunmed.com

CareData Solutions Corp.
Tonya Clausen
800-775-6709
Tony@caredata-biz
www.caredata.med.pro

Carefx
Andrew Hurd
866-922-7339
ahurd@carefx.com
www.carefx.com

CareVoyant (Formerely 'Infosys)
Vernon Mathias
888-463-6797
www.carevoyant.com
www.carevoyant.com

Catalis
Ed Taylor
888-241-1325
info@TheCatalis.com
www.thecatalis.com

Cerner
Michele Connors
866-221-0054
mconnors@cerner.com
www.cerner.com

CHARTCARE EMR
Brent Mitchell
800-438-1277
marketing@chartcare.com
www.chartcare.com

ChartLogic
Eric Sorenson
888-337-4441
ericsorenson@chartlogic.com
www.chartlogic.com

ChartStar/Asystar
Janice Charko
888-294-5372
support@asystar.com
www.asystar.com

ChartWare
Daniel Essin
800-652-4278
sales@chartware.com
www.chartware.com

Cimplify
Stryker Warren jr
888-812-5171
swarren@cimplify-net
www.cimplify.net

Clinic Pro
John Bartos
888-271-9898
jbartos@clinicpro.com
www.clinicpro.com

Clinical Insight
Stan Beal
585-419-3912
info@clinicalinsight.com
www.clinicalinsight.com

Clinical Research Information System
A. Deo Garlock
919-303-9704
www.mindlinc.com

Clinicare Corp.
Fred Chapman
800-5630579
marketing@clinicare.com
www.clinicare.com

CliniComp
Susan Yamamoto
800-350-8202
susany@clinicomp.com
www.clinicomp.com

ClinicPro
Marilyn Gard
866-333-2776
info@clinicpro.com
www.clinicpro.com

CliniMed Systems
800-764-3033
solutions@clinimed.com
www.clinimed.com

Clinix Medical Information Services (formerly MedicWare)
Jerry Killough
866-254-6496
jkillough@clinixmis.com
www.clinixmis.com

CMHC Systems
Zachary Zettler
800-528-9025
zzettler@cmhc.com
www.cmhcsys.com

CMR Complete Medical Record
Cris Mandry
225-751-8501
cmrinfo@cm-med
www.cmr.med.net

CodoniX
Stephens Speights
800-495-7270
stephens@codonix.com
www.codonix.com

Cognecy Solutions
Mark Shipp
214-206-8910
mark@cognecy.com
www.cognecy.com

ComChart
Hayward Zwerling, MD
978-407-0101
hzmd@me.com
www.ComChart.com

Community EHR
Dr. David Jones
800-516-1516
djones@community-emr.com
www.community-emr.com

CompassCare
David Bermingham
847-815-0031
dbermingham@compass-care.com
www.compasscare.info

Complex Corporation
Andrew Cohen
516-466-1942
ac@complexcorp.com
www.complexcorp.com

Compulink (formerly Richware)
Rich Rohde
800-456-4522
rich@richware.net
www.oms2000.com

CompuMed Systems
Joyce Crawley
502-292-2891
jcrawley@advantachart.com
www.advantachart.com

Conceptual Mindworks
Catherine Huddle
877-777-2298
chuddle@sevocity.com
www.conceptualmindworks.com

CorEMR
Jonathan Burton
801-225-0317
JBurton@CorEMR.com
www.CorEMR.com

Cornucopia Software
Phil Manfield
510-528-7000
support@practicemagic.com
www.practicemagic.com

CPSI
Sean Nicholas
800-711-2774
sales@cpsinet.com
www.cpsinet.com

Creative Concepts
Marilyn
866-333-2776
marilyn@clinicpro.com
www.clinicpro.com

Crowell Systems
Sally Crowell
800-366-4564
admin@crowellsystems.com
www.crowellsystems.com

CureMD
Bilal Hashmat
212-509-6200
bilal.hashmat@curemd.com
www.curemd.com

Cyber Records
Henry Klotz
516-612-7223
klotz@cyberrecordsmd.com
www.cyberrecordsmd.com

Cygnus
Shawn L. Peterson
231-347-5404
slp@cygnusinc-net
www.cygnusinc.net

Cylink Solutions (Healthcare)
Michael Hall
410-931-7500
mhall@cylink.com
www.safenet-inc.com

Data Tec
Andrew J. Grant
info@ezmedsoft.com
www.ezmedsoft.com

Database Constructs
Steve Welch
steve@databaseconstructs.com
www.databaseconstructs.com

Databases for Doctors
Rick D'Antonio
410-825-3103
rdantdfd@aol.com
www.databasesfordoctors.com

Datamed Systems
James Baker
703-385-3333
info@datamedsystems.com
www.datamedsystems.com

DataNet Systems Corporation
Robert Nathan
202-496-1122
info@dnscorp.com
www.dnscorp.com

DavLong Business Solutions
Ben Levonius
800-413-7764
blevonius@davlong.com
www.davlong.com

Daw Systems
Adam Forman
866-755-1500
Aforman@dawsystems.com
www.dawsystems.com

dbMotion
412-605-1952
www.dbmotion.com

DescriptMED
R. Terry Ellis
800-358-6479
questions@descriptmed.com
www.descriptmed.com

digiChart
Harris Gilbert
877-634-2727
support@digichart.com
www.digichart.com

Digital Documents
Sales Manager
866-992-5323
www.DigitalDocumentsLLC.com

Digital MD Systems
Danny Allison
817-545-2869
dannya@digitalmd.com
www.digitalmd.com

Dinmar (Oacis Healthcare)/Emergis
Jason Huckaby
707-778-3030
jhuckaby@dinmar.com
www.emergis.com

DMBI
Ash Patel
908-834-1608
ashpatel22@gmail.com
www.digidms.com

DocPad
954-781-3073
bob@docpad.com
www.docpad.com

DOCS
Randall Oates
800-455-7627
roates@soapware.com
www.docs.com

DocSite
John Haughton MD
919-256-9500
info@docsite.com
www.docsite.com

Doc-tor-com
Jim Smith
877-505-1888
sales@doc-tor.com
www.doctor.com

DoctorsPartner
Naveen
800-779-1723
sales@doctorspartner.com
www.emr-electronicmedicalrecords.com

Doc-U-Chart for the Tablet PC
Jill Spain
903-561-7096
jspain@docuchart.com
www.docuchart.com

DocuMed
Les Bloom
800-321-5595
lbloom@documed.com
www.documed.com

DocumentPlus
Hale
800-642-0600
hale@docplus.net
www.docplus.net

DocuSYS
Teecie Cozad
888-465-9903
info@docusys.net
www.docusys.net

DocuTAP
Dusty Schroeder
877-697-4696
Sales&Marketing@docutap.com
www.docutap.com

DocuTrac
Arnie Schuster
800-850-8510
Sales@quicdoc.com
www.quicdoc.com

DOMA Technologies
Leticia Feliciano
757-306-4920
info@domaonline.com
www.domatechnologies.com

DOX Podiatry
Bart Ripperger
866-301-7700
info@doxemr.com
www.doxemr.com

DrFirst-com
James F. Chen
301-231-9510
jchen@drfirst.com
www.clinicpro.com

Dr-Notes
Carlos Saradinia
888-679-2123
csaradinia@drnotes.com
www.drnotes.com

DSS
Mark Byers
561-227-0207
mbyers@dssinc.com
www.docstorsys.com

EasyChart
Walter Graff
800-430-0290
wgraff@softwareperformance.com
www.softwareperformance.com

EasyMD Systems
Randy Farr
615-294-3837
easemd@easemd.com
www.easemd.com

eCast Corporation
Martin Frazier
919-833-8999
mfrazier@ecastcorp.com
www.ecastcorp.com

eClinicalWorks
Heather Caouette
866-888-6929
heather.c@eclinicalworks.com
www.eclinicalworks.com

Eclipsys Corp.
Don Shoen
800-869-8300
dschoen@medinotes.com
www.eclipsys.com

EdgeMed Solutions
Gary Kurstin
800-832-3274
edgemed@edgemed.com
www.edgemed.com

Edims
Scott Serbin
973-251-1075
serbins@edims.net
www.edims.net

Egton Medical Information Systems
Peter Anderson
866-443-3647
peter-anderson@emis.ca
www.emis.ca

eHealthSolutions
Stephen Pacicco
877-432-5858
sales@sigmacare.com
www.ehealthsolutions.com

Electronic Healthcare Systems
W. Sanders Pitman
888-879-7302
marketing@ehsmed.com
www.ehsmed.com

Electronic Pediatrician
Andrew Schuman, MD
603-626-8016
ajs@electronicpediatrician.com
www.electronicpediatrician.com

Elekta IMPAC Software
Jay Hoey
408-830-8000
jhoey@elekta.com
www.impac.com

Elysium
Veri Croce
888-296-5685 x 5
sales@axolotl.com
www.axolotl.com

Emageon
Noel Gartman
205-980-7602
noel-gartman@emageon.com
www.emageon.com

eMDfix
Michelle Greiver
201-392-1727
support@emdfix.com
www.emdfix.com

e-MDs
David Winn
888-344-9836
dlwinn@e-mds.com
www.e-mds.com

e-Medical Solutions
Laurence Cohen
732-599-5686
lcohen@emedicalsolutions.net
www.emedicalsolutions.net

Emedical
Son H. Le, MD
626-572-9791
info@ezmedicaloffice.com
www.ezmedicaloffice.com

e-MedRecords
Wendy Frieling, MD
973-726-4444
www.compukid.com

e-MedSoft.com
Steve Erickson
800-653-0350
steveerickson@emedsoft.com
www.emedsoft.com

Emergis
Dan Polomark
800-661-1659
dan@ebill.ca
www.emergis.com

Emergisoft
Jose Lugo
800-682-7729
jlugo@emergisoft.com
www.emergisoft.com

EMIS
Heather Linkletter
866-443-3647
Heather-Linkletter@emis.ca
www.emis.ca

EMR Solutions
Carol Goddard
cgoddard@emr2.com
www.emr2.com

EMR4 Doctors
800-758-9539
sales@emr4doctors.com
www.emr4doctors.com

EMRnetwork
Dustin LeBleu
support@emrnetwork.com
www.emrnetwork.com

EMRWorks
Jason Centrella
866-775-7779
sales@medstarsystems.com
www.medstarsystems.com

Encite
Jock Putney
800-714-7199
jputney@encite.us
www.encite.us

EncounterNotes
866-289-6298
sales3@encounternotes.com
www.encounternotes.com

EncounterPro Healthcare Resources
Greg Vacca
800-677-5653
greg-vacca@jmjtech.com
www.encounterpro.com

Enterprise Healthcare Systems
Phil Krieg
480-998-5452
sales@ehsiplus.com
www.ehsiplus.com

Epic Systems Corporation
Judith R. Faulkner
608-271-9000
judy@epicsystems.com
www.epicsystems.com

Epocrates
Robert J. Quinn
650-227-1750
rquinn@epocrates.com
www.epocrates.com

Ergo Partners
Peter King-Smith
800-631-4052
pkingsmith@ergopartners.com
www.ergopartners.com

Essence Healthcare
Bryan Dieter
866-935-5469
Bdieter@essencehealthcare.com
www.purkinje.com

esurg.com
Cindi Pendergraft
877-443-7874
info@esurg.com
www.esurg.com

Ethidium Health Systems
Matias Klein
800-842-0873
matias@ethidium.com
www.ethidium.com

Excelcare
724-238-9599
www.excelcare.com

EXmedic
Harry Berstein
206-331-4009
hbmd@exmedic.com
www.exmedic.com

Experior Corp.
Richard Presser
800-595-2020
rpresser@experior.com
www.experior.com

Exscribe
Ranjan Sachdev MD
866-870-1521
ranjan@exscribe.com
www.exscribe.com

FertiSoft
Ginette DeRepentigny
819-275-2117
info@OrdinateursLaval.ca
www.FertiSoft.com

FlexMedical
Matt Price
256-694-2650
sales@oceris.com
www.flexmedical.com

Fox Meadows Software
Ronnie Spell
800-754-7213
salesfms@foxmeadows.com
www.foxmeadows.com

GE Healthcare
Sunny Sanyal
800-558-5120
sunny.sanyal@med-ge.com
www2.gehealthcare.com

GEMMS
Brian Bromberek
800-773-3111
bbromber@gemmsnet.com
www.gemmsnet.com

GeniusDoc
Sunil Nemani
866-443-6362
info@geniusdoc.com
www.geniusdoc.com

gloStream
Michael Sappington
877-456-3671
mike@glostream.com
www.glostream.com

gMed
Marc Shapiro
888-577-8801
marcs@gmed.com
www.gmed.com

Greenway Medical Technologies
Rebekah Green
866-242-3805
RebekahGreen@greenwaymedical.com
www.greenwaymedical.com

Gscribe
Rakesh Sharma
651-494-7413
GSCRIBE@igsp.com
www.gscribe.com

Health Care Software
Joseph J. Fahey
800-524-1038
jfahey@hcssupport.com
www.hcsinteractant.com

Health Data Services
Chris Brancato
800-800-4021
cbrancato@healthdataservices.com
www.healthdataservices.com

Health Probe
Sales
765-346-3332
sales@healthprobe.com
www.healthprobe.com

Healthcare Management Systems HMS
Michael Freeman
800-383-3317
mfreeman@hmstn.com
www.hmstn.com

HealthIS
Michael Plaia
205-972-1222
mplaia@healthis.com
www.healthis.com

Healthland
Angie Franks
800-323-6987
angie-franks@healthland.com
www.healthland.com

Healthlink
James Adams
713-852-2117
james-adams@healthlinkinc.com

HealthPac Computer Systems
Lindy Backner
800-831-9419
lindy@healthpac.net
www.healthpac.net

HealthPort
Hadiya Reynolds
800-367-1500
hadiya.reynolds@healthport.com
www.healthport.com

HealthTek Solutions
Mary L. cherry
757-625-0800
business@healthtek.com
www.healthtek.com

HEALTHvision
James Elder
877-446-1800
www.healthvision.com

HemiData
Sam Pendleton
435-216-5346
spendle@hemidata.com
www.hemidata.com

Henry Schein Medical Systems
Susan Vassallo
800-624-8832
susan.vassallo@henryschein.com
www.henryschein.com

Hill-Rom Div- of Hillenbrand Industry
Mike Harmon
812.934.7777
www.hill-rom.com

Holt Systems
Brendon Holt
561-272-1640
sales@edocrec.com
www.holtsystems.com

i2i Systems
Janice Nicholson
866-820-2212
contact@i2isys.com
www.i2isys.com

Iatroware, Division of Medical Dental
Building
Edgar Anders
800-816-8370
edgar@iatroware.com
www.iatroware.com

ICS Software
516-766-2129
sales@icssoftware.net
www.icssoftware.net

IDX Corp. Div GE Healthcare
Jeffrey Kao
617-519-2822
jeff_kao@ge.com
www.idx.com

iHealth
Jason Willett
415-644-3926
jason-willett@medem.com
www.medem.com

iKnowMed
Elizabeth Larricq
866-216-5053
ikm@usoncology.com
www.iknowmed.com

iMDsoft
781-449-5567
www.imd-soft.com

iMed Software
Glenn Jumonville
886-379-7930
info@imedemr.com
www.imedemr.com

iMedx
Kevin Ross
866-840-4354
sales@imedx.com
www.imedx.com

IMRAC Corp.
Doug Vincent
615-777-8070
Dvincent@imrac.com
www.imrac.com

Infinite Software Solutions dba MD-REPORTS
Srikanth Gosike
718-982-1315
info@md-reports.com
sales@md-reports.com
www.infinitesoftsol.com

Informatics Corporation of America
C. Thomas Smith
615-866-1500
thomas.smith@icainformatics.com
www.icainformatics.com

InforMed Corporation
Praxis EMR
Sales & Marketing
800-985-6016
sales@praxisemr.com
www.infor-med.com

Ingenious Med
Jennifer Errico
404-815-0862
jerrico@ingeniousmed.com
www.ingeniousmed.com

Integrated Digital Systems (MedDocs)
Bob Deuby
800-283-0999
ldhunt@idsscan.com
www.idss.net

Integrated Healthcare
John Bradbury
888-813-7575
jbradbury@ihealthware.com
www.ihealthware.com

Integrated Systems Management
Divan Dave
914-332-5590
ddave@omnimd.com
www.ismnet.com

IntegriMED
Traci Detchon
866-440-4863
tdetchon@integrimed.com
www.integrimed.com

Integritas
David Price
203-438-4357
dprice3@integritas.com
www.integritas.com

Intelligent Medical Systems
Anthony Sforza
800-747-4154
asforza@smartdoctor.com
www.smartdoctor.com

InterCare DX
Russ Lyon
213-627-8878
rlyon@intercare.com
www.intercare.com

IntrinsiQ
Brent Clough
800-565-2279
info@intrinsiq.com
www.intrinsiq.com

Intuitive Medical Software
Howard Follis
877-570-8721
info@intuitivemedical.com
www.intuitivemedical.com

iSalus Healthcare
Mark A. Day
866-575-6678
markday@isalushealthcare.com
www.isalushealthcare.com

I-Scribe
David Levison
877-483-1324
service@iscribe.com
www.iscribe.com

Isoft
Laurie Giles
0-9-985-3200
laurie-giles@isoftaus.com-au
www.isoftplc.com

iSprit
Dick Aderman
317-767-7630
mediarelations@isprit.com
www.isprit.com

Jonoke Software Development
Jody Bevan
800-254-0739
info@jonoke.com
www.jonoke.com

KeyMedical Software
Susan Jones
888-953-9633
susanjones@keymedical.net
www.keymedical.net

Lakes Health Systems
Swandoyo Hartono
888-746-5995
swandoyo-hartono@weblakes.com
www.lakeshealth.com

LeonardoMD
858-450-6611
customer.service@leonardomd.com
www.leonardomd.com

Life Record
Michael Pike
877-577-3727
mike@liferecord.com
emr.liferecord.com

Lighthouse Medical Management
William Scatchard III
401-331-5300
wsatchard@lhmm.com
www.lhmm.com

Lille Corp.
Jordan Rosen
866-372-7423
info@lillecorp.com
www.lillecorp.com

LMS Medical Systems
514-488-3461
info@lmsmedical.com
www.lmsmedical.com

LoginClinic
Pratap Chudasama
773-267-7777
pc@loginclinic.com
www.loginclinic.com

LSS/Meditech
Ken Carlson
952-941-1000
kcarlson@lssdata.com
www.lssdata.com

Lynx CosmetiSoft
Larry Peterson
530-852-0306
sales@cosmetisoft.com
www.cosmetisoft.com

M E Computer Systems
Wendy Gaston
800-532-3543
info@MECSNet.com
www.mecsnet.com

M2 Information Systems
800-598-6647
www.m2is.com

MacPractice
Mark Hollis
402-420-2430
MarkHollis@MacPractice.com
www.macpractice.com

Macro Doctor
Wayne Bryan
804-726-6500
support@macrodoctor.com
www.macrodoctor.com

Mardon Healthcare Information Systems
Don McKeny
800-877-9257
don@mardon2000.com
www.mardon2000.com

Mars Medical Systems/Noteworthy
Mark Conner
888-627-7633
markc@marsmedical.com
www.noteworthymedical.com

McKesson
Tom Leonard
415-983-8300
tom.leonard@mckesson.com
www.mckesson.com

MD Logic
VP Sales
770-497-1560
marketing@mdlogic.com
www.mdlogic.com

MD Tablet
Robbin Hunter
888-989-1965
rhunter@mdtablet.com
www.mdtablet.com

MD Technologies/Medtopia
William Davis
225-343-7169
sales@mdtechnologies.com
www.medtopia.com

MDanywhere Technologies
Dina Feinstein
877-632-4488
dina@mdanywhere.com
www.mdanywhere.com

MDI Achieve
Tom Lalonde
800-869-1322
tom.lalonde@achievehealthcare.com
www.mdiachieve.com

MDLAND
212-363-8000
www.mdland.com

MDoffice
Jay Lodhia
732 744 2700
JayL@mdoffice.com
www.mdoffice.com

MD-Reports / Infinite Software Solutions
Srikanth Gosike
718-982-1315
sales@md-reports.com
www.md-reports.com

MDServe
Jock Putney
973-573-9100
info@mdserve.com
www.mdserve.com

MDSyncEMR
Stephen K. Miyasato
miyasat@flex.com
www.mdsync.net

MDTablet
Keith Marks
888-989-1965
info@mdtablet.com
www.mdtablet.com

MED3000 (InteGreat)
David Koeller
800-676-1360
jhoutz@igreat.com
www.igreat.com

Medamation
Jeffrey Gersbach
843-559-0109
sales@medamation.com
www.medamation.com

Medappz
Brian Lichtlin
877-633-2779
info@MedAppz.com
www.medappz.com

MedAZ
Sonia S. Sharmeen
888-633-2972
sonia@medaz-net
www.medaz.net

Medcere
888-573-1233
info@medcereint.com
www.medcere.com

Medcom Information Systems
Mark Steward
800-213-2161
msteward@emirj.com
www.emirj.com

MEDecision
Danielle Russella
610-540-0202
salesinfo@medecision.com
www.medecision.com

MedePresence
David J. Dugan
847-337-1501
info@medepresence.com
www.medepresence.com

Medfusion
Stephen Malik
877-599-5123
smalik@medfusion.net
www.medfusion.net

Medhost
Craig Herrod
888-218-4678
info@medhost.com
www.medhost.com

Medical Communication Systems (MCS)
David Payne
877-8-MED-DATA
info@medcomsys.com
www.medcomsys.com

Medical Informatics Engineering
Doug Horner
888-498-3484
dhorner@mieweb.com
www.mieweb.com

Medical Information Systems
Ted Itzkowitz
800-487-9135
titzkowitz@sticomputer.com
www.hksys.com

Medical Information
David Jones
800.516.1516
djones@xeniamed.org
www.community.emr.com

Medical Management Resources
John Pennisi
800-289-3390
Sales@mmriny.com
www.mmri.ny.com

Medical Merlin
321-821-5369
sales@MedMerlin.com
www.MedMerlin.com

Medical Office Online
John B. Costello
866-995-9889
jcostello@medicalofficeonline.com
www.medicalofficeonline.com

Medical Technology International
John Sprankle
800-777-7684
info@medtec.net
www.harmonymedical.net

MedicalNotes-com
Kent S. Kapitan
217-726-8892
info@medicalnotes.com
www.medicalnotes.com

Medicat
Dr. Stacy Kottman
866-633-4053
sales@medicat.com
www.medicat.com

Medicity
Kipp Lassetter
888-830-1022
publicrelations@medicity.com
www.medicity.com

Medico Systems
Sheila Bahrami
425-268-0174
info@medicosystem.com
www.medicosystem.com

Medi-EMR
Matthew D'Alesandro
888-633-1367
mdalessandro@mediemr.com
www.mediemr.com

Medigrate
Lancy Allyn
877-633-4472
sales@medigrate.com
www.medigrate.com

MedInformatix
Tom McGonigle
866-277-8735
info@medinformatix.com
www.medinformatix.com

MediNotes
Dave Fotiadis
866-792-6900
www.bondclinician.com

MediSync (E&M Coding)
Charlie Hardtke
513-533-1199
www.medisync.com

Meditab Software
Amos Lim
866-994-6367
AmosL@Meditab.com
www.meditab.com

Mediture
Dan Vatland
800.430.2045
dan_vatland@mediture.com
www.mediture.com

Mediware Information Systems
Blood Bank Med Mgmt
George Barry
913-307-1000
sales@mediware.com
www.mediware.com

MedLink International
Ray Vuono
631-342-8800
rvuono@medlinkus.com
www.medlinkus.com

Mednet System
John Schaeffer
877-633-6384
info@mednetsystem.com
www.mednetsystem.com

MedPlexus
Prabhakar Muppidi
408-878-6263
muppidi@medplexus.com
www.medplexus.com

Medrium
John Martin
877-6337486
sales@medrium.com
www.medrium.com

Medscribbler
Michael Milne
866-350-6337
frontdesk@medscribbler.com
www.medscribbler.com

MedSeek
John Mark Taylor
888-medseek
Johnmark-Taylor@accessptinc.com
www.accessptinc.com

Medsphere Systems (OpenVistA)
Rick Jung
760-692-3700
rick.jung@medsphere.com
www.medsphere.com

MedStar Systems
Ian Bjorsvik
866-775-7779
info@drworks.com
www.medstarsystems.com

Medtuity
Brandon Chase
614-259-2000
bbchase@medtuity.com
www.medtuity.com

MeridianEMR
Larry Drappi
877-411-4367
ldrappi@meridianEMR.com
www.meridianEMR.com

MICA Information Systems
Scott Yingling
800-344-6422
syingling@micamedical.com
www.micamedical.com

MicroFour
Brett Taylor
800-235-1856
mbtaylor@micro4.com
www.micro4.com

MicroMD
Richard Yonis
800-624-8832
www.micromd.net

MobileMD a division of Intraprise Solutions
John Skinner
908-232-7816
jskinner@mobileMD.com
www.mobilemd.com

Momentum Healthware
Victoria Paine-Mantha
877-231-3836
info@momentumhealthware.com
www.momentumhealthware.com

Mountain Medical Technologies
Stefan Dragitsch
800-595-9373
sdragitsch@mountainmeditech.com
www.visualmed.net

Mountainside Software
Leonard Hampton
800-868-8423
lhampton@mountainsidesoftware.com
www.mtnsdsoft.com

MRO Corp
John Walton
888-252-4146
sales@mrocorp.com
www.mrocorp.com

MyMedicalRecords.com
Robert H. Lorsch
310-887-0663
rhl@mmrmail.com
MyMedicalRecords.com

NexTech
Kamal Majeed
800-829-0580
support@nextech.com
www.nextech.com

NextGen Healthcare Information Systems
Patrick Cline
215-657-7010
pcline@nextgen.com
www.nextgen.com

NextMed Systems
info@nextmedsystems.com
www.nextmedsystems.com

Nightingale Informatix
Jennifer Morgano
jmorgano@vantagemed.com
800-343-5737
916-638-4744
www.nightingale.md

NorthBase
Joseph Landau
jlandau@northbase.com
www.northbase.com

Northrop-Grumman Information
Wm. Lovell
703-713-4000
healthsolutions@ngc.com
www.logicon.com

Noteworthy Medical Systems
Greg Jewell
800-224-9740
greg@chartconnect.com
www.noteworthyemr.com

Nuesoft
678-303-1140
www.nuesoft.com

OBEverywhere
Ed Klimas
440-925-2800
sales@OBEverywhere.com
obeverywhere.com

OCERIS
Ryan McGinty
256-694-2650
sales@oceris.com
www.oceris.com

OmniMD
Hitender Soni
914-332-5590 ext.107
Soni@OmniMD.com
www.omnimd.com

OneHealthPort
Richard Rubin
800-973-4797
info@OneHealthPort.com
www.onehealthport.com

Optimus EMR System
Tim Quarberg
888-242-9080 ext. 217
tquarberg@optimusemr.com
www.optimusemr.com

Optio Software
603-436-0300
www.optiosoftware.com

Opus Healthcare Solutions
Fred Beck
800-643-6439
sales@opushealthcare.com
www.opushealthcare.com

Orion Health - USA
Kelly Weinstein
310-526-4049
weinstein@orionhealth.com
www.orionhealth.com

Patient Care Technologies
John Festa
404-4257828
john_festa@ptct.com
www.ptct.com

Patient Keeper
Stephen S. Hau
617-987-0300
shau@patientkeeper.com
www.patientkeeper.com

Patient NOW
Jerry Jacobson
800-436-3150
jjacobson@patientnow.com
www.patientnow.com

PBF Online (formerly Medcomsoft)
Shawn Long
800-699-5533
@pbfonline.com
www.medcomsoft.com

PCTS Patient Care Technology Systems
Stephen Armstrong
949-367-6698
inquiry@pcts.com
www.pcts.com

Pearle Computer Services
Earle Eidenire
888-253-0412
sales@pearlecomputer.com
www.pearlecomputer.com

Penn Medical Informatics
Kevin Doyle
888-942-4430
info@pennmedical.com
www.pennmidical.com

PeopleMed.com
Steven M. Schmidt
888-806-8400
steve@peoplemed.com
www.peoplemed.com

PersonalMD
925-460-1337
comms@PersonalMD.com
www.personalmd.com

Petra Systems
Sales & Marketing
dawny@aspectx.com
www.petrasystems.com

PhyMD
Eric Fritschler
301-315-6330
EricF@PhyMD.com
www.phymd.com

Physician Computer Company
John Canning
800-7227708
john@pcc.com
www.pcc.com

Physicians Information Exchange
W. Ernest Rutherford
ernie@piexchange.com
www.piexchange.com

Physicians Practice
Scott Weber
800-781-2211
info@physicianspractice.com
www.physicianspractice.com

Physicians Trust
Scott Belcher
949-234-1881
www.physicianstrust.net

Picis
Todd C. Cozzens
781-557-3300
todd_cozzens@picis.com
www.picis.com

Plexis Healthcare Systems
Jorge Yant
877-475-3947
info@plexisweb.com
www.plexisweb.com

Point and Click Solutions
Jeff Gleis
781-272-9800
jgleis@pointnclick.com
www.pointnclick.com

Poseidon Group
888-291-0401
www.poseidongroup.com

PowerMed
Bill Zellman
888-621-5565
info@powermed.com
www.powermed.com

Practical Medical Record
Andrew J. Schuman, MD
603-623-2229
ajs@electronicpediatrician.com
www.electronicpediatrician.com

Practice Expert
Mark Richards
888-294-6070
mrichards@pxpert.com
www.practicexpert.com

Practice Fusion
Matthew Douglass
415-344-4467
matthew@practicefusion.com
www.practicefusion.com

Practice Insight
Houston Johnson
713-333-6000
hjohnson@practiceinsight.com
www.practiceinsight.com

Practice Partner
Hedge Stahm
800-770-7674
hstahm@practicepartner.com
www.practicepartner.com

Practice Solutions
Larry Mohr
800-361-9151
practice.solutions@cma.ca

Practice Today
Carroll
888-881-0038
carroll@legacypress.com
www.practicetoday.com

Practice Velocity
David E. Stern, MD
815-544-7480
info@practicevelocity.com
www.practicevelocity.com

PracticeAdmin.com
Fred Taute
888-294-9255
tautef@practiceadmin.com

Practicehwy.com
Jamshid Rahimi
927-247-3483
Jamshid@practicehwy.com
www.practicehwy.com

PracticeOne
Dan Schulman
877-363-3797
Dan.Schulman@PracticeOne.com
www.PracticeOne.com

PracticeXpert
Stephen Dart
sdart@pxpert.com
www.pxpert.com

Praxis Electronic Medical Record
Sales & Marketing
800-985-6016
sales@praxisemr.com
www.praxisemr.com

Primaris
Amber Lear
800-735-6776
alear@moqio.sdps.org
www.mprcf.org

Prime Clinical Systems
Barry Ardelan
877-444-1156
barry@primeclinical.com
www.primeclinical.com

PrimeCare Systems
W. Jordan Fitzhugh
800-774-7898
info@pcare.com
www.pcare.com

Primetime Medical Software
Dr. Matthew R. Ferrante
803-796-7980
ferrante@medicalhistory.com
www.medicalhistory.com

Prodata Systems
Brian Goertz
866-4878346
Brian.Goertz@prodata.com
www.prodata.com

Professional Data Services
Michelle Bogner
800-282-7543
mbogner@pdsmed.com
www.pdsmed.com

ProPractica
Sean M. Mullen
866-406-2224
Sales@StreamlineMD.com
www.propractica.com

Protomed Corporation
800-648-4836
www.protomed.com

ProVation Medical
612-313-1504
support@ProVationMedical.com
www.provationmedical.com

ProVox Technologies Corp.
Kelly Hardy
888-776-8691
kellyhandy@provox.com
www.provox.com

Psych Notes EMR
Wendla Schwartz
877-693-6704
www.psychnotesemr.com

Pulse Systems
316.636.5900
www.pulseinc.com

Purkinje
Andrew Shea
866-935-8069
ashea@purkinje.com
www.purkinje.com

Quadax
Catherine Sicker
440-777-6300
sales@quadax.com
www.quadax.com

Quadramed
Randy Parker
703-709-2300
rparker@quadramed.com
www.quadramed.com

QualTimeMed Software
sales@ezsoap.com
www.ezSOAP.com

Quick Notes
Ken Schenley
800-899-2468
www.qnotes.com

Quincy Systems
Chuck Leider
888-346-6842
chuckleider@yahoo.com
quincysys.com

Quovadx
Harvey A. Wagner
469-420-2500
harvey.wagner@quovadx.com
www.quovadx.com

Raintree Systems
Richard Welty
800-333-1033
enhancements@raintreeinc.com
www.raintreeinc.com

Reliance Software Systems
Alicia Brown
877-735-9273
abrown@relware.com
www.relware.com

RemedyMD
Gary Kennedy
877-736-3399
gkennedy@remedymd.com
www.remedymd.com

Rosch Visionary Systems
Dr. Rosch
800-307-3320
rvssales@roschmd.com
rvssales@roschvisionary.com

Sage Software
Healthcare Division
Lynne Durham
877-932-6301
lynne.durham@sage.com
www.sagehealth.com

Sajix
Prasada Pyala
925-218-7370
info@sajix.com
www.sajix.com

SecureChart
Mike O'Neal
888-741-1113
www.securechart.com

SeeBeyond
Sun Microsystems
Suzi Lambourne
415-856-5100
slambourne@bando.com
www.blancandotus.com

Sequel Systems
Irfan Iqbal
800-9652728
info@sequelsys.com
www.sequelsys.com

Sevocity
Elaine Mendoza
877-777-2298
emendoza@teamcmi.com
www.sevocity.com

Siemens Healthcare
Sam Brandt M.D.
610-219-5701
hannelore.kahles@siemens.com
www.siemens.com

Sigmund Software
Marcus Sharpe
800-448-6975
msharpe@sigmundsoftware.com
www.sigmundsoftware.com

SmartEMR
Lorn Leitman
305.227.7780
executive@smartemr.com
www.smartemr.com

SOAPware
Randell Oates
800-455-7627
roates@soapware.com
www.soapware.com

SoftAid Medical Management Systems
Jim Clark
877-763-8243
jclark@softaid.com
www.soft-aid.com

SoftMed Systems
Kerry Waltrip
301-572-3800
kwaltrip@softmed.com
www.SoftMed.com

Software Performance Specialists
Walter Graff
800-430-0290
wgraff@softwareperformance.com
www.softwareperformance.com

Solcom
Marv Addink
888-335-0815
info@solcominc.com
www.solcominc.com

Sonix Healthcare Solutions
Richard Wilson
888-779-3440
info@sonixhealthcaresolutions.com
www.sonixhealthcaresolutions.com

Source Medical Solutions
Aaron Basil
800-562-7069
aaron.basil@sourcemed.net
www.sourcemed.net

Spring Medical Systems
SpringCharts EHR
Jack B. Smyth
281-453-2310
Jack.Smyth@SpringMedical.com
www.springmedical.com

SRS Software
Evan Steele
201-802-1300
ESteele@srssoft.com
www.srssoft.com

SSIMED EMRge
Cheryl Pederzoli
800-276-6992
sales@ssimed.com
www.ssimed.com

STAT! Systems
Frederick Dietrich
877-424-2787
dietrich@statsystems.com
www.statsystems.com

Streamline Health
Melissa Vincent
866-639-7541
Melissa.Vincent@streamlinehealth.net
www.streamlinehealth.net

Stryker Imaging
Private Label
Bojan Gospavic
972-410-5092
bojan.gospavic@stryker.com
www.stryker.com

Surgical Information Systems
800-930-0895
info@sisfirst.com
www.sisfirst.com

SynaMed
Holly Demuro
866-796-2633
holly.demuro@synamed.com
www.synamed.com

Systemedx
Kevin Bonner
888-499-8324
kbonner@systemedx.com
www.systemedx.com

Sytec Health
800-824-2365
www.systechealth.com

TetriDyn Solutions
Antoinette Knapp
888-895-7115
info@tetridyn.com
www.aeromd.com

TheraManager
Mike Tompsett
800-913-4294
mike@TheraManager.com
www.theramanager.com

T-System
Suzette M. Wier-Thornby
800-667-2482
suzette@tsystem.com
www.tsystem.com

Turbo-Doc
Ward Clark
800-977-4868
TurboDoc@TurboDoc.com
www.turbodoc.net

Versaform
Joseph Landau
800-678-1111
jrl@versaform.com
www.versaform.com

VersaSuite
Rodney Brown
800-903-8774
sales@versasuite.com
www.versasuite.com

VIP Medicine
Dr. Jack M Berdy
201-891-9463
Mdceo@aol.com
www.vipmedicine.com

Vipa Health
Jessica Lemoine
305-227-7780
jlemoine@vipahealth.com
www.smartemr.com

Virtual Software Systems
Tom Palmquist
tip@vss3.com
www.vss3.com

Visionary Medical Systems
Jason Patchen
888-895-2466
jpatchen@visionarymed.com
www.visionarymed.com

Visual Data
800-218-9916
info@officepracticum.com
www.officepracticum.com

VisualMED Clinical Solutions Corp.
Gerard Dab
888-333-0243
gdab@visualmedsolutions.com
www.visualmedsolutions.com

VitalWorks
Office Based Phys. Division
Peter McClennen
617-779-7878
info@amicas.com
www.vitalworks.com

Vox2Data
medvoice@comcast.net
www.vox2data.com

Waiting Room Solutions
Diane Unger
866-977-4367
sales@waitingroomsolutions.com
www.WaitingRoomSolutions.com

WebeDoctor
Anwer Siddiqi
714-990-3999
asiddiqi@webedoctor.com
www.webedoctor.com

Wellmed
Brad Bowman, MD
503-279-9010
ebradb@wellmed.com
www.wellmed.com

Wellogic
Sumit Nagpal
617-621-9775
info@wellogic.com
www.wellogic.com

Wellsoft EDIS
Denise Helfand
800-597-9909
dhelfand@wellsoft.com
www.wellsoft.com

WIMcare
Cheryl Advocat
800-616-5008
support@wimcare.com
www.wimcare.com

WinMedStat
Thomas Riggs
800-788-2845
sales@winmedstat.com
www.winmedstat.com

zCHART EMR
866-924-2787
www.zchart.com

APPENDIX II

List of Conferences to View EMRs/EHRs

The conferences listed in the following table are attended by a subset of EMR developers each year. Check the announcements published on the organization's Web site for a list of exhibiting vendors. Compare those to the list of EMR developers in Appendix I to see which EMR developers will be attending the conference of interest to you.

Figure A2.1 List of Annual Conferences Attended by EMR Developers

Conferences to Attend to View EMRs/EHRs	Time/Location	http://www.
AAAAI American Academy of Allergy, Asthma and Immunology	2-26 to 3-2, 2010 New Orleans	aaaai.org
AAO American Academy of Ophthalmology	10-16 to 19, 2010 Chicago	aao.org
AAOS American Academy of Orthopedic Surgeons	3-10 to 13, 2010 New Orleans	aaos.org
AAPM American Academy of Pain Medicine	2-3 to 6, 2010 San Francisco	painmed.org
AAPMR American Academy of Physical Medicine & Rehab	11-3 to 7, 2010 Seattle	aapmr.org
AAD American Academy of Dermatology	2-26 to 3-3, 2010 Miami	aad.org
AAP American Academy of Pediatrics	10-2 to 10, 2010 San Francisco	aap.org
AAFP American Academy of Family Physicians	9-29 to 10-02, 2010 Denver	aafp.org
AAO American Academy of Otolaryngology	9-26 to 29, 2010 Boston	entnet.org
AASM American Academy of Sleep Medicine	6-5 to 9, 2010 San Antonio	sleepmeeting.org
AACE American Association of Clinical Endocrinologists	4-21 to 25, 2010 Boston	aace.com
AAPS American Association of Plastic Surgeons	3-20 to 23, 2010 San Antonio	aaps1921.org
AATS American Association of Thoracic Surgeons	5-1 to 5, 2010 Toronto	aats.org
ACA American Chiropractic Association	10-30 to 11-1, 2010 Chicago	acatoday.org
ACC American College of Cardiology	3-13 to 16, 2010 Atlanta	acc.org

Successfully Choosing Your EMR: 15 Crucial Decisions. By © Arthur Gasch and Betty Gasch. Published 2010 by Blackwell Publishing

Conferences to Attend to View EMRs/EHRs	Time/Location	http://www.
ACCP American College of Chest Physicians	10-30 to 11-4, 2010 Vancouver, BC	chestnet.org
ACEP American College of Emergency Physicians	9-28 to 10-1, 2010 Las Vegas	acep.org
ACOG American College of Obstetricians and Gynecologists	5-15 to 19, 2010 San Francisco	acog.org
ACP American College of Physicians	4-22 to 24, 2010 Toronto	acponline.org
ACR American College of Rheumatology	11-6 to 11, 2010 Atlanta	rheumatology.org
ACS American College of Surgeons	10-3 to 10, 2010 Washington, DC	facs.org
ADA American Dental Association	10-8 to 11, 2010 Orlando	ada.org
AGA American Gastroenterological Association	5-2 to 5, 2010 New Orleans	gastro.org
AGS American Geriatrics Society	5-12 to 15, 2010 Orlando	americangeriatrics.org
AHIMA American Health Information Management Association	9-25 to 30, 2010 Orlando	ahima.org
AMIA American Medical Informatics Association	11-14 to 17, 2010 Washington, DC	amia.org
AMSSM American Medical Society for Sports Medicine	4-17 to 22, 2010 Cancun, MX	newamssm.org
APA American Psychiatric Association	5-21 to 26, 2010 New Orleans	psych.org
ASA American Society of Anesthesiology	10-16 to 20, 2010 San Diego	asahq.org
ASCO American Society of Clinical Oncology	6-4 to 8, 2010 Chicago	asco.org
ASCP American Society for Clinical Pathology	10-27 to 31, 2010 San Francisco	ascp.org
ASH American Society of Hematology	12-4 to 11, 2010 Orlando	hematology.org
AUA American Urological Association	5-29 to 6-10, 2010 San Francisco	auanet.org
HIMSS Healthcare Information and Management System Society	3-1 to 4, 2010 Atlanta	himss.org
IDSA Infectious Disease Society of America	10-21 to 24, 2010 Vancouver, BC	idsociety.org
MGMA Medical Group Management Association	10-24 to 27, 2010 New Orleans	mgma.com
RPA Renal Physicians Association	3-12 to 15, 2010 Baltimore	renalmd.org
RSNA Radiology Society of North America	11-28 to 12-3, 2010 Chicago	rsna.org
SNM Society of Nuclear Medicine	6-5 to 9, 2010 Salt Lake City	www.snm.org

APPENDIX III

Using the MSP EHR Selector to Compare EMRs

The MSP EHR Selector™ and the MSP ESP Portal™

Depending upon your level of technological expertise, this book may be all that you need to choose a suitable EMR product. If you want more assistance, we invite you to visit the MSP ESP portal (www.ehrselector.com). There you will find the MSP EHR Selector and a variety of accounting, legal, consulting and financial services, as well as paper record conversion and archiving, installation and post-deployment support, learning and other resources. The MSP EHR Selector can quickly narrow the field from many EMR products to a short list of three to five well-qualified products that meet (or come closest to meeting) your specific EMR requirements.

The MSP EHR Selector was conceived by Dr. Caroline Samuels, a physician practicing in the Washington D.C. area. MSP has expanded it to include more features and supplementary services for physicians.

Power of the MSP EHR Selector

The MSP EHR Selector currently has around 700 criteria that can be displayed and asserted individually, grouped into related categories. For example, the PQRI Quality-Measures Category has 70 criteria, the Medication-Content Category has 36 criteria, and so on. These criteria cover all care settings and practice specialities supported by the MSP EHR Selector.

The extensive scope of selection criteria provides a highly-granular view of EMR product capabilities, yet the Selector's category organization and keyword search capabilities make it a simple-to-use tool. In selecting your EMR, you will probably only interact with 300 to 400 criteria, unless you are choosing an EMR for more than one medical specialty and practice setting.

Ease-of-use features include "Flags" for individual criterion that indicate if the feature is vetted (V), recommended (hp) or required (HP) for HIPAA compliance, helpful in achieving certification for Meaningful Use (MU) functionality, or have legal (LA) implications for RFPs and contracting language.[1] Coupled with

---

[1] The legal alerts are provided by a large law firm with a healthcare focus. You will find contact information by mousing over the EMR Solutions & Resources area.

Successfully Choosing Your EMR: 15 Crucial Decisions. By © Arthur Gasch and Betty Gasch. Published 2010 by Blackwell Publishing

the embedded Help (?) screens, these flags draw attention to features that require particular consideration. Figure A3.1 shows the MSP EHR Selector homepage.

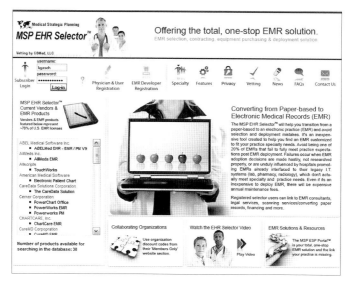

Figure A3.1 MSP EHR Selector Homepage (www.ehrselector.com)

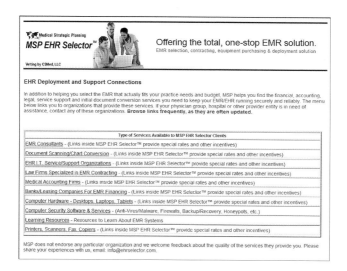

Figure A3.2 Table of EMR-Related Resources

Clicking on any link in Figure A3.2 reveals a list of providers, as shown in Figure A.3.3, in this case EMR Consultants.

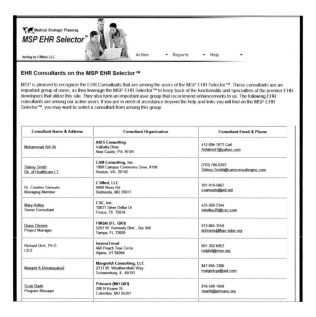

Figure A3.3 Selected EMR Consultants Found at MSP ESP

Each provider listed is an independent entity that offers services and sets their own fees. Some are high-profile, well-known and more expensive; while others have lower profiles and may be a bit more affordable and available. The goal of the portal is to provide a cross-section of professionals and services.

Selecting an EMR is Like Buying a House

The different criteria on the MSP EHR Selector are analogous to different photographs of a house being purchased. Each picture tells you something distinctive about the house. The first pictures are the outside orientation shots; the curb view and perhaps the view from the backyard and from each side. These shots give you a sense of the house shape, lot size, roof design, windows, finish and landscaping. From these few pictures you can reject some houses. If the house you have in mind is a three-bedroom ranch and the picture is of a two-story colonial, you can presume that this isn't a house you want to consider further, even without seeing the inside shots. In this way you don't waste your time looking at houses that don't match your purchase requirements.

If the outside of the house looks suitable, you proceed to explore the interior, learning about room layouts, traffic flow patterns, electrical service, kitchen appliances and so on. These pictures let you decide which houses you want to visit personally.

The same is true as you explore EMR product alternatives using the MSP EHR Selector. If you want an EMR that is installed in your office, you can immediately reject those that operate remotely over the Web, or vice versa. If you choose an in-office EMR deployment, then the MSP EHR Selector will display additional features and criteria related to EMRs installed in your office. If you don't know what you want, or don't care about where your EMR is deployed, you simply don't specify either preference as one of your requirements.

Help Screens Provide a Learning Tool

Because most features have "Help" screens, indicated by the '?' symbol next to each criterion, the MSP EHR Selector is also a useful learning resource. Key EMR-specific words and concepts are linked to a "Glossary." Inside the Glossary, keywords, terms and phrases are defined and Web links are provided to other Web sites where supplemental information is available. This helps you become acquainted with EMR terminology without having to search all over the Internet, or reveal your identity by visiting a vendor's Web site.

Limiting Criteria to Practice Setting and Interests

Some users jump right in and wade through all Selector criteria. Others find it helpful to limit the information the tool provides to the general capabilities they want in their EMR. You can use the Criteria menu shown in Figure A3.4 to do either.

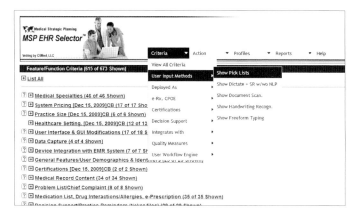

Figure 3.4   Using the Criteria Menus Prior to Assert Features

Methods of Using the Selector

Use the "Click Here to Show Instructions" link for a fast orientation to the Selector's controls. There are three basic ways to assert your criteria.

1 In the "Classic" method, click any ⊞ sign by a category to display all of the EMR features it contains. Next, select any criteria you desire. Finally, submit them and see which EMRs match your requirements. This method was created for the original MSP EHR Selector, when the total number of criteria were small. The disadvantage of this mode is that it requires you to work through every category to find all the criteria that may be of interest.

2 In the "Search and Assert" method, you enter keywords and then the EHR Selector finds all criteria that contain those keywords. You then assert any criteria desired. Since a keyword (like medication) can appear in multiple categories, you don't have to open all of the categories to find and assert criteria about medication. The disadvantage is that you have to think of keywords to search on.

3 In the "Global Profiles" (GP) method, you can assert dozens of criteria in just one mouse click by choosing the Profiles already created by MSP. A few of the profiles available relate to "Meaningful Use" and "HIPAA compliance," and there are others for particular practice specialties such as gastroenterology.

Most users employ a combination of these methods when working with the MSP EHR Selector. Each method is briefly illustrated in the following sections.

Indicating Criteria Of Interest

To use the Classic Method, select a category and click on its ⊞ Button to expand it to show the individual criterion it contains. You can see the first few categories shown in Figure A3.5.

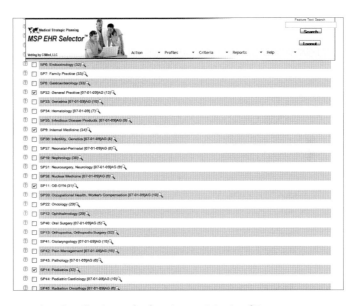

Figure A3.5 Using the Classic Method to Assert Criteria of Interest

Work through each category until you have chosen all the criteria you need by clicking the ⊞ Button next to each individual criterion. Then use the menus to retrieve the EMR products that match all of your checked criteria. Figure A3.5 also illustrates many of the 46 different practice specialties supported by the MSP EHR Selector.

The Keyword Search and Assert Method

Reviewing each category can be tedious and navigating hundreds of criteria can also be daunting. In the Search and Assert method, you enter a keyword in the search box located on the upper-right side of the floating toolbar. The search feature is the fastest way to find all criteria that share a common keyword, such as: medication, quality, alert or many other words. Type in the keyword and click the "Search Button." Doing this builds a list of criteria containing this keyword from across all categories of the Selector. Just check off any you wish to assert as criteria, as shown in Figure A3.6.

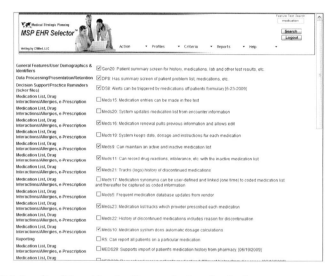

Figure A3.6 Results of Searching for Keyword = "medication"

From the 30 criteria found by the "medication" keyword search, nine criteria have been checked and submitted as capabilities wanted in an EMR. These criteria come from several different categories of the MSP EHR Selector. Without the keyword search feature, you would need to visit a category to find and click the criteria of interest, and then go to the next category and repeat the process until you have finished with your choices.

The Global Profile Method

Global Profiles (GP) are available on the "Profile" menu, as shown in Figure A3.7. Select the GP you want to assert and "Add" it to other criteria you've chosen. You might choose the GI (gastroenterology) global profile for example, if GI is of interest to you, as it has over 100 assertions created by the AGA Institute, an MSP EHR Selector collaborating organization. Using the GI Profile asserts GI-specific features in a single mouse click. This saves a lot of time compared to searching for all these individual criteria and asserting them individually.

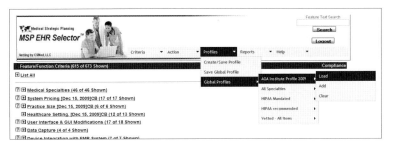

Figure A3.7 Accessing the Global Profiles

User-Created Profiles

The Profile Menu also supports "User-Defined" Profiles. These are much like the "file save as" function of a conventional Windows application. User-defined profiles allow you to save the state of your work on the MSP EHR Selector at any point and to give it a name. You create User Profiles by clicking the "Save Profile" button and entering a profile name of your choice. This immediately adds your Profile name to the User Profile menu, making it easy to find and reload later. This is the normal way to save your work at the end of a session. User profiles also allow you to evaluate more than one set of criteria, so that you can determine whether the EMR you choose today will also meet your future needs, for example.

Think of the house-buying metaphor again. Are you planning on having a family? Will one of those bedrooms work as a nursery? On the other hand, if your kids are leaving for college, can their room be converted to an office or otherwise repurposed after they're gone?

Profiles and iterative selections on the MSP EHR Selector help you evaluate current and future practice needs. Do you plan to add another physician to your practice? Will that introduce a new practice specialty? Will you open another office at a different location in the community? Profiles let you to break down criteria into groups of related features that can be asserted independently or in combinations. All criteria on the MSP EHR Selector are logically combined ("ANDed" together).

This illustrates the power of profiles as an EMR planning and decision-support resource.

Finding All Matches to Any Set of User Criteria

Each new feature asserted narrows the group of EMR products that meet all asserted criteria. To submit your criteria and immediately receive a returned list of matching vendors, use the "Select Matching Vendors" menu item shown in Figure A3.8.

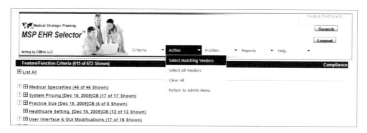

Figure A3.8 Select Matching EMR Products From the Action Menu

Figure A3.9 shows the list of EMR products matching all asserted features.

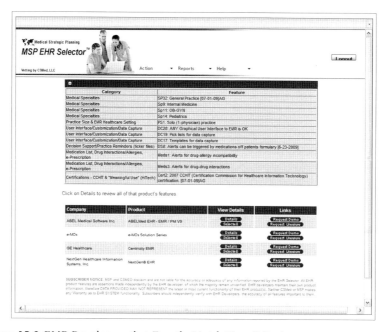

Figure A3.9 EMR Developers that Exactly Match User Criteria

Once you have your list of matching EMR products, you could do any of the following:

• Modify and continue your search by asserting more criteria;
• Request literature for an EMR of interest;
• Request a demo of any EMR product;
• Review the Klas Research satisfaction rating of any rated EMR(s);
• Print out all selection criteria and attach them to an RFP (or RFI).

The Null-Match Case

In some cases, no EMR solution is returned (e.g. no EMR has all the features you specified). When this happens, use the "Select All Vendors" menu option to force all EMR products to show what percentage of the user-asserted criteria they were able to match. This approach is also helpful when a particular vendor you are interested in does NOT come up on your initial list of matching vendors. In both cases you can go back and use the "Match All Vendors" menu choice to generate a list like that shown in Figure A3.10.

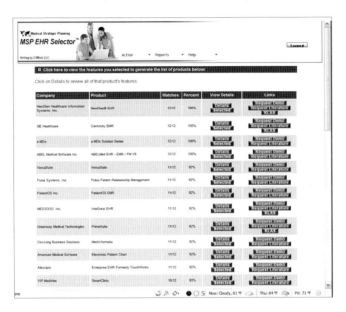

Figure A3.10 The "Select All Vendors" Menu Provides Percentage Matching

The EMR products on the Select All Vendors report are shown in the percentage matched column. The list is sorted in declining percentage of features matched to all of your asserted criteria. Since all vendors are included in this report, the degree of match for any vendor can be easily determined. Suppose you want to see how well GEMMS matched the asserted criteria. Simply run down the list until you find GEMMS, and then look at the percentage matched column. In this case, GEMMS matched 67 percent of the criteria submitted.

Want to know what criteria GEMMS didn't match? OK, click on the "Selected" button to the right of GEMMS. The display (see Figure A3.11) shows that GEMMS didn't match all practice specialties because GEMMS focuses on cardiology as its primary specialty and that wasn't the specialty asserted in this case. However, if it met all the other user requirements and had templates for the specialty asserted, GEMMS might still be a good EMR candidate to consider.

This is a very useful function for helping your practice compare EMR products that different personnel like but that offer varying characteristics. It can highlight criteria trade-offs that can lead to a compromise choice when no one EMR product satisfies everyone's diverse product needs. Only when you are armed with all the data can you see such compromise opportunities.

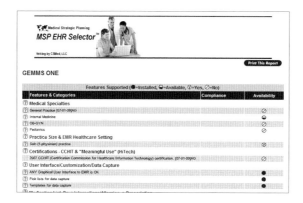

Figure A3.11 Not Matched Criteria (Slashed-Through Circles)

The colored circles (red and green) on the EHR Selector make the matches (or not) obvious. In Figure A3.11 above, the black circles are really green, meaning the EMR matches this feature as part of its basic functionality. The half-black circles are actually half green. That means the EMR provides the feature as an option available at extra cost. The circles with the line through them indicate that the functionality is not available from that vendor.

Wrap Up

This chapter has introduced you to an additional resource that could prove useful in your search for an EMR, no matter what care setting you are looking to equip. We are pleased to offer readers of this book a discount on subscriptions to the MSP EHR Selector (www.ehrselector.com) of approximately 15 percent. Simply indicate "Wiley" as your organization source and put in "Crucial15" as the password (both case sensitive) when you register. If you run into any issues, e-mail info@ehrselector.com.

If you use the MSP EHR Selector take the optional user survey and let us know what other resources you've used (EMR consultant, accountant, lawyer, document scanning firm, after-sale I.T. support organization). It is of particular interest to us to know whether or not these were organizations listed on our site. Each consultant/service has to maintain good client feedback in order to remain on the site, so filling out the survey is your way of letting us know how they're doing. It also gives us a better idea of the total cost of actually selecting and deploying an EMR, something that remarkably, hasn't been closely studied yet.

Your feedback concerning your experience in using the MSP EHR Selector is most helpful in guiding our on-going product enhancement priorities. Most innovative changes have come from user suggestions and critiques. Finally, we hope that you found this book to be a valuable investment of your time and that it keeps you on the path to successful selection and deployment of your EMR. Any feedback you have to offer on the book is welcome. E-mail it to agasch@ehrselector.com.

Index

Symbols

A